Marine Drug Discovery through Computer-Aided Approaches

Marine Drug Discovery through Computer-Aided Approaches

Editors

Susana P. Gaudencio
Florbela Pereira

MDPI

Basel • Beijing • Wuhan • Barcelona • Belgrade • Novi Sad • Cluj • Manchester

Editors
Susana P. Gaudencio
NOVA University of Lisbon
Lisbon, Portugal

Florbela Pereira
NOVA University of Lisbon
Caparica, Portugal

Editorial Office
MDPI
St. Alban-Anlage 66
4052 Basel, Switzerland

This is a reprint of articles from the Special Issue published online in the open access journal *Marine Drugs* (ISSN 1660-3397) (available at: https://www.mdpi.com/journal/marinedrugs/special_issues/computer-aided_MD).

For citation purposes, cite each article independently as indicated on the article page online and as indicated below:

Lastname, A.A.; Lastname, B.B. Article Title. *Journal Name* **Year**, *Volume Number*, Page Range.

ISBN 978-3-0365-9911-3 (Hbk)
ISBN 978-3-0365-9912-0 (PDF)
doi.org/10.3390/books978-3-0365-9912-0

Contents

About the Editors

Susana P. Gaudencio

Susana P. Gaudêncio (S.P.G.) is the leader of the Blue Biotechnology and Biomedicine Lab at UCIBIO, FCT-NOVA, Portugal. Her research focuses on the discovery of Natural Products from marine-derived actinomycetes (Actinobacteria) as lead-like agents for drug discovery and other biotechnological applications. These bacteria are obtained from marine sediments collected off the coast of Portugal and off the Atlantic Macaronesia ecoregion, which comprises the Azores, Madeira and Cape Verde archipelagos and the Canary Islands. Her actinomycetes Biobank collection is the biggest in Portugal. In 2019, she hosted the XVI MaNaPro and XI ECMNP joint conferences, in Peniche, Portugal. She is an MC member, WG leader and STSM committee member of the European Transdisciplinary Networking Platform for Marine Biotechnology OCEAN4BIOTECH CA18238. She has been a part of the Editorial Board for the following Scientific Journals: Natural Product Reports, Marine Drugs, and Frontiers in Marine Science.

Florbela Pereira

Florbela Pereira (FP) is a team member of the Cheminformatics Lab at LAQV@REQUIMTE, FCT-NOVA, and her research focuses on the development of computational methods for drug discovery and materials (e.g., QSAR, QSPR, virtual screening, molecular docking). FP is very interested in machine-learning (ML)-based discovery from data pre-calculated using DFT methods to predict properties of atoms, bonds, and molecules very quickly and accurately. She has been a part of the Editorial Board for the following Scientific Journals: Computational and Structural Biotechnology Journal; In silico Methods and Artificial Intelligence for Drug Discovery (Frontiers in Drug Discovery); and Editorial Board Member for the section 'Synthesis and Medicinal Chemistry of Marine Natural Products' of Marine Drugs.

marine drugs

MDPI

Editorial

Marine Drug Discovery through Computer-Aided Approaches

Susana P. Gaudêncio [1,2,*] and Florbela Pereira [3]

1 Associate Laboratory i4HB, Institute for Health and Bioeconomy, NOVA Faculty of Sciences and Technology, NOVA University of Lisbon, 2819-516 Lisbon, Portugal
2 UCIBIO, Applied Molecular Biosciences Unit, Chemistry Department, NOVA Faculty of Sciences and Technology, NOVA University of Lisbon, 2819-516 Lisbon, Portugal
3 LAQV, Chemistry Department, NOVA Faculty of Sciences and Technology, NOVA University of Lisbon, 2819-516 Lisbon, Portugal; florbela.pereira@fct.unl.pt
* Correspondence: s.gaudencio@fct.unl.pt

1. Blue Biotechnology Framework

Besides the importance of our oceans as oxygen factories, food providers, shipping pathways, and tourism enablers, oceans hide an unprecedented wealth of opportunities [1]. Marine organisms and microorganisms are valuable sources of primary and secondary metabolites, biopolymers, and enzymes, which can be used as lead agents for drug discovery, filling in the pharmaceutical industry pipeline and improving their development processes (e.g., drug discovery, drug repurposing, absorption, distribution, metabolism, elimination, and toxicity (ADMET) prediction, drug delivery, among others), especially when applying computer-aided tools and methods, and also as a source of bio-inspired material for numerous medical and biotechnological applications. The field of computer-aided ligand- and structure-based methodologies for marine drug lead discovery is still developing. By assisting in the structure elucidation of secondary metabolites, repurposing known marine natural products (MNPs) for new therapeutic purposes, and identifying novel hits or leads against selected therapeutic targets, computational approaches and chemistry simulation methods can be successfully used in the discovery, design, and development of new chemical agents for therapeutic applications [2–4]. The eminent marine (blue) biotechnology field has gained visibility worldwide in many complementary scientific fields, inspiring the creation of several legislative, infrastructural, and scientific collaborative networks [5,6]. With computer-aided approaches playing a crucial role in advancing this scientific field, the computational tools could ultimately become a significant driver in economic development, the formation of innovative biotechnological applications, and in the accomplishment of sustainable drug discovery approaches worldwide.

Citation: Gaudêncio, S.P.; Pereira, F. Marine Drug Discovery through Computer-Aided Approaches. *Mar. Drugs* **2023**, *21*, 452. https://doi.org/10.3390/md21080452

Received: 11 August 2023
Accepted: 16 August 2023
Published: 17 August 2023

2. Objective of Marine Drug Discovery through Computer-Aided Approaches Special Issue

The Special Issue "Marine Drug Discovery through Computer-Aided Approaches" was created with the objective of mapping the current scientific actors in the field of computer-aided approaches applied to blue biotechnology, and of providing a comprehensive overview of the great variety of advanced computer-aided methods for the discovery and identification of molecular agents with added value and health-promoting properties for the development of medical and biotechnological applications. This Special Issue invited the blue biotechnology community working with computer-aided technology to submit original research, reviews, and perspectives in all steps of the marine biotechnology development pipeline including computer-aided methods; from blue biotechnology, drug discovery, drug repurposing, chemoinformatics, bioinformatics, dereplication, MNPs databases, machine learning techniques, biological and chemical space, Quantitative Structure–Activity Relationship (QSAR), molecular docking, Computer-Aided Drug Design (CADD), and Computer-Assisted Structure Elucidation (CASE), generating a compilation of processes and technologies. The aim was also to develop a "guidebook" for maximizing the impact of marine biotechnology development that can be used to start, improve, and facilitate collaborations between related and complementary scientific fields, by providing information, expert contacts, and their expertise that will, both directly and indirectly, improve the discovery and innovation in blue biotechnology and boosting blue bioeconomy using computing methodologies.

3. Topics of the Participating Research Community

The Special Issue "Marine Drug Discovery through Computer-Aided Approaches" comprises nine articles reporting original research. These range from using computer software, machine learning, molecular docking, in silico modelling and animal modelling for dereplication, aiding MNPs structure elucidation, and the prediction of MNPs bioactivities and protein binding targets. This Special Issue is a must read for those who want to start using computer methods in marine biotechnology research. The nine contributions are described below by publication date.

3.1. Predicting Antifouling Activity and Acetylcholinesterase Inhibition of Marine-Derived Compounds Using a Computer-Aided Drug Design Approach

A CADD strategy combining ligand- and structure-based approaches was used for predicting the antifouling properties of MNPs. The QSAR classification model was constructed using antifouling screening data from 141 organic compounds that were taken from the ChEMBL database and the literature using the CADD ligand-based technique, attaining a highest prediction accuracy score of up to 71%. The best QSAR model created was also used to conduct a virtual screening campaign on 14,492 MNPs from Encinar's website and 14 MNPs that are currently in the clinical pipeline. The 125 MNPs chosen by the QSAR approach were employed in molecular docking tests against the acetylcholinesterase enzyme in the CADD structure-based approach. The most promising marine drug-like leads as antifouling agents were identified as 16 MNPs, including macrocyclic lactam, macrocyclic alkaloids, indole, and pyridine derivatives [7].

3.2. Uncovering the Bioactive Potential of a Cyanobacterial Natural Products Library Aided by Untargeted Metabolomics

Numerous cyanobacteria are kept in the Blue Biotechnology and Ecotoxicology Culture Collection (LEGE-CC), but little is known about their chemical diversity. A library of natural compounds was created to speed up its bioactivity screening. Sixty strains were examined for their cytotoxic potential against 2D and 3D models of human colon cancer (HCT 116) and the non-cancerous cell line hCMEC/D3. Their metabolome was analyzed and annotated using MolNetEnhancer and processed with MetaboAnalyst, allowing the selection of seven out of sixty cyanobacterial strains for the discovery of anticancer drug leads while dereplicating the chemical content of these cyanobacteria [8].

3.3. Application of Networking Approaches to Assess the Chemical Diversity, Biogeography, and Pharmaceutical Potential of Verongiida Natural Products

A review of all isolated natural products (NPs) identified in the sponge's order Verongiida from 1960 to May 2020 was performed compiling detailed information on their physico-geographical characteristics. Pharmacokinetic characteristics and possible medicinal potential of NPs from Verongiida were inferred using physico-chemical data. To comprehensively study the chemical space interactions between taxonomy, secondary metabolites, and drug score variables, a network analysis was used for the NPs made by Verongiida sponges, allowing the detection of differences and correlations within a dataset. Bipartite connection networks and scaffold networks provided a platform for investigating chemical diversity, and chemical similarity networks linking pharmacokinetic features with structural similarities, which can be used for other sponge orders or families [9].

3.4. Investigation of Marine-Derived Natural Products as Raf Kinase Inhibitory Protein (RKIP)-Binding Ligands

Numerous illnesses, including cancer, Alzheimer's, and diabetic nephropathy, are associated with the aberrant expression of RKIP. RKIP also functions as a tumor suppressor, making it a desirable therapeutic target. Only a few small molecules have been identified to alter the activity of RKIP. A pharmacophore model was created to investigate the characteristics of locostatin, the most effective RKIP modulator. A MNPs library was then obtained after the generated model was put through a screening process. The in silico hits may serve as strong RKIP modulators and disrupt interactions with RKIP's binding proteins [10].

3.5. Saliniquinone Derivatives, Saliniquinones G—I and Heraclemycin E, from the Marine Animal-Derived *Nocardiopsis aegyptia* HDN19-252

The Antarctic marine-derived actinomycete *Nocardiopsis aegyptia* HDN19-252 was used as a resource to produce four novel anthraquinone derivatives, including saliniquinones G–I (**1**–**3**) and heraclemycin E (**4**). Extensive NMR, MS, and ECD investigations revealed their structures, including absolute configurations. Saliniquinones **1** and **2** demonstrated encouraging inhibitory action against six tested bacterial strains, including methicillin-resistant coagulase-negative staphylococci (MRCNS), with MIC values ranging from 3.1 to 12.5 μM [11].

3.6. Efficacy of Chondroprotective Food Supplements Based on Collagen Hydrolysate and Compounds Isolated from Marine Organisms

The prevalence of osteoarthritis is higher in older individuals and is one of the most prevalent joint diseases in both humans and animals. The bioactivities of collagen hydrolysates, sulfated glucosamine, and specific fatty-acid-enriched dog rations were examined as prospective therapeutic options for early osteoarthritis using 52 dogs. The possibility that these well-characterized compounds may function as efficient nutraceuticals is supported by biophysical, biochemical, cell biology, and molecular modeling techniques. Animal model and molecular modeling for the receptor proteins MMP-3, TIMP-1 and ADAMTS-5 of intermolecular interactions strongly validated the applied collagen hydrolysates as well as sulfated glucosamine compounds from marine organisms. Molecular modeling simulations were employed to further evaluate the contact efficacy of collagen fragments and glucosamines with protein receptor architectures. There are potential advantages of using lipids, particularly eicosapentaenoic acid (extracted from fish oil), sulfated glycans (such as sulfated glucosamine from crabs and mussels), and collagen hydrolysates on biochemical and physiological processes for applications in dietary supplements for human and veterinary medicine [12].

3.7. Solid-Phase Extraction Embedded Dialysis (SPEED), an Innovative Procedure for the Investigation of Microbial Specialized Metabolites

In situ physical separation of the mycelium of filament-forming microorganisms, such as actinomycetes and fungi, and the XAD-16 resin used to trap the secreted specialized metabolites was accomplished using the novel solid-phase extraction embedded dialysis (SPEED) technology. SPEED is made up of an internal dialysis tube holding XAD resin and an exterior nylon cloth. The dialysis barrier chooses the molecular weight of the trapped chemicals and stops biomass or macromolecules from accumulating on the XAD beads. SPEED is a cultivation procedure assisted by a microbial biofilm since the external nylon encourages its creation. Marine *Streptomyces albidoflavus* 19-S21, isolated from a core of a submerged Kopara sampled at 20 m from a saltwater pond border, was subjected to SPEED technology. Using dereplication techniques based on molecular networking and thorough chemical analysis, the chemical space of this strain was successfully studied, demonstrating the influence of the culture support on the molecular profile of the secondary metabolites produced by *Streptomyces albidoflavus* 19-S21 [13].

3.8. Potency- and Selectivity-Enhancing Mutations of Conotoxins for Nicotinic Acetylcholine Receptors Can Be Predicted Using Accurate Free-Energy Calculations

Nicotinic acetylcholine receptor (nAChR) subtypes are important therapeutic targets, however, because of their striking similarity in sequence identities, it is difficult to pharmacologically distinguish between them. Additionally, nAChR problems may be successfully treated by using -conotoxins (-CTXs), which are naturally occurring selective and competitive antagonists for nAChRs. The primary goal of most -CTX mutagenesis investigations is to identify selectivity-enhancing mutations, although doing so with conventional docking techniques is challenging due to the lack of crystal structures for -CTX and nAChR. This study anticipates the structures of -CTXs bound to the nAChR subtypes 3 and 4 using homology modeling and re-predicts the relative potency and selectivity of -CTX mutants at these subtypes using free-energy perturbation (FEP). First, we employ the three crystal structures of the acetylcholine-binding protein, a homologue of the nAChR. The relative affinities of twenty point mutations made to the -CTXs LvIA, LsIA, and GIC using three crystal structures of the nAChR homologue, acetylcholine-binding protein (AChBP) was re-predicted, with an overall root mean square error (RMSE) of 1.08 $\pm$ 0.15 kcal/mol and an R^2 of 0.62, equivalent to experimental uncertainty. Then, with an overall RMSE of 0.85 $\pm$ 0.08 kcal/mol and an R^2 of 0.49, we employ AChBP as a template for 32 and 34 nAChR homology models linked to the -CTX LvIA and re-predict the potencies of eleven point mutations at both subtypes. The commonly used molecular mechanics–generalized born/surface area (MM-GB/SA) approach, which yields an RMSE of 1.96 $\pm$ 0.24 kcal/mol and an R^2 of 0.06 on the identical data, is substantially worse than this. Moreover, in contrast to MM-GB/SA, FEP correctly categorizes 32 nAChR selective LvIA mutants. FEP was used to undertake a thorough scan for amino acid alterations in LvIA. Fifty-two of these mutations will have greater than 100X selectivity for the 32 nAChR. FEP is ideally adapted to properly forecast mutations that will increase the potency and selectivity of -CTXs for nAChRs and to find alternative methods for discovering selective α-CTXs drugs [14].

3.9. In Vitro and In Silico Characterization of G-Protein Coupled Receptor (GPCR) Targets of Phlorofucofuroeckol-A and Dieckol

Polyphenolic substances called phlorotannins are obtained from marine algae, particularly brown algae. Dieckol and phlorofucofuroeckol-A (PFF-A) are the two main phlorotannins among many others, and although possessing a greater range of biological activities, less is known about the G protein-coupled receptors (GPCRs) that these phlorotannins target. Twenty major protein targets were predicted by in silico proteocheminformatics modeling, and in vitro functional assays demonstrated that two phlorotannins' primary GPCR targets had good agonist and antagonist effects at the 2C adrenergic receptor (2CAR), adenosine 2A receptor (A2AR), glucagon-like peptide-1 receptor (GLP-1R), and 5-hydroxytryptamine 1A receptor (5-TH1AR). Additionally, PFF-A had a promising agonist action at the cannabinoid 1 receptor and an antagonist effect at the vasopressin 1A receptor (V1AR) while dieckol demonstrated an antagonist effect at the V1AR. In silico molecular docking simulation enables the analysis and pinpointing of specific binding characteristics of these phlorotannins to the target proteins. According to the docking data, dieckol and PFF-A bind to the proteins' crystal structures with good affinity and important interplaying amino acid residues equivalent to reference ligands. The primary receptors for dieckol and PFF-A are the 2CAR, A2AR, -OPR, GLP-1R, 5-TH1AR, CB1R, and V1AR [15].

Author Contributions: Conceptualization, S.P.G.; validation, S.P.G.; formal analysis, S.P.G.; writing—original draft preparation S.P.G.; writing—review and editing, S.P.G. and F.P.; visualization, S.P.G. and F.P.; project administration, S.P.G.; funding acquisition, S.P.G. and F.P. All authors have read and agreed to the published version of the manuscript.

Acknowledgments: This work is financed by national funds from FCT—Fundação para a Ciência e a Tecnologia, I.P., in the scope of the project UIDP/04378/2020 of the Research Unit on Applied Molecular Biosciences—UCIBIO, the project LA/P/0140/2020 of the Associate Laboratory Institute for Health and Bioeconomy—i4HB. We also thank the project UIDB/50006/2020 of the Associated Laboratory for Green Chemistry (LAQV) of the Network of Chemistry and Technology (REQUIMTE).

Conflicts of Interest: The authors declare no conflict of interests.

References

1. Rotter, A.; Barbier, M.; Bertoni, F.; Bones, A.M.; Cancela, M.L.; Carlsson, J.; Carvalho, M.F.; Cegłowska, M.; Chirivella-Martorell, J.; Conk Dalay, M.; et al. The Essentials of Marine Biotechnology. *Front. Mar. Sci.* **2021**, *8*, 629629. [CrossRef]
2. Gaudêncio, S.P.; Pereira, F. Dereplication: Racing to speed up the natural products discovery process. *Nat. Prod. Rep.* **2015**, *32*, 779–810. [CrossRef] [PubMed]
3. Pereira, F.; Aires-De-Sousa, J. Computational Methodologies in the Exploration of Marine Natural Product Leads. *Mar. Drugs* **2018**, *16*, 236. [CrossRef] [PubMed]
4. Gaudêncio, S.P.; Bayram, E.; Bilela, L.L.; Cueto, M.; Díaz-Marrero, A.R.; Haznedaroglu, B.Z.; Jimenez, C.; Mandalakis, M.; Pereira, F.; Reyes, F.; et al. Advanced Methods for Natural Products Discovery: Bioactivity Screening, Dereplication, Metabolomics Profiling, Genomic Sequencing, Databases and Informatic Tools, and Structure Elucidation. *Mar. Drugs* **2023**, *21*, 308. [CrossRef] [PubMed]
5. Rotter, A.; Gaudêncio, S.P.; Klun, K.; Macher, J.-N.; Thomas, O.P.; Deniz, I.; Edwards, C.; Grigalionyte-Bembič, E.; Ljubešić, Z.; Robbens, J.; et al. A New Tool for Faster Construction of Marine Biotechnology Collaborative Networks. *Front. Mar. Sci.* **2021**, *8*, 685164. [CrossRef]
6. Rotter, A.; Bacu, A.; Barbier, M.; Bertoni, F.; Bones, A.M.; Cancela, M.L.; Carlsson, J.; Carvalho, M.F.; Cegłowska, M.; Dalay, M.C.; et al. A New Network for the Advancement of Marine Biotechnology in Europe and Beyond. *Front. Mar. Sci.* **2020**, *7*, 278. [CrossRef]
7. Gaudêncio, S.P.; Pereira, F. Predicting Antifouling Activity and Acetylcholinesterase Inhibition of Marine-Derived Compounds Using a Computer-Aided Drug Design Approach. *Mar. Drugs* **2022**, *20*, 129. [CrossRef] [PubMed]
8. Ferreira, L.; Morais, J.; Preto, M.; Silva, R.; Urbatzka, R.; Vasconcelos, V.; Reis, M. Uncovering the Bioactive Potential of a Cyanobacterial Natural Products Library Aided by Untargeted Metabolomics. *Mar. Drugs* **2021**, *19*, 633. [CrossRef] [PubMed]
9. Lever, J.; Brkljača, R.; Rix, C.; Urban, S. Application of Networking Approaches to Assess the Chemical Diversity, Biogeography, and Pharmaceutical Potential of Verongiida Natural Products. *Mar. Drugs* **2021**, *19*, 582. [CrossRef] [PubMed]
10. Parate, S.; Kumar, V.; Hong, J.C.; Lee, K.W. Investigation of Marine-Derived Natural Products as Raf Kinase Inhibitory Protein (RKIP)-Binding Ligands. *Mar. Drugs* **2021**, *19*, 581. [CrossRef]
11. Zhou, L.; Chen, X.; Sun, C.; Chang, Y.; Huang, X.; Zhu, T.; Zhang, G.; Che, Q.; Li, D. Saliniquinone Derivatives, Saliniquinones G−I and Heraclemycin E, from the Marine Animal-Derived *Nocardiopsis aegyptia* HDN19-252. *Mar. Drugs* **2021**, *19*, 575. [CrossRef]
12. Eckert, T.; Jährling-Butkus, M.; Louton, H.; Burg-Roderfeld, M.; Zhang, R.; Zhang, N.; Hesse, K.; Petridis, A.K.; Kožár, T.; Steinmeyer, J.; et al. Efficacy of Chondroprotective Food Supplements Based on Collagen Hydrolysate and Compounds Isolated from Marine Organisms. *Mar. Drugs* **2021**, *19*, 542. [CrossRef] [PubMed]
13. Mai, P.-Y.; Le Goff, G.; Poupon, E.; Lopes, P.; Moppert, X.; Costa, B.; Beniddir, M.A.; Ouazzani, J. Solid-Phase Extraction Embedded Dialysis (SPEED), an Innovative Procedure for the Investigation of Microbial Specialized Metabolites. *Mar. Drugs* **2021**, *19*, 371. [CrossRef] [PubMed]
14. Katz, D.; DiMattia, M.A.; Sindhikara, D.; Li, H.; Abraham, N.; Leffler, A.E. Potency- and Selectivity-Enhancing Mutations of Conotoxins for Nicotinic Acetylcholine Receptors Can Be Predicted Using Accurate Free-Energy Calculations. *Mar. Drugs* **2021**, *19*, 367. [CrossRef] [PubMed]
15. Paudel, P.; Seong, S.H.; Park, S.E.; Ryu, J.H.; Jung, H.A.; Choi, J.S. In Vitro and In Silico Characterization of G-Protein Coupled Receptor (GPCR) Targets of Phlorofucofuroeckol-A and Dieckol. *Mar. Drugs* **2021**, *19*, 326. [CrossRef]

marine drugs

Article

Predicting Antifouling Activity and Acetylcholinesterase Inhibition of Marine-Derived Compounds Using a Computer-Aided Drug Design Approach

Susana P. Gaudêncio [1,2] and Florbela Pereira [3,*]

1 Associate Laboratory i4HB—Institute for Health and Bioeconomy, NOVA School of Science and Technology, NOVA University of Lisbon, 2819-516 Caparica, Portugal; s.gaudencio@fct.unl.pt
2 UCIBIO—Applied Molecular Biosciences Unit, Department of Chemistry, Blue Biotechnology and Biomedicine Lab, NOVA School of Science and Technology, NOVA University of Lisbon, 2819-516 Caparica, Portugal
3 LAQV, Department of Chemistry, NOVA School of Science and Technology, NOVA University of Lisbon, 2829-516 Caparica, Portugal
* Correspondence: florbela.pereira@fct.unl.pt

Abstract: Biofouling is the undesirable growth of micro- and macro-organisms on artificial water-immersed surfaces, which results in high costs for the prevention and maintenance of this process (billion €/year) for aquaculture, shipping and other industries that rely on coastal and off-shore infrastructure. To date, there are still no sustainable, economical and environmentally safe solutions to overcome this challenging phenomenon. A computer-aided drug design (CADD) approach comprising ligand- and structure-based methods was explored for predicting the antifouling activities of marine natural products (MNPs). In the CADD ligand-based method, 141 organic molecules extracted from the ChEMBL database and literature with antifouling screening data were used to build the quantitative structure–activity relationship (QSAR) classification model. An overall predictive accuracy score of up to 71% was achieved with the best QSAR model for external and internal validation using test and training sets. A virtual screening campaign of 14,492 MNPs from Encinar's website and 14 MNPs that are currently in the clinical pipeline was also carried out using the best QSAR model developed. In the CADD structure-based approach, the 125 MNPs that were selected by the QSAR approach were used in molecular docking experiments against the acetylcholinesterase enzyme. Overall, 16 MNPs were proposed as the most promising marine drug-like leads as antifouling agents, e.g., macrocyclic lactam, macrocyclic alkaloids, indole and pyridine derivatives.

Keywords: marine natural products (MNPs); blue biotechnology; quantitative structure–activity relationship (QSAR); machine learning (ML) techniques; computer-aided drug design (CADD); molecular docking; virtual screening; antifouling activity; acetylcholinesterase enzyme (AChE)

Citation: Gaudêncio, S.P.; Pereira, F. Predicting Antifouling Activity and Acetylcholinesterase Inhibition of Marine-Derived Compounds Using a Computer-Aided Drug Design Approach. *Mar. Drugs* **2022**, *20*, 129. https://doi.org/10.3390/md20020129

Academic Editor: Orazio Taglialatela-Scafati

Received: 13 December 2021
Accepted: 6 February 2022
Published: 8 February 2022

1. Introduction

Marine biofouling is the undesired accumulation of micro-organisms, e.g., bacteria, cyanobacteria, unicellular algae and protozoa, and macro-organisms, e.g., seaweeds, barnacles, mussels and shells, on artificial water-immersed surfaces in a dynamic process that starts immediately after water submersion and can be a fast or slow process taking only hours or months to develop, respectively [1]. Marine biofouling creates risks to various industries, such as aquaculture and shipping, as well as for non-marine industries, e.g., paper manufacturing, food processing, underwater construction, power plants and others [2,3]. Settlement on the vessel's hull results in damage to the rudder and propulsion systems [2,4], leads to an increasing drag of up to 60%, as well as a fuel consumption increase by 40%, increasing carbon dioxide and sulfur dioxide emissions [5] and the spread of nonindigenous marine species into ecosystems worldwide, leading to environmental imbalances [6–10]. The most effective antifouling (AF) coatings contained biocides, such as tributyltin (TBT) and tributyltin oxide (TBTO), which were found to be harmful to non-target organisms and the environment [11] and thus were prohibited by the International Maritime Organization from Ship Surfaces in 2008, generating the demand for new generations of non-toxic or environment-friendly AF solutions [12–14].

Natural alternatives including primary or secondary metabolites isolated from marine organisms have been reported in several reviews to inhibit the settlement of different biofouling species [15–24]. The search for AF agents from marine sources began with bromo-derived metabolites, among the 2-furanone bromine derivatives extracted from red algae, which have been reported to prevent fouling [25], as well as bromopyrrole alkaloid derivatives with AF activity isolated from sponges (oroidin), inspiring the design of more than 50 synthetic analogues [26,27], and, more recently, antifouling bromotyrosine derivatives of the synoxazolidinone and the pulmonarin families [28]. Several studies reported MNPs with antifouling activity comprising the 2,5-diketopiperazine scaffold isolated from the marine sponge *Geodia barretti* [29], 6-benzyl and 6-isobutyl 2,5-diketopiperazine derivatives from marine-derived actinomycete *Streptomyces praecox* [30] and five diketopiperazines, cyclo-(L-Leu-L-Pro), cyclo-(L-Phe-L-Pro), cyclo-(L-Val-L-Pro), cyclo-(L-Trp-L-Pro) and cyclo-(L-Leu-L-Val), from deep-sea *Streptomyces fungicidicus* [31]. Comprising a meroterpenoid scaffold, napyradiomycin derivatives, isolated from marine-derived actinomycetes *Streptomyces aculeolatus*, were investigated by our group as antifouling inhibitors, having the advantage of inhibiting both micro- (antibiofilm activity) and macrofouling [32–34].

Computer-aided drug design (CADD) approaches have been used to guide decisions concerning the in vivo and in vitro testing of isolated NPs and extracts [35–39], to assist in the design of bioactive NP derivatives [40,41] and to virtually screen databases of known or proposed NPs [40,42–44]. To the best of our knowledge, the antifouling activity was quantitative structure–activity relationship (QSAR) modeled in only two previous works for the settlement of *Mytilus galloprovincialis* larvae [45,46]. Almeida et al. built two QSAR models using multilinear regression methods with, respectively, 19 and 16 nature-inspired (thio)xanthone [46] and chalcone [45] derivatives, including in vitro antifouling activity screening assays for the settlement of *Mytilus galloprovincialis* larvae.

Acetylcholinesterase (AChE) inhibitors are a class of drugs used for the treatment of Alzheimer's disease, glaucoma and autoimmune disorders [47–49]. The enzymes AChE [28] and tyrosinase (Tyr) were associated with the adhesive processes in the settlement of different biofouling species [28,46,50]. Almeida et al. reported a molecular docking study conducted by modulation of *Electrophorus electric* (fish) AChE of the two most promising (thio)xanthone antifouling agents [46]. Recently, Arabshahi et al. [50] reported an extensive virtual *Tetronarce californica* (fish) AChE homology screening campaign for 10,000 small organic molecules from the Chembridge library. The authors also reported the experimental screening of the most promising AChE inhibitors proposed by the in silico model, against five microfouling marine bacteria and marine microalgae macrofouling tunicate *Ciona savignyi*, discovering a potent novel inhibitor of tunicate settlement [50].

Herein, we report comprehensive computational modeling for the prediction of antifouling activities from two MNP libraries, by employing structure- and ligand-based CADD methodologies. The two libraries comprised 14,492 MNP from Prof. Encinar (http://docking.umh.es/downloaddb, accessed on 25 October 2021) and 14 MNPs from the clinical pipeline of MNPs (eight drugs approved and six MNPs in Phase II and III clinical trials). All the MNPs from the virtual screening libraries that were predicted to belong to the active class, i.e., 125 MNPs, were selected to proceed to the CADD structure-based method, where 125 MNPs selected by QSAR approach were screened by molecular docking against the AChE enzyme. In this CADD approach, a virtual screening hit list comprising 19 MNPs was assented based on some established thresholds, such as the probability of being active in the best antifouling model and the prediction of affinity between the AChE of selected MNPs by molecular docking. A total of 16 MNPs have been proposed as the most promising marine drug-like leads as antifouling agents.

2. Results and Discussion

2.1. Chemical Space of the Antifouling Model

The whole data set (i.e., 141 small organic molecules) was randomly divided into a training set of 127 molecules (comprising 57 active and 70 inactive molecules) and a test set of 14 molecules (comprising six active and eight inactive molecules), which were used for the development and external validation of the QSAR classification models, respectively. The whole data set comprised seven structural classes or scaffold types, which are represented in Table 1 along with their antifouling activity classes and scaffold representative.

Table 1. Structural clusters and antifouling activity class counts within the seven structural clusters.

Clusters [1]	# [2] (Active Class)		Average MW (Da) [3]		Average ALogP [4]	
	Tr	Te	Tr	Te	Tr	Te
I—acyclic derivative 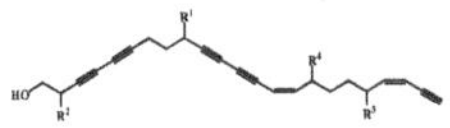	11 (11)	0 (0)	361.65	0	2.86	0
II—*O*-heterocyclic derivative 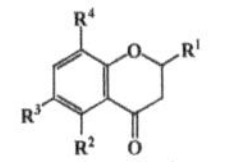 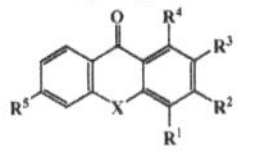	28 (9)	3 (1)	328.09	334.64	3.18	3.22
III—*N*-heterocyclic derivative 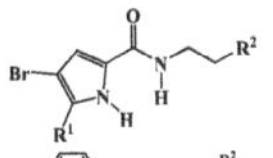 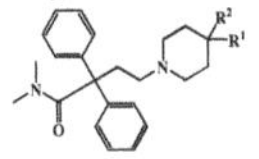	19 (14)	1 (0)	363.92	493.04	2.50	3.65
IV—terpenoid derivative 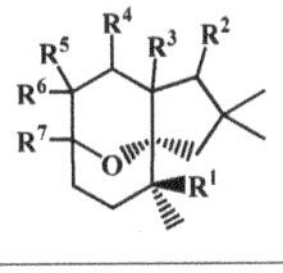	22 (5)	6 (3)	264.64	341.76	3.00	4.49
V—diketopiperazine derivative 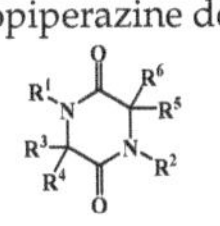	15 (10)	3 (2)	392.54	415.15	3.06	3.10

Table 1. *Cont.*

Clusters [1]	# [2] (Active Class)		Average MW (Da) [3]		Average ALogP [4]	
	Tr	Te	Tr	Te	Tr	Te
VI—chalcone derivative 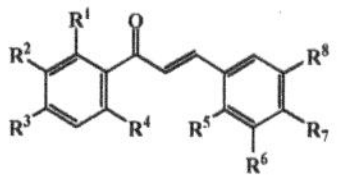	16 (3)	0 (0)	352.37	0	4.56	0
VII—miscellaneous	16 (5)	1 (0)	1164.53	975.69	−0.88	−1.57

[1] Cluster code and chemical structure of the cluster scaffold. [2] Number of molecules in the training (Tr) and the test (Te) sets. [3] Molecular weight (MW) within the cluster for the training and test sets. [4] Octanol–water partition coefficient prediction within the cluster for the training and test sets.

All seven structural clusters (I, acyclic derivative, II, *O*-heterocyclic derivative, III, *N*-heterocyclic derivative, IV, terpenoid derivative, V, diketopiperazine derivative, VI, chalcone derivative, and VII, miscellaneous) were well represented in the training set, each comprising more than 10 molecules per class. The active class was more represented in three structural clusters with a percentage higher than 50%, namely I—acyclic derivative (100%), III—*N*-heterocyclic derivative (74%) and V—diketopiperazine derivative (67%). In the test set, only five structural clusters were represented, II-V and VII. In Table 1, the most representative scaffolds of the structural cluster are highlighted—for instance, for cluster I, a polyacetylene derivative; II, a chromone and a xanthone derivative; III, a pyrrole and a piperidine derivative; IV, a sesquiterpene derivative; V, a diketopiperazine, VI, a chalcone derivative; and VII, various scaffolds such as peptides and nature-inspired sulfated compounds. All clusters for the training and test sets, except for cluster VII, had an average MW value of less than 500 Da.

2.2. Establishment of QSAR Classification Model

Random Forests (RF) [51] were used to build models for antifouling prediction, exploring well-established PaDEL fingerprints (FPP and descriptors, e.g., five different types of FPs with different sizes (166 MACCS, MACCS keys; 307 Substructure; 881 PubChem fingerprints; 1024 CDK, circular fingerprints; 1024 CDK Ext, extended circular fingerprints with additional bits describing ring features) and 1376 1D&2D molecular descriptors (including electronic, topological and constitutional descriptors)) [52]. The performance of the models was successfully evaluated by internal validation (out-of-bag, OOB, estimation on the training set); see Table 2.

Table 2. Evaluation of the predictive performance of FPs and 1D&2D molecular descriptors for modeling the antifouling activity using the RF algorithm for the training set with an OOB estimation. The best models are highlighted in bold.

Descriptors (#)	TP [1]	TN [2]	FN [3]	FP [4]	SE [5]	SP [6]	Q [7]	MCC [8]
MACCS (166) [9]	41	51	16	19	0.719	0.729	0.724	0.446
Sub (307) [9]	41	53	16	17	0.719	0.757	**0.740**	**0.476**
PubChem (881) [9]	43	48	14	22	0.754	0.686	0.717	0.438
CDK (1024) [9]	42	47	15	23	0.737	0.671	0.701	0.406
ExtCDK (1024) [9]	41	49	16	21	0.719	0.700	**0.709**	**0.417**
1D&2D (1376)	40	53	17	17	0.702	0.757	**0.732**	**0.459**

[1] True positive. [2] True negative. [3] False negative. [4] False positive. [5] Sensitivity, the ratio of true positive to the sum of true positive and false positive. [6] Specificity, the ratio of true negative to the sum of true negative and false negative. [7] Overall predictive accuracy, the ratio of the sum of true positive and true negative to the sum of true positive, true negative, false positive and false negative. [8] Matthews correlation coefficient. [9] Fingerprints, FPs.

From the seven sets of FPs and descriptors used to build the QSAR classification model, the best set for each type, fragment FPs (Sub), circular FPs (ExtCDK) and molecular descriptors (1D&2D), were selected for further investigations; see Table 2. The 3D descriptors had a well-established relationship with biological activity and were expected to increase both the accuracy and robustness of the predictive models. After the exploration of models derived with molecular descriptors and FPs, we investigated the inclusion of 3D descriptors such as radial distribution function (RDF) descriptors (using a range of 128 and partial atomic charge as an atomic property) and the selection of descriptors using the RF descriptor importance parameter for the best three sets (Sub FPs, ExtCDK FPs and 1D&2D descriptors). Three sets of descriptors (Sub + RDF, ExtCDK + RDF and 1D&2D + RDF) as well as their selection were explored for modeling the antifouling activity using the RF algorithm in Table 3, where the results for the training set in OOB estimation are presented.

Table 3. Evaluation of the predictive performance of RDF descriptors and descriptor selection for modeling the antifouling activity using the RF algorithm for the training set with an OOB estimation. The best models are highlighted in bold.

Model	#	SE [1]	SP [2]	Q [3]	MCC [4]
Sub + RDF	691	0.667	0.714	0.693	0.380
Selection [5]	50	0.667	0.714	0.693	0.380
Selection [5]	100	0.684	0.757	0.724	0.442
Selection [5]	150	0.702	0.786	**0.748**	**0.489**
Selection [5]	200	0.684	0.757	0.724	0.442
ExtCDK + RDF	1408	0.667	0.743	0.709	0.410
Selection [5]	12	0.754	0.729	0.740	0.481
Selection [5]	25	0.737	0.786	**0.764**	**0.523**
Selection [5]	50	0.702	0.771	0.740	0.474
Selection [5]	100	0.684	0.771	0.732	0.457
1D&2D + RDF	1760	0.719	0.714	0.717	0.432
Selection [5]	50	0.807	0.800	0.803	0.605
Selection [5]	100	0.825	0.786	0.803	0.607
Selection [5]	150	0.807	0.800	0.803	0.605
Selection [5]	200	0.842	0.786	**0.811**	**0.625**
Selection [5]	250	0.772	0.800	0.787	0.571

[1] Sensitivity, the ratio of true positive to the sum of true positive and false positive. [2] Specificity, the ratio of true negative to the sum of true negative and false negative. [3] Overall predictive accuracy, the ratio of the sum of true positive and true negative to the sum of true positive, true negative, false positive and false negative. [4] Matthews correlation coefficient. [5] The descriptor selection was evaluated based on the importance assigned by the RF model with the R program.

The 200 most important descriptors selected by the MeanDecreaseAccuracy parameter of the 1D&2D + RDF model were identified by the RF algorithm and enabled the training of a new RF model with better prediction accuracy in accordance with the Q and MCC values than the model trained with the whole set of descriptors (Table 3). A comparison of three machine learning (ML) techniques using the Weka software (support vector machines, SVM), R software (RF) and Keras software (deep learning multilayer perceptron networks, $_{d}$MLP) for building the antifouling models with the 200 descriptors that were selected by the RF is shown in Table 4 for the test set.

Table 4. Exploration of different ML algorithms using the 200 selected descriptors.

Model	SE [1]	SP [2]	Q [3]	MCC [4]
RF	0.667	0.750	0.714	0.417
SVM	0.830	0.500	0.643	0.344
$_{d}$MLP	0.670	0.750	0.714	0.417

[1] Sensitivity, the ratio of true positive to the sum of true positive and false positive. [2] Specificity, the ratio of true negative to the sum of true negative and false negative. [3] Overall predictive accuracy, the ratio of the sum of true positive and true negative to the sum of true positive, true negative, false positive and false negative. [4] Matthews correlation coefficient.

The best models were accomplished with the RF and $_{d}$MLP algorithms using the 200 1D&2D + RDF selected descriptors, which achieved, for both models, a Q and MCC of 0.714 and 0.417 for the external test set. Majority voting predictions (consensus) were obtained by the RF, SVM and $_{d}$MLP models (the consensus model, CM), and did not improve the results, with a Q and MCC of 0.571 and 0.167 for the test set; thus, in the next step of the virtual screening, we used the best model obtained, RF, with the 200 selected descriptors; see Tables 3 and 4).

The results obtained by the RF for the training and test sets that were in accordance with the seven structural clusters (I–VII), reported in Table 1, are shown in Table 5.

Table 5. The predictions of the best RF model by the seven structural clusters for the training and test sets. The best models are highlighted in bold.

Cluster	#	SE [1]	SP [2]	Q [3]	MCC [4]
		Training set			
I	11	1.000	-	**1.000**	**1.000**
II	28	0.889	0.789	**0.821**	**0.640**
III	19	1.000	0.400	0.842	0.574
IV	22	0.800	0.941	**0.909**	**0.741**
V	15	0.900	0.000	0.600	-
VI	16	0.000	1.000	0.813	-
VII	16	0.400	0.812	0.688	0.234
All		0.842	0.786	0.811	0.625
		Test set			
II	3	1.000	1.000	**1.000**	**1.000**
III	1	-	1.000	**1.000**	**1.000**
IV	6	0.333	1.000	0.667	0.447
V	3	1.000	0.000	0.667	-
VII	1	-	0.000	0.000	-
All		0.667	0.750	0.713	0.417

[1] Sensitivity, the ratio of true positive to the sum of true positive and false positive. [2] Specificity, the ratio of true negative to the sum of true negative and false negative. [3] Overall predictive accuracy, the ratio of the sum of true positive and true negative to the sum of true positive, true negative, false positive and false negative. [4] Matthews correlation coefficient.

There were three structural clusters (I, II and IV, bold highlighted in Table 5) in which the predictions obtained were better than those obtained for the overall training set simultaneously considering the Q and MCC values. An improvement in the RF model prediction accuracies (Q = 0.821–1 and MCC = 0.64–1) was achieved for these three clusters of the training set, when compared with the prediction accuracy obtained for all the molecules of the training set (Q = 0.811 and MCC = 0.625). For the clusters II and V-VII, lower prediction accuracies were obtained, Q = 0.6–0.842 and MCC = 0.234–0.574. Interestingly, the best achieved predictions for structural clusters I and II were related to the best performance obtained for the active class prediction, with SE values of 1 and 0.889, respectively, compared to the SE value of 0.842 for all training sets. For example, for the test set, the average of the Prob_active (a_Prob_active) obtained by the active molecules predicted by the model as active, i.e., true positive (TP), was 0.59, which compares with the value of a_Prob_active of 0.54 obtained by the predicted molecules by the model as false positives (FP). The same relationship was obtained for molecules predicted as true negatives (FN) and false negatives (FN), with an a_Pro_active of 0.44 and 0.48, respectively. Additionally, it appears that, with a Prob_active higher than 0.59, there was no error in the prediction and all molecules predicted as active were active.

2.3. Analysis of Fingerprints and Descriptors Identified as Relevant for Modeling the Antifouling Activity

The selected 200 descriptors included 164 1D&2D (115 topological descriptors, 48 count type descriptors and one constitutional descriptor (Mannhold LogP, logarithm of the octanol–water partition coefficient)) and 36 RDF 3D descriptors (12 of type a (a positive and a negative charge), 12 of type b (two positive charges) and 12 of type c (two negative charges)). The 1D&2D descriptors comprised 72 autocorrelation topological descriptors, which were 50 Broto–Moreau, 12 Moran and 10 Geary autocorrelation descriptors, weighted by mass, charges, van der Waals volumes, Sanderson electronegativities, polarizabilities, first ionization potential or I-state. Other topological descriptors, such as 6 Barysz matrices, 24 Burden-modified eigenvalues, 1 Detour matrix, 2 MDEs, 2 path counts, 3 topological charges, 3 distance matrices, 1 walk count descriptor and 1 weighted path descriptor, were also presented. The count type descriptors included 28 electrotopological state atom types, 10 extended topochemical atoms and 10 information content descriptors. A comparison of the best twenty 1D&2D + RDF molecular descriptors selected by descriptor importance of RF was used to build the QSAR classification models, which are presented in Tables 3 and 4, and these were analyzed and are presented in Figure 1.

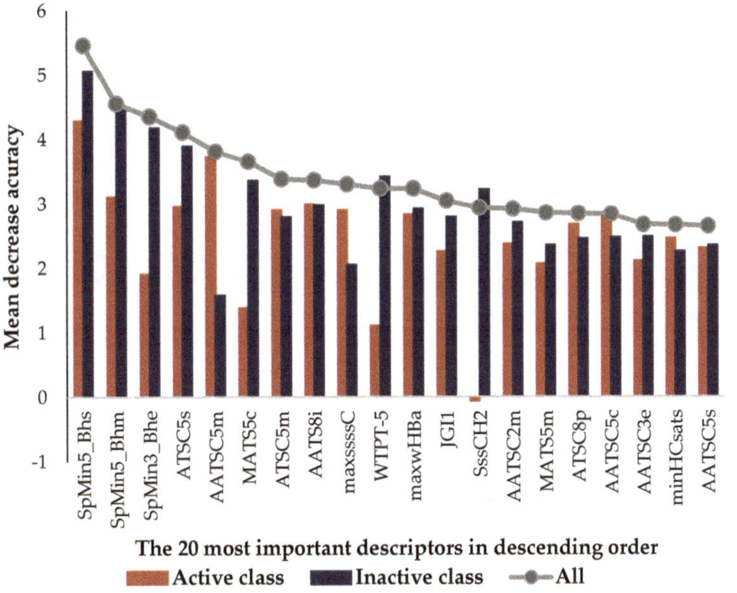

Figure 1. The twenty most important 1D&2D +RDF descriptors selected in RF classification models, where the first three descriptors in terms of importance are three Burden-modified eigenvalue descriptors weighted by relative I-state, mass and Sanderson electronegativities, respectively; there are several Broto–Moreau autocorrelations 4th–5th, 7th–8th, 14th, 16th–18th, 20th weighted by I-state, mass, mass, first ionization potential, mass, polarizabilities, charge, Sanderson electronegativities and I-state; two Moran autocorrelation descriptors, 6th and 15th weighted by charge and mass, respectively; four electrotopological state atom type descriptors, 9th (>C<), 11th (weak hydrogen bond acceptors), 13th (-CH2-), 19th (H bonded to B, Si, P, Ge, As, Se, Sn or P); one PaDEL weighted path descriptor, 10th (sum of path lengths starting from nitrogens); and one topological charge descriptor, 12th (mean topological charge index of order 1).

Interestingly, no 3D RDF descriptor appeared in the list of the twenty most important descriptors and the first RDF descriptor appeared only in the 30th position (two positive charges). Moreover, there were only seven out the twenty most important descriptors that were more relevant in discriminating the active class, namely AATSC5m (5th), ATSC5m (7th), AATS8i (8th), maxssssC (9th), ATSC8p (16th), AATSC5c (17th) and minHCsats (19th). Of the nine Broto–Moreau autocorrelation descriptors existing in the list of the top 20, five of them were more relevant to discriminate the active class and, on the other hand, they also presented a lag higher than or equal to 5, which was related to a greater distance between the structural features of interest. In contrast, the four Broto–Moreau autocorrelation descriptors that were more relevant for the inactive class presented a lag lower than or equal to 5. The three most important descriptors in the top 20 list were three Burden-modified eigenvalue descriptors and all of them were most relevant in the inactive class discrimination. This eigenvalue was suggested as an index of molecular branching, the smallest values corresponding to chain graphs (SpMin3_Bhe) and the highest to the most branched graphs (SpMin5_Bhs and SpMin5_Bhm) [53]. A very interesting behavior was observed with the two electrotopological state atom types, maxssssC (maximum atom-type E-state: >C<) and SssCH2 (sum of atom-type E-state: -CH_2-), which were more relevant for the active and inactive classes, respectively. The maxssssC descriptor encodes the maximum number of quaternary or asymmetric carbon atoms and could be seen as encoding structural complexity. On the other hand, the SssCH2 descriptor encoded the saturation of the molecule. Another very important descriptor to discriminate mainly the inactive class is the PaDEL weighted path descriptor, WTPT-5, which is the sum of all path weights starting from nitrogen atoms, revealing nitrogen-specific branching information. In agreement with the present work, the two QSAR studies reported by Almeida et al. highlighted the descriptors related to the branching, complexity and the influence of the molecule's interatomic distance for the modeling of the antifouling activity [45,46].

2.4. Application of the In Silico Antifouling QSAR Model in Virtual Screening

A virtual screening campaign was carried out to search for new lead-like antifouling inhibitors. The best QSAR model, the RF model, was selected for the virtual screening procedure using 14,492 MNPs from Prof. Encinar's website and 14 MNPs in the pharmaceutical pipeline (eight approved drugs and six MNPs in Phase II and III of clinical trials). The antifouling virtual screening of the MNP library in the pharmaceutical pipeline allowed us to assess the possibility of repurposing drugs of marine origin. Of these 14 MNPs from the pharmaceutical pipeline, only one MNP in Phase II of clinical trials presented activity against AChE, GTS-21 (DMXBA), a derivative of the NP, 2,4-dimethoxybenzylidene anabaseine dihydrochloride. There were 13,902 MNPs that were predicted to be active by the best QSAR model, of which 8349 MNPs were predicted to be active with a Prob_active greater than 0.59 (limit defined for the test set for which there are no prediction errors). From these MNPs, 5 (one approved drug and four MNPs in Phase II and III of clinical trials) and 8344 MNPs were from the pharmaceutical pipeline and from Encinar's database, respectively. Interestingly, of the five MNPs from the MNP pharmaceutical pipeline predicted to be active with the highest Prob_active was DMXBA with a value of 0.658. A more demanding limit has been defined for the CADD structure-based approach: all the MNPs from the virtual screening libraries that were predicted as belonging to the active class with a Prob_active greater than or equal to 0.68 were selected for molecular docking experiments. In the CADD structure-based method, the 125 MNPs selected by the QSAR classification approach were screened by molecular docking against acetylcholinesterase enzyme (AChE).

The list of eleven lead-like AChE inhibitors against antifouling activity generated from the AChE homology virtual screening, which were experimentally screened in in vitro and micro- and macrofouling assays reported by Arabshahi et al. [50], was used in this study as a second virtual screening library (Supplementary Data, Table S5). Only one out of the eleven lead-like AChE inhibitors was predicted to have antifouling activity with a Prob_active higher than 0.59 (Table S5), the morpholine derivative (Figure 2), in which experimental antifouling activity IC_{50} = 16 μg/mL was reported (51.7 μM) [50]. However, none of the eleven compounds passed the established threshold, which was more demanding (Prob_active $\geq$ 0.68), to be selected for the molecular docking experiments.

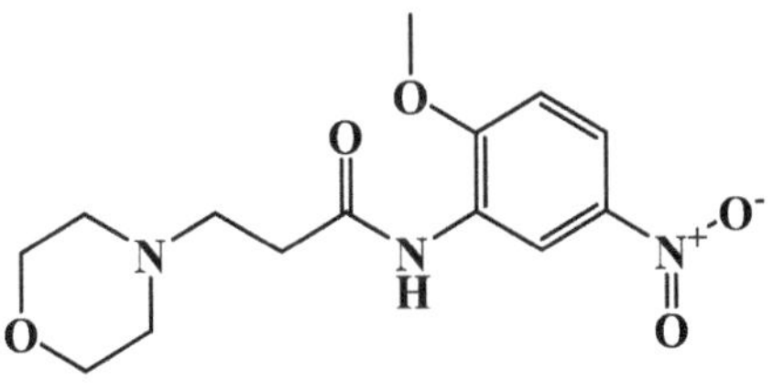

Figure 2. Chemical structure of the morpholine derivative.

2.5. Molecular Docking against AChE Enzyme

The 125 MNPs from Encinar's database selected by the QSAR classification approach were screened by molecular docking against AChE enzyme (PDB ID: 6TT0) [54]. The antifouling agents, synoxazolidinone A, synoxazolidinone C and donepezil, known as AChE inhibitors [28], were used as positive controls and the phenolic derivative that was predicted to not have antifouling activity in virtual screening was used as a negative control in the molecular docking experiments. A list of virtual screening hits comprising 19 MNPs was approved based on molecular docking experiments, in which a threshold of $\Delta GB \leq -7$ kcal/mol was established for predicting the affinity between AChE and selected MNPs. To prioritize the best marine drug-like leads as antifouling AChE inhibitors from the list of 19 selected MNPs by the antifouling QSAR model and molecular docking of AChE enzyme, the absorption, distribution, metabolism, excretion and toxicity (ADMET) properties were predicted via in silico methods using the pKCSM software (http://biosig.unimelb.edu.au/pkcsm/, accessed on 25 October 2021) [55]. Sixteen MNPs, a macrocyclic lactam (CAS 156310-18-8), seven macrocyclic alkaloids (CAS 126622-63-7, 126622-64-8, 156310-18-8, 155944-26-6, 157536-35-1, 105305-54-2 and 105418-77-7), seven indole derivatives (CAS 142677-10-9, 134029-43-9, 134029-44-0, 134029-45-1, 142677-09-6, 223596-72-3, 134779-34-3) and a pyridine derivative (CAS 59697-14-2) were proposed as marine drug-like leads as antifouling AChE inhibitors. Three MNPs were excluded due to their predicted toxicity to fish, namely against flathead minnows. The Autodock Vina software (http://vina.scripps.edu/, accessed on 25 October 2021) [56] was used to perform the flexible virtual screening of the 125 MNPs to find the most favorable binding interactions, and the calculated free binding energies by the set of search space coordinates are reported in Table 6 for the 16 MNPs selected, and the positive (synoxazolidinone A and C; donepezil, an AChE inhibitor used for Alzheimer disease therapy) and the negative (phenolic derivative derivative) controls.

Table 6. Structures and calculated free binding energies (ΔG_B, in kcal/mol) of the sixteen selected MNPs, the positive (synoxazolidinone A and C; donepezil) and negative (phenolic derivative) controls.

CAS	Chemical Structure	Name/Structural Category	Natural Source	Prob_A	ΔG_B (kcal/mol) [1]
147362-39-8	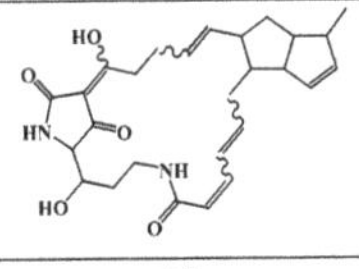	cylindramide/lactam	marine sponge [2]	0.684	−11.3
126622-63-7	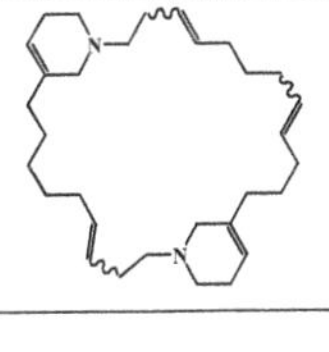	haliclamine B/macrocyclic alkaloid	marine sponge [3]	0.682	−8.2

Table 6. *Cont.*

CAS	Chemical Structure	Name/Structural Category	Natural Source	Prob_A	ΔG_B (kcal/mol) [1]
126622-64-8	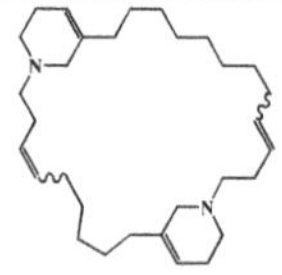	haliclamine A/macrocyclic alkaloid	marine sponge [3]	0.682	−7.8
156310-18-8	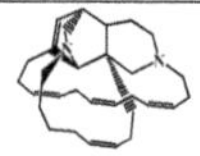	ingamine B/macrocyclic alkaloid	marine sponge [4]	0.682	−7.8
155944-26-6	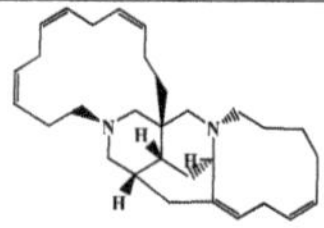	madangamines A/macrocyclic alkaloid	marine sponge [4]	0.694	−7.7
105305-54-2	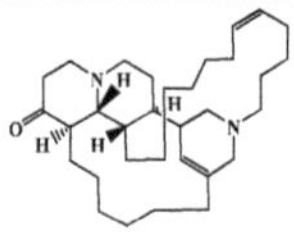	serain 3/ macrocyclic alkaloid	marine sponge [5]	0.686	−7.5
142677-10-9	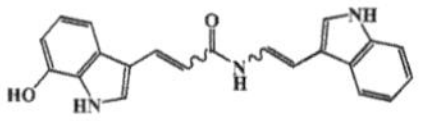	chondriamide B/indole	red alga [6]	0.682	−7.5
134029-43-9	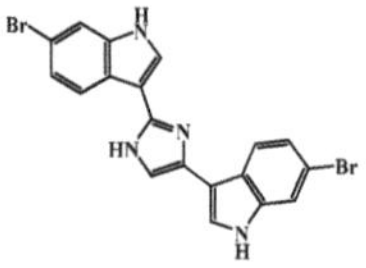	nortopsentin A/indole	marine sponge [7]	0.702	−7.3
134029-44-0	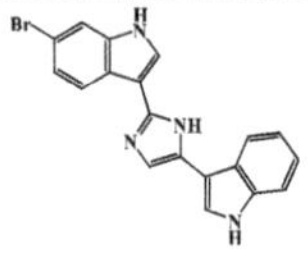	nortopsentin B/indole	marine sponge [7]	0.698	−7.3
134029-45-1	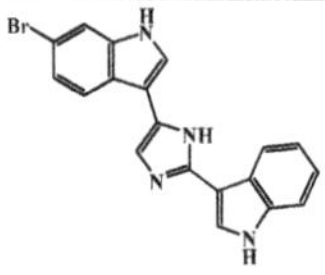	nortopsentin C/indole	marine sponge [7]	0.700	−7.3
105418-77-7	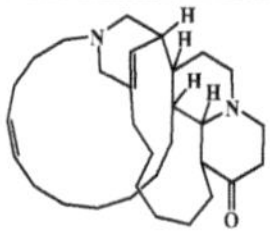	serain 1/ macrocyclic alkaloid	marine sponge [5]	0.686	−7.2
142677-09-6	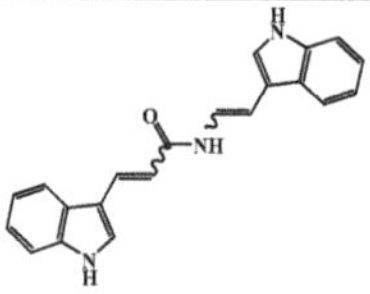	chondriamide A/indole	red alga [6]	0.682	−7.2

Table 6. *Cont.*

CAS	Chemical Structure	Name/Structural Category	Natural Source	Prob_A	ΔG_B (kcal/mol) [1]
223596-72-3	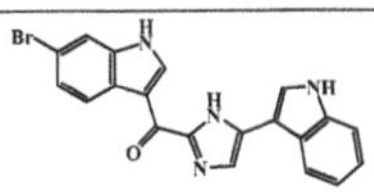	isobromodeoxytopsent/ indole	marine sponge [8]	0.680	−7.2
134779-34-3	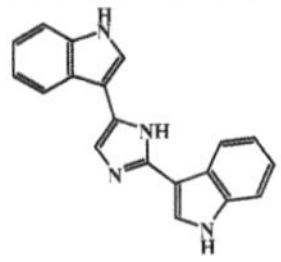	nortopsentin D/indole	marine sponge [7]	0.688	−7.1
157536-35-1	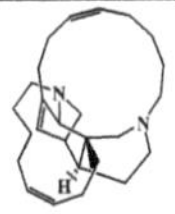	keramaphidin B/macrocyclic alkaloid	marine sponge [9]	0.684	−7.1
59697-14-2	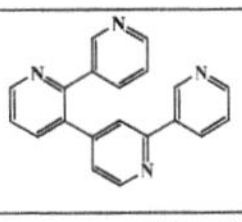	nemertelline/ pyridine	marine worm [10]	0.680	−7.0
positive control	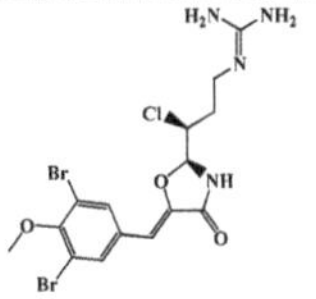	synoxazolidinone A	-	-	−6.5
positive control	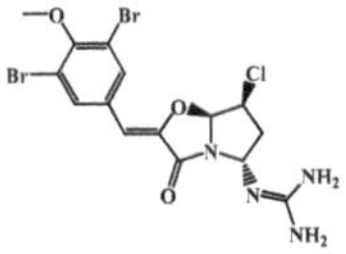	synoxazolidinone C	-	-	−6.7
positive control	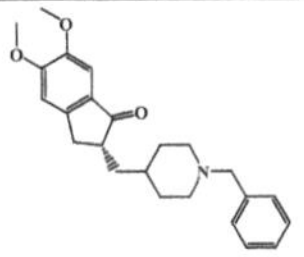	donepezil	-	-	−6.5
negative control	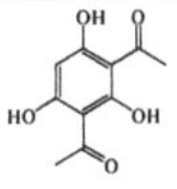	phenolic	-	-	−5.1

[1] AChE enzyme: center X: 25.435 Y: 69.621 Z: 278.986; [2] *Halichondria cylindrata*; [3] *Haliclona* sp.; [4] *Xestospongia ingens*; [5] *Reniera sarai*; [6] *Chondria* sp.; [7] *Spongosorites ruetzleri* and *Haliclona* sp.; [8] *Spongosorites* sp.; [9] *Amphimedon* sp.; [10] *Amphiporus angulatus*.

The prediction of the ADMET properties of the sixteen selected MNPs by the antifouling QSAR model and molecular docking of AChE enzyme is presented in Table S1, in the Supplementary Materials. In Figure 3, the interaction profile of the best-docked pose for the two most probable lead-like antifouling AChE inhibitors, a lactam derivative—cylindramide—and a macrocyclic alkaloid—haliclamine B—is represented.

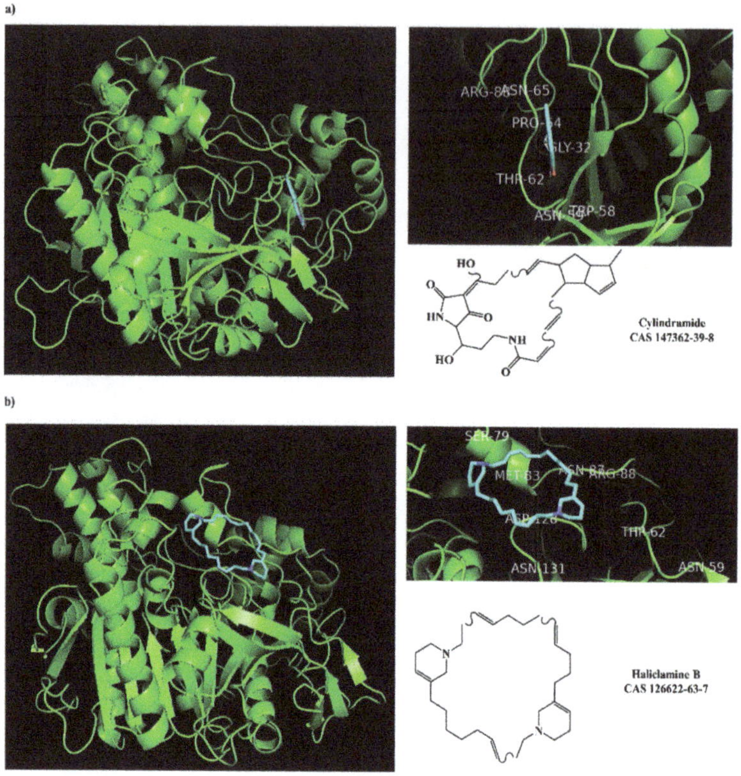

Figure 3. Interaction profiles of the best-docked poses for the two hits (**a**) cylindramide and (**b**) haliclamine B.

New scoring functions based on more precise physics-based descriptors to better represent the protein–ligand recognition process have been developed. DockThor, a web service for molecular docking simulation (https://dockthor.lncc.br/v2/, accessed on 6 January 2022), was used to perform molecular docking of the two best macrocycle hits (cylindramine and haliclamine B), the best non-macrocycle hit (indole derivative, CAS 142677-10-9) and the positive and negative controls against the AChE enzyme (PDB ID: 6TT0). In DockThor, a set of new empirical scoring functions to estimate protein–ligand binding affinity were developed by explicitly accounting for physics-based interaction terms based on the MMFF94S force field combined with ML [57]. The DockThor scores obtained for the two best macrocycle hits (cylindramine and haliclamine B), the best non-macrocycle hit (indole derivative, CAS 142677-10-9) and the positive (synoxazolidinone A and C; donepezil) and negative (phenolic derivative) controls were −8.508 kcal/mol (−11.3 kcal/mol using Autodock Vina), −7.008 kcal/mol (−8.2 kcal/mol using Autodock Vina), −8.634 kcal/mol (−7.5 kcal/mol using Autodock Vina), −7.749 kcal/mol (−6.5 kcal/mol using Autodock Vina), −7.56 kcal/mol (−6.7 kcal/mol using Autodock Vina) and −6.416 kcal/mol (−5.1 kcal/mol using Autodock Vina), respectively. The interaction profiles of the best-docked poses predicted by DockThor for the two best macrocycle hits, the best non-macrocycle hit and the positive and negative controls are presented in Figure 4.

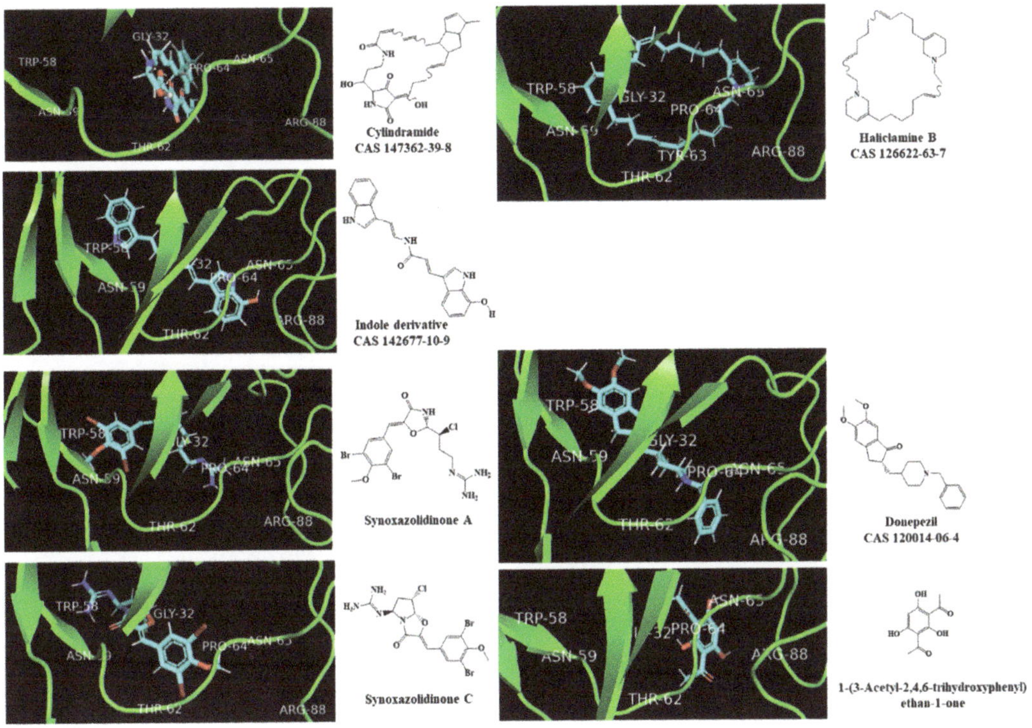

Figure 4. Interaction profiles of the best-docked poses for the two macrocyclic hits (cylindramide and haliclamine B), the best non-macrocycle hit (indole derivative) and the positive (synoxazolidinone A and C; donepezil) and negative (phenolic derivative) controls.

The peripheral anionic site (PAS) of AChE is composed of five residues (TYR-70, ASP-72, TYR-121, TRP-279 and TYR-334) and is involved in the allosteric modulation of catalysis at the active center [46]. This site is the target of various anti-cholinesterase inhibitors. In this work, other residues (e.g., ARG-88, ASN-65, PRO-64, GLY-32, THR-62, TRP-58 and ASN-59) forming the hydrophobic interactions in the PAS pocket are highlighted in Figures 3 and 4. The binding of donepezil to the PAS of AChE is in accordance with its proposed peculiar inhibitory mechanism, which involves a reversible double-binding site interaction with the catalytic anionic site and PAS of the enzyme [54]. Unlike our approach and in other reported studies [46,54], Arabshahi et al. [50] performed a virtual screening by molecular docking of AChE at the catalytic anionic site and not at the PAS. Although none of the 11 reported compounds [50] passed the QSAR model threshold to be subjected to molecular docking, we still performed the molecular docking and the docking scores are presented in Table S5 (Supplementary Data). It was verified that none of these compounds exceeded the established threshold in the molecular docking experiments, $\Delta GB \leq -7$ kcal/mol.

3. Materials and Methods

3.1. Data Sets/Selection of Training and Test Sets

The antifouling data set comprising 142 molecules, 63 and 79 organic molecules, was extracted from the ChEMBL (https://www.ebi.ac.uk/chembl/, accessed on 21 July 2021) [58] and by searching in the literature indexed in the Web of Science Core Collection until June 2021, respectively. The ChEMBL data set was obtained by searching for marine organisms with antifouling activity, such as barnacles (e.g., *Balanus amphitrite*), mussels (e.g., *Mytilus galloprovincialis*), bushy bryozoan (e.g., *Bugula neritina*) and marine algae (e.g., *Ulva conglobata*). The antifouling activity was classified using two activity classes: (A, active)—inhibition % > 52% and EC_{50}, $IC_{50} \leq 25$ µg/mL; (B, inactive)—inhibition % $\leq$ 52% and EC_{50}, IC_{50} > 25 µg/mL. After collecting these data sets, the duplicates were removed based on the IUPAC international chemical identifier (InChI) codes; however, the chirality was considered, and racemic compounds (or cases where no stereochemistry was indicated) were considered as one of the possible stereoisomers. Thereafter, the final data set comprised 141 organic molecules and was divided into a training set comprising 127 molecules (class A, 57 molecules and class B, 70 molecules) and a test set comprising 14 molecules (class A, 6 molecules and class B, 8 molecules). The partitioning of the data set into training and testing sets was performed randomly according to the composition of the antifouling classes (active and inactive). The composition of the 10 structural categories shown in Table 1 was not considered. The built QSAR models were developed and externally validated using the training and test sets, respectively.

The virtual data set comprised 14,492 MNPs from Prof. Encinar's website (http://docking.umh.es/downloaddb, accessed on 25 October 2021) saved in the MDL SDF data format and 14 MNPs from the pharmaceutical pipeline set (eight approved drugs and six MNPs in Phase II and III of clinical trials). Three duplicates with the training and test sets were removed and the final virtual data set comprised 14,503 molecules.

A second virtual library comprising eleven lead-like AChE inhibitors against antifouling activity reported by Arabshahi et al. [50] was also used.

SMILES strings of the data sets, and the corresponding experimental and predicted activities, are available as Supplementary Data, Tables S2, S3 and S5.

3.2. Calculation of Descriptors

The molecular structures of molecules in all data sets were standardized by normalizing tautomeric and mesomeric groups and by removing small disconnected fragments using the JChem Standardizer tool, version 5.7.13.0 (ChemAxon Ltd., Budapest, Hungary). The optimization of the three-dimensional molecular structures was carried out with CORINA version 2.4 (Molecular Networks GmbH, Erlangen, Germany). PaDEL-Descriptor (Pharmaceutical Data Exploration Laboratory, Singapore) version 2.21 (http://www.yapcwsoft.com/dd/padeldescriptor/, accessed on 21 July 2021) [52] was used to calculate empirical molecular fingerprints (FPs) and 1D&2D molecular descriptors. FPs of various types were calculated and exploited to build QSAR models, namely 166 MACCS (MACCS keys), 307 Substructure (presence and count of SMARTS patterns for Laggner functional group classification—Sub), 881 PubChem fingerprints (ftp://ftp.ncbi.nlm.nih.gov/pubchem/specifications/pubchem_fingerprints.txt, accessed on 21 July 2021), 1024 CDK (circular fingerprints) and 1024 CDK extended (Ext circular fingerprints with additional bits describing ring features). The 1D&2D molecular descriptors comprised descriptors of various types, including electronic, topological and constitutional descriptors, in a total of 1376 descriptors. Radial distribution function (RDF) pair descriptors [59] and 3D RDF descriptors were calculated by sampling the function of Equation (1) at 128 equally distributed values of r between 0 and 12.8 Å:

$$RDF(r) = \sum_{i=1}^{N-1} \sum_{j=1+1}^{N} p_i p_j e^{-B\,(r-r_{ij})^2} \quad (1)$$

where N is the number of atoms in the molecule, p_i is the charge of atom i, B is a fuzziness parameter (it was 100 in this study), and r_{ij} is the 3D distance between atoms i and j. The *RDF* descriptors were separated into three sets of 128 descriptors per pair of atoms with (a) one positive and one negative charge, (b) two positive charges and (c) two negative charges. The partial atomic charges—natural bond orbital (NBO) partial atomic charges—were estimated using an ML tool developed by Aires-de-Sousa and co-workers (http://joao.airesdesousa.com/charges, accessed on 21 July 2021) [60].

3.3. Selection of Descriptors and Optimization of QSAR Models

In the quest for QSAR models with the minimum possible number of descriptors, descriptor selection was performed based on the importance of descriptors assessed by the RF (computeAttributeImportance) algorithm [51] implemented in the R program [61]. Selection of descriptors was accomplished using this procedure, with the importance of descriptors assessed by RF within an OOB methodology using the 12, 25, 50, 100, 150, 200 and 250 most important descriptors and RF algorithm as an ML technique employing the following statistical metrics: true positives (TP), true negatives (TN), false positives (FP), false negatives (FN), sensitivity (SE, prediction accuracy for active antifouling molecules), specificity (SP, prediction accuracy for inactive antifouling molecules), overall predictive accuracy (Q) and Matthews correlation coefficient (MCC).

3.4. Class Balancer

In general, class imbalance is more demanding for ML algorithms and this imbalance introduces a bias due to their preference for the majority class [62]. Our antifouling activity training set was unbalanced, and the imbalance ratio was 1:1.22 for the A: active and B: inactive classes, respectively. To solve this problem, the classes were balanced using the RF *sampsize* parameter with R version 3.6.1. [61]. This parameter was set to be of the same size as the minority class (active class). With this parameter, some molecules belonging to the minority class were used more than once.

3.5. Machine Learning (ML) Methods

3.5.1. Random Forest (RF)

The RF model [51,63] was built from a set of unpruned classification trees, which were created using bootstrap samples from the training set. For each individual tree, the best split at each node was defined using a randomly selected subset of descriptors. Each of the individual classification trees was created using different training and validation sets. The final prediction of the model resulted from the majority vote of classification trees in the forest. Model performance was evaluated internally with the prediction error for molecules left out in the bootstrap procedure (OOB estimation). The method quantifies the importance of a descriptor by the increase in misclassification that occurs when descriptor values are randomly permuted, correlated with the mean decrease in the precision parameter. RFs also assigned a probability to every prediction based on the number of votes obtained by the predicted class. RFs were grown with the R program [61], version 3.6.1, using the random forest library [64]. As a result of the nature of the two-class imbalance, this problem was alleviated by defining the class weight ranges of 1–57 and 1–57 for classes A and B, respectively, using the *sampsize* parameter.

3.5.2. Support Vector Machines (SVMs)

SVMs [65] map the training data into a hyperspace through a nonlinear mapping (a boundary or hyperplane) and then separate the classes of objects in this space. The examples of the training set—the support vectors—allowed us to position the boundary. To transform data into a hyperspace where classes become linearly separable, kernel functions were used. In this study, SVMs were implemented with Scikit-learn [66] using the LIBSVM package [67]. The type of SVM was set to C-SVM-classification and the radial basis function was used for the kernel function. Hyperparameter tuning was performed using ten-fold cross-validation with the GridSearchCV tool. C and γ values varied in the range of 1×10^{-2} to 1×10^{13} and 1×10^{-9} to 1×10^{13}, respectively. In total, 10,000 experiments were performed. The C and γ values were finally set to 1×10^{7} and 1×10^{-8}, respectively, and the other parameters were used with default values. To alleviate the imbalanced two-class problem, the class_weight parameter was set to be "balanced", in which the smaller class was replicated until it had as many molecules as in the larger one class.

3.5.3. Deep Learning Multilayer Perceptron Networks ($_d$MLP)

The feed-forward neural networks were implement using the open-source software library Keras [68] version 2.2.5 based on the Tensorflow numerical backend engine [69]. These popular software tools, written in Python, make it easy to develop and apply deep neural networks; however, the main challenge in applying $_d$MLP is the design of an adequate network architecture. After several experiments, the final optimal hyperparameter settings were selected for our study based on 10-fold cross-validation experiments with the training set and are listed in Table 7.

Table 7. Hyperparameter settings of the best $_d$MLP model.

Hyperparameter	Setting
Initializer	Glorot uniform
Number of hidden layers	2
Number of neurons in the 1st and 2nd layers	200
Number of neurons in the 3rd	2
Activation 1st–2nd layers	Relu
Activation 3rd layer	Sigmoid
Batch size	36
Optimizer	Adadelta
Loss	Binary crossentropy
Epochs	100

3.6. Molecular Docking

The virtual screening using the best QSAR model, the RF classification model using the 200 most important 1D&2D + RDF molecular descriptors, allowed the prioritization of a list of the 125 MNP virtual screening hits. OpenBabel software (version 2.3.1, freely available under an open-source license from http://openbabel.org, accessed on 21 July 2021) [70] was used to convert mol2 files into PDBQT files. PDBQT files were used for coupling to the AChE enzyme with Autodock Vina (version 1.1, Center for Computational Structural Biology, Scripps Research Institute, CA, USA) [56]. The macromolecule coupling target was the AChE enzyme from *Tetronarce californica* (PDB ID: 6TT0) [54]. Water molecules, carbohydrate molecules and ligands (1R, 3S-cis- and 1S, 3R-cis-donepezil derived enantiomers) were removed from 6TT0 [54] prior to docking using AutoDockTools (http://mgltools.scripps.edu/, accessed on 21 July 2021). During enzyme preparation, GTT0, explicit hydrogen atoms and Gasteiger charges for each atom were added. Autodock Vina performed a flexible molecular docking in which the target's conformation was considered a rigid unit while the ligands were flexible and adaptable to the target. Autodock Vina looked for the lowest binding affinity conformations and returned ten different conformations for each ligand. The search space coordinates of the AChE enzyme were maximized to allow the entire macromolecule to be considered for docking. The search space coordinates were center X: 25.179 Y: 72.212 Z: 281.175; dimensions X: 20,000 Y: 20,000 Z: 20,000. AchE enzyme ligand tethering was performed by regulating the parameters of the genetic algorithm (GA), using 10 runs of the GA criteria. DockThor, a web service for molecular docking simulation (https://dockthor.lncc.br/v2/, accessed on 6 January 2022), was used to perform molecular docking of the two best macrocycle hits (cylindramine and haliclamine B), the best non-macrocycle hit (indole derivative, CAS 142677-10-9) and the positive and negative controls against AChE enzyme (PDB ID: 6TT0) [57]. The search space coordinates were center X: 25.179 Y: 72.212 Z: 281.175; dimensions X: 20,000 Y: 20,000 Z: 20,000. AChE enzyme ligand tethering was performed by regulating the parameters of the GA, using 12,750 and 500,000 runs, population size and number of evaluations of the GA criteria, respectively.

The docking binding poses were visualized with PyMOL Molecular Graphics System, Version 2.0 (Schrödinger, LLC). Docking scores of 125 virtual hits against the AChE enzyme are shown in Table S4, Supplementary Data.

4. Conclusions

A CADD approach relying on ligand- and structure-based methodologies was successfully used to predict new inhibitory MNPs against antifouling AChE. Two MNPs, cylindramide (CAS 147362-39-8) and haliclamine B (CAS 126622-63-7), were proposed as the most promising marine drug-like leads as antifouling AChE inhibitors. To the best of our knowledge, the CADD ligand-based study using a QSAR classification model, developed here in this study, is the largest study ever performed with regard both to the number of molecules involved and to the number of structural families involved in the modeling of the antifouling activity, and the best model achieved an overall predictive accuracy score of up to 71% for both test and training sets. In future works, the proposed sixteen marine drug-like leads against antifouling AChE enzyme may be validated experimentally. These results enabled us to build virtual libraries of marine-derived drug-like leads, which may be virtually screened using the best antifouling QSAR model and molecular docking against the AChE enzyme. In addition, for MNPs that are experimentally confirmed to have antifouling activity, the AChE inhibitory mechanism will be studied to determine the type of action, e.g., reversible interaction with both the catalytic anionic site and the PAS, sterically blocking ligands from entering and leaving the active site gorge and allosteric alteration of the catalytic triad conformation.

Supplementary Materials: The following data are available online at https://www.mdpi.com/article/10.3390/md20020129/s1, Tables S1–S5 (XLSX). The following files are available free of charge. SMILES strings of the data set (training and test sets), the corresponding experimental and predicted activities are available as Supplementary Materials, Tables S2 and S3, respectively. Moreover, SMILES strings of the 14,492 MNPs from Encinar's website and MNPs clinical pipeline sets, for the virtual screening data set, the corresponding predicted activities are available as Supplementary Materials, Table S4. Predictions of ADMET properties with in silico methods, using the pKCSM software for a list of 16 selected MNPs by QSAR antifouling model and molecular docking of AChE enzyme are available as Supplementary Materials, Table S1. The list of eleven lead-like AChE inhibitors by Arabshahi et al. [50], the corresponding experimental, predicted activities and docking scores against the AChE enzyme are available as Supplementary Materials, Table S5.

Author Contributions: Conceptualization: F.P. and S.P.G.; Methodology: F.P.; Software: F.P.; Validation: F.P. (in silico modeling), S.P.G. (pharmaceutical pipeline data); Formal Analysis: F.P. (in silico modeling); Investigation: F.P. (in silico modeling) and S.P.G. (pharmaceutical pipeline data and MNP meroterpenoid library); Resources: F.P. (in silico modeling) and S.P.G. (pharmaceutical pipeline data and MNP meroterpenoid library); Writing—Original Draft Preparation: F.P. and S.P.G.; Writing—Review and Editing: F.P. and S.P.G.; Funding Acquisition: F.P. and S.P.G. All authors have read and agreed to the published version of the manuscript.

Funding: Financial support from Fundação para a Ciência e Tecnologia (FCT) Portugal, under grant UIDB/50006/2020 (provided to the Associate Laboratory for Green Chemistry LAQV), is greatly appreciated. F.P. thanks Fundacão para a Ciência e a Tecnologia, MCTES, for the Norma transitória DL 57/2016 Program Contract. This work is financed by national funds from FCT—Fundação para a Ciência e a Tecnologia, I.P., in the scope of the project UIDP/04378/2020 of the Research Unit on Applied Molecular Biosciences—UCIBIO and the project LA/P/0140/2020 of the Associate Laboratory Institute for Health and Bioeconomy—i4HB.

Data Availability Statement: Data are contained within the article or Supplementary Material.

Acknowledgments: We thank ChemAxon Ltd. for access to JChem and Marvin.

Conflicts of Interest: The authors declare no conflict of interest.

References

1. Magin, C.M.; Cooper, S.P.; Brennan, A.B. Non-toxic antifouling strategies. *Mater. Today* **2010**, *13*, 36–44. [CrossRef]
2. Schultz, M.P.; Bendick, J.A.; Holm, E.R.; Hertel, W.M. Economic impact of biofouling on a naval surface ship. *Biofouling* **2011**, *27*, 87–98. [CrossRef] [PubMed]
3. Schultz, M.P. Effects of coating roughness and biofouling on ship resistance and powering. *Biofouling* **2007**, *23*, 331–341. [CrossRef]

4. Schultz, M.P.; Walker, J.M.; Steppe, C.N.; Flack, K.A. Impact of diatomaceous biofilms on the frictional drag of fouling-release coatings. *Biofouling* **2015**, *31*, 759–773. [CrossRef] [PubMed]
5. Bhushan, B. Biomimetics: Lessons from nature—An overview. *Philos. Trans. Royal Soc. A* **2009**, *367*, 1445–1486. [CrossRef] [PubMed]
6. Ware, C.; Berge, J.; Sundet, J.H.; Kirkpatrick, J.B.; Coutts, A.D.M.; Jelmert, A.; Olsen, S.M.; Floerl, O.; Wisz, M.S.; Alsos, I.G. Climate change, non-indigenous species and shipping: Assessing the risk of species introduction to a high-Arctic archipelago. *Divers. Distrib.* **2014**, *20*, 10–19. [CrossRef]
7. Ashton, G.V.; Davidson, I.C.; Geller, J.; Ruiz, G.M. Disentangling the biogeography of ship biofouling: Barnacles in the Northeast Pacific. *Glob. Ecol. Biogeogr.* **2016**, *25*, 739–750. [CrossRef]
8. Pettengill, J.B.; Wendt, D.E.; Schug, M.D.; Hadfield, M.G. Biofouling likely serves as a major mode of dispersal for the polychaete tubeworm Hydroides elegans as inferred from microsatellite loci. *Biofouling* **2007**, *23*, 161–169. [CrossRef]
9. Piola, R.F.; Johnston, E.L. The potential for translocation of marine species via small-scale disruptions to antifouling surfaces. *Biofouling* **2008**, *24*, 145–155. [CrossRef]
10. Yamaguchi, T.; Prabowo, R.E.; Ohshiro, Y.; Shimono, T.; Jones, D.; Kawai, H.; Otani, M.; Oshino, A.; Inagawa, S.; Akaya, T.; et al. The introduction to Japan of the Titan barnacle, *Megabalanus coccopoma* (Darwin, 1854) (Cirripedia: Balanomorpha) and the role of shipping in its translocation. *Biofouling* **2009**, *25*, 325–333. [CrossRef] [PubMed]
11. Sonak, S.; Pangam, P.; Giriyan, A.; Hawaldar, K. Implications of the ban on organotins for protection of global coastal and marine ecology. *J. Environ. Manag.* **2009**, *90*, S96–S108. [CrossRef]
12. Callow, J.A.; Callow, M.E. Trends in the development of environmentally friendly fouling-resistant marine coatings. *Nat. Commun.* **2011**, *2*, 244. [CrossRef] [PubMed]
13. Kirschner, C.M.; Brennan, A.B. Bio-Inspired Antifouling Strategies. *Annu. Rev. Mater. Res.* **2012**, *42*, 211–229. [CrossRef]
14. Chambers, L.D.; Stokes, K.R.; Walsh, F.C.; Wood, R.J.K. Modern approaches to marine antifouling coatings. *Surf. Coat. Technol.* **2006**, *201*, 3642–3652. [CrossRef]
15. Othmani, A.; Bunet, R.; Bonnefont, J.L.; Briand, J.F.; Culioli, G. Settlement inhibition of marine biofilm bacteria and barnacle larvae by compounds isolated from the Mediterranean brown alga *Taonia atomaria*. *J. Appl. Phycol.* **2016**, *28*, 1975–1986. [CrossRef]
16. Satheesh, S.; Ba-akdah, M.A.; Al-Sofyani, A.A. Natural antifouling compound production by microbes associated with marine macroorganisms—A review. *Electron. J. Biotechnol.* **2016**, *21*, 26–35. [CrossRef]
17. Almeida, J.R.; Vasconcelos, V. Natural antifouling compounds: Effectiveness in preventing invertebrate settlement and adhesion. *Biotechnol. Adv.* **2015**, *33*, 343–357. [CrossRef] [PubMed]
18. Qian, P.-Y.; Li, Z.; Xu, Y.; Li, Y.; Fusetani, N. Mini-review: Marine natural products and their synthetic analogs as antifouling compounds: 2009-2014. *Biofouling* **2015**, *31*, 101–122. [CrossRef] [PubMed]
19. Qian, P.-Y.; Xu, Y.; Fusetani, N. Natural products as antifouling compounds: Recent progress and future perspectives. *Biofouling* **2010**, *26*, 223–234. [CrossRef]
20. Dobretsov, S.; Dahms, H.U.; Qian, P.Y. Inhibition of biofouling by marine microorganisms and their metabolites. *Biofouling* **2006**, *22*, 43–54. [CrossRef]
21. Wang, K.-L.; Wu, Z.-H.; Wang, Y.; Wang, C.-Y.; Xu, Y. Mini-Review: Antifouling Natural Products from Marine Microorganisms and Their Synthetic Analogs. *Mar. Drugs* **2017**, *15*, 266. [CrossRef]
22. Qi, S.-H.; Ma, X. Antifouling Compounds from Marine Invertebrates. *Mar. Drugs* **2017**, *15*, 263. [CrossRef] [PubMed]
23. Dahms, H.U.; Dobretsov, S. Antifouling Compounds from Marine Macroalgae. *Mar. Drugs* **2017**, *15*, 265. [CrossRef] [PubMed]
24. Moodie, L.W.K.; Sepcic, K.; Turk, T.; Frangez, R.; Svenson, J. Natural cholinesterase inhibitors from marine organisms. *Nat. Prod. Rep.* **2019**, *36*, 1053–1092. [CrossRef]
25. Dworjanyn, S.A.; de Nys, R.; Steinberg, P.D. Chemically mediated antifouling in the red alga *Delisea pulchra*. *Mar. Ecol. Prog. Ser.* **2006**, *318*, 153–163. [CrossRef]
26. Richards, J.J.; Ballard, T.E.; Huigens, R.W., III; Melander, C. Synthesis and screening of an oroidin library against *Pseudomonas aeruginosa* biofilms. *Chembiochem* **2008**, *9*, 1267–1279. [CrossRef]
27. Melander, C.; Moeller, P.D.R.; Ballard, T.E.; Richards, J.J.; Huigens, R.W., III; Cavanagh, J. Evaluation of dihydrooroidin as an antifouling additive in marine paint. *Int. Biodeterior. Biodegradation* **2009**, *63*, 529–532. [CrossRef] [PubMed]
28. Trepos, R.; Cervin, G.; Hellio, C.; Pavia, H.; Stensen, W.; Stensvag, K.; Svendsen, J.-S.; Haug, T.; Svenson, J. Antifouling Compounds from the Sub-Arctic Ascidian Synoicum pulmonaria: Synoxazolidinones A and C, Pulmonarins A and B, and Synthetic Analogues. *J. Nat. Prod.* **2014**, *77*, 2105–2113. [CrossRef] [PubMed]
29. Sjogren, M.; Goransson, U.; Johnson, A.L.; Dahlstrom, M.; Andersson, R.; Bergman, J.; Jonsson, P.R.; Bohlin, L. Antifouling activity of brominated cyclopeptides from the marine sponge Geodia barretti. *J. Nat. Prod.* **2004**, *67*, 368–372. [CrossRef] [PubMed]
30. Cho, J.Y.; Kang, J.Y.; Hong, Y.K.; Baek, H.H.; Shin, H.W.; Kim, M.S. Isolation and Structural Determination of the Antifouling Diketopiperazines from Marine-Derived *Streptomyces praecox* 291-11. *Biosci. Biotechnol. Biochem.* **2012**, *76*, 1116–1121. [CrossRef]
31. Li, X.; Dobretsov, S.; Xu, Y.; Xiao, X.; Hung, O.S.; Qian, P.-Y. Antifouling diketopiperazines produced by a deep-sea bacterium, *Streptomyces fungicidicus*. *Biofouling* **2006**, *22*, 201–208. [CrossRef] [PubMed]
32. Prieto-Davo, A.; Dias, T.; Gomes, S.E.; Rodrigues, S.; Parera-Valadezl, Y.; Borralho, P.M.; Pereira, F.; Rodrigues, C.M.P.; Santos-Sanches, I.; Gaudencio, S.P. The Madeira Archipelago As a Significant Source of Marine-Derived Actinomycete Diversity with Anticancer and Antimicrobial Potential. *Front. Microbiol.* **2016**, *7*, 1594. [CrossRef] [PubMed]

33. Bauermeister, A.; Pereira, F.; Grilo, I.R.; Godinho, C.C.; Paulino, M.; Almeida, V.; Gobbo-Neto, L.; Prieto-Davo, A.; Sobral, R.G.; Lopes, N.P.; et al. Intra-clade metabolomic profiling of MAR4 Streptomyces from the Macaronesia Atlantic region reveals a source of anti-biofilm metabolites. *Environ. Microbiol.* **2019**, *21*, 1099–1112. [CrossRef] [PubMed]
34. Pereira, F.; Almeida, J.R.; Paulino, M.; Grilo, I.R.; Macedo, H.; Cunha, I.; Sobral, R.G.; Vasconcelos, V.; Gaudencio, S.P. Antifouling Napyradiomycins from Marine -Derived Actinomycetes *Streptomyces aculeolatus*. *Mar. Drugs* **2020**, *18*, 63. [CrossRef] [PubMed]
35. Cruz, S.; Gomes, S.E.; Borralho, P.M.; Rodrigues, C.M.P.; Gaudencio, S.P.; Pereira, F. In Silico HCT116 Human Colon Cancer Cell-Based Models En Route to the Discovery of Lead-Like Anticancer Drugs. *Biomolecules* **2018**, *8*, 56. [CrossRef]
36. Dias, T.; Gaudencio, S.P.; Pereira, F. A Computer-Driven Approach to Discover Natural Product Leads for Methicillin-Resistant *Staphylococcus aureus* Infection Therapy. *Mar. Drugs* **2019**, *17*, 16. [CrossRef] [PubMed]
37. Wang, M.; Carver, J.J.; Phelan, V.V.; Sanchez, L.M.; Garg, N.; Peng, Y.; Don Duy, N.; Watrous, J.; Kapono, C.A.; Luzzatto-Knaan, T.; et al. Sharing and community curation of mass spectrometry data with Global Natural Products Social Molecular Networking. *Nat. Biotechnol.* **2016**, *34*, 828–837. [CrossRef]
38. Lang, G.; Mayhudin, N.A.; Mitova, M.I.; Sun, L.; van der Sar, S.; Blunt, J.W.; Cole, A.L.J.; Ellis, G.; Laatsch, H.; Munro, M.H.G. Evolving trends in the dereplication of natural product extracts: New methodology for rapid, small-scale investigation of natural product extracts. *J. Nat. Prod.* **2008**, *71*, 1595–1599. [CrossRef]
39. Camp, D.; Davis, R.A.; Campitelli, M.; Ebdon, J.; Quinn, R.J. Drug-like Properties: Guiding Principles for the Design of Natural Product Libraries. *J. Nat. Prod.* **2012**, *75*, 72–81. [CrossRef]
40. Gaudencio, S.P.; Pereira, F. A Computer-Aided Drug Design Approach to Predict Marine Drug-Like Leads for SARS-CoV-2 Main Protease Inhibition. *Mar. Drugs* **2020**, *18*, 633. [CrossRef]
41. Wang, L.; Le, X.; Li, L.; Ju, Y.C.; Lin, Z.X.; Gu, Q.; Xu, J. Discovering New Agents Active against Methicillin-Resistant *Staphylococcus aureus* with Ligand-Based Approaches. *J. Chem. Inf. Model.* **2014**, *54*, 3186–3197. [CrossRef] [PubMed]
42. Pereira, F.; Aires-de-Sousa, J. Computational Methodologies in the Exploration of Marine Natural Product Leads. *Mar. Drugs* **2018**, *16*, 236. [CrossRef] [PubMed]
43. Pereira, F. Have marine natural product drug discovery efforts been productive and how can we improve their efficiency? *Expert Opin. Drug Discov.* **2019**, *14*, 717–722. [CrossRef] [PubMed]
44. Llanos, M.A.; Gantner, M.E.; Rodriguez, S.; Alberca, L.N.; Bellera, C.L.; Talevi, A.; Gavernet, L. Strengths and Weaknesses of Docking Simulations in the SARS-CoV-2 Era: The Main Protease (Mpro) Case Study. *J. Chem. Inf. Model.* **2021**, *61*, 3758–3770. [CrossRef]
45. Almeida, J.R.; Moreira, J.; Pereira, D.; Pereira, S.; Antunes, J.; Palmeira, A.; Vasconcelos, V.; Pinto, M.; Correia-da-Silva, M.; Cidade, H. Potential of synthetic chalcone derivatives to prevent marine biofouling. *Sci. Total Environ.* **2018**, *643*, 98–106. [CrossRef] [PubMed]
46. Almeida, J.R.; Palmeira, A.; Campos, A.; Cunha, I.; Freitas, M.; Felpeto, A.B.; Turkina, M.V.; Vasconcelos, V.; Pinto, M.; Correia-da-Silva, M.; et al. Structure-Antifouling Activity Relationship and Molecular Targets of Bio-Inspired(thio)xanthones. *Biomolecules* **2020**, *10*, 1126. [CrossRef] [PubMed]
47. Tadesse, M.; Svenson, J.; Sepicic, K.; Trembleau, L.; Engqvist, M.; Andersen, J.H.; Jaspars, M.; Stensvag, K.; Haug, T. Isolation and Synthesis of Pulmonarins A and B, Acetylcholinesterase Inhibitors from the Colonial Ascidian Synoicum pulmonaria. *J. Nat. Prod.* **2014**, *77*, 364–369. [CrossRef]
48. Kaur, J.; Zhang, M.Q. Molecular modelling and QSAR of reversible acetylcholinesterase inhibitors. *Curr. Med. Chem.* **2000**, *7*, 273–294. [CrossRef]
49. Munoz-Torrero, D. Acetylcholinesterase Inhibitors as Disease-Modifying Therapies for Alzheimer's Disease. *Curr. Med. Chem.* **2008**, *15*, 2433–2455. [CrossRef]
50. Arabshahi, H.J.; Trobec, T.; Foulon, V.; Hellio, C.; Frangez, R.; Sepcic, K.; Cahill, P.; Svenson, J. Using Virtual AChE Homology Screening to Identify Small Molecules With the Ability to Inhibit Marine Biofouling. *Front. Mar. Sci.* **2021**, *8*, 762287. [CrossRef]
51. Breiman, L. Random forests. *Mach. Learn.* **2001**, *45*, 5–32. [CrossRef]
52. Yap, C.W. PaDEL-Descriptor: An Open Source Software to Calculate Molecular Descriptors and Fingerprints. *J. Comput. Chem.* **2011**, *32*, 1466–1474. [CrossRef]
53. Todeschini, R.; Consonni, V. *Molecular Descriptors for Chemoinformatics*; WILEY-VCH: Weinheim, Germany, 2009; Volumes 1–2.
54. Catto, M.; Pisani, L.; de la Mora, E.; Belviso, B.D.; Mangiatordi, G.F.; Pinto, A.; De Palma, A.; Denora, N.; Caliandro, R.; Colletier, J.-P.; et al. Chiral Separation, X-ray Structure, and Biological Evaluation of a Potent and Reversible Dual Binding Site AChE Inhibitor. *ACS Med. Chem. Lett.* **2020**, *11*, 869–876. [CrossRef]
55. Pires, D.E.V.; Blundell, T.L.; Ascher, D.B. pkCSM: Predicting Small-Molecule Pharmacokinetic and Toxicity Properties Using Graph-Based Signatures. *J. Med. Chem.* **2015**, *58*, 4066–4072. [CrossRef] [PubMed]
56. Trott, O.; Olson, A.J. Software News and Update AutoDock Vina: Improving the Speed and Accuracy of Docking with a New Scoring Function, Efficient Optimization, and Multithreading. *J. Comput. Chem.* **2010**, *31*, 455–461. [CrossRef]
57. Guedes, I.A.; Barreto, A.M.S.; Marinho, D.; Krempser, E.; Kuenemann, M.A.; Sperandio, O.; Dardenne, L.E.; Miteva, M.A. New machine learning and physics-based scoring functions for drug discovery. *Sci. Rep.* **2021**, *11*, 1–19. [CrossRef]
58. Mendez, D.; Gaulton, A.; Bento, A.P.; Chambers, J.; De Veij, M.; Felix, E.; Magarinos, M.P.; Mosquera, J.F.; Mutowo, P.; Nowotka, M.; et al. ChEMBL: Towards direct deposition of bioassay data. *Nucleic Acids Res.* **2019**, *47*, D930–D940. [CrossRef]
59. Selzer, P.; Ertl, P. Identification and classification of GPCR ligands using self-organizing neural networks. *QSAR Comb. Sci.* **2005**, *24*, 270–276. [CrossRef]

60. Zhang, Q.; Zheng, F.; Fartaria, R.; Latino, D.A.R.S.; Qu, X.; Campos, T.; Zhao, T.; Aires-de-Sousa, J. A QSPR approach for the fast estimation of DFT/NBO partial atomic charges. *Chemom. Intell. Lab. Syst.* **2014**, *134*, 158–163. [CrossRef]
61. *R: A Language and Environment for Statistical Computing*. R Foundation for Statistical Computing: Vienna, Austria. 2014. Available online: http://www.R-project.org (accessed on 21 July 2021).
62. Jain, S.; Kotsampasakou, E.; Ecker, G.F. Comparing the performance of meta-classifiers-a case study on selected imbalanced data sets relevant for prediction of liver toxicity. *J. Comput.-Aided Mol. Des.* **2018**, *32*, 583–590. [CrossRef]
63. Svetnik, V.; Liaw, A.; Tong, C.; Culberson, J.C.; Sheridan, R.P.; Feuston, B.P. Random forest: A classification and regression tool for compound classification and QSAR modeling. *J. Chem. Inform. Comput. Sci.* **2003**, *43*, 1947–1958. [CrossRef] [PubMed]
64. Liaw, A.; Wiener, M. Classification and Regression by randomForest. *R News* **2002**, *2*, 18–22.
65. Cortes, C.; Vapnik, V. Support-Vector Networks. *Mach. Learn.* **1995**, *20*, 273–297. [CrossRef]
66. Pedregosa, F.; Varoquaux, G.; Gramfort, A.; Michel, V.; Thirion, B.; Grisel, O.; Blondel, M.; Prettenhofer, P.; Weiss, R.; Dubourg, V.; et al. Scikit-learn: Machine Learning in Python. *J. Mach. Learn. Res.* **2011**, *12*, 2825–2830.
67. Chang, C.-C.; Lin, C.-J. LIBSVM: A Library for Support Vector Machines. *ACM Trans. Intell. Syst. Technol.* **2011**, *2*. [CrossRef]
68. Chollet, F.K. GitHub, Seattle, WA, USA. 2015. Available online: https://github.com/fchollet/keras (accessed on 21 July 2021).
69. Abadi, M.; Agarwal, A.; Barham, P.; Brevdo, E.; Chen, Z.; Citro, C.; Corrado, G.S.; Davis, A.; Dean, J.; Devin, M.; et al. TensorFlow: Large-Scale Machine Learning on Heterogeneous Distributed Systems. *arXiv* **2016**, arXiv:1603.04467.
70. O'Boyle, N.M.; Banck, M.; James, C.A.; Morley, C.; Vandermeersch, T.; Hutchison, G.R. Open Babel: An open chemical toolbox. *J. Cheminform.* **2011**, *3*, 33. [CrossRef]

marine drugs

Article

Uncovering the Bioactive Potential of a Cyanobacterial Natural Products Library Aided by Untargeted Metabolomics

Leonor Ferreira [1], João Morais [1,2], Marco Preto [1], Raquel Silva [1], Ralph Urbatzka [1], Vitor Vasconcelos [1,2] and Mariana Reis [1,*]

1 CIIMAR/CIMAR, Interdisciplinary Centre of Marine and Environmental Research, Terminal de Cruzeiros do Porto de Leixões, University of Porto, 4450-208 Matosinhos, Portugal; lferreira@ciimar.up.pt (L.F.); jmorais@ciimar.up.pt (J.M.); mpreto@ciimar.up.pt (M.P.); rssilva@ciimar.up.pt (R.S.); rurbatzka@ciimar.up.pt (R.U.); vmvascon@fc.up.pt (V.V.)
2 Departamento de Biologia, Faculdade de Ciências, Universidade do Porto, Rua do Campo Alegre, Edifício FC4, 4169-007 Porto, Portugal
* Correspondence: mreis@ciimar.up.pt

Abstract: The Blue Biotechnology and Ecotoxicology Culture Collection (LEGE-CC) holds a vast number of cyanobacteria whose chemical richness is still largely unknown. To expedite its bioactivity screening we developed a natural products library. Sixty strains and four environmental samples were chromatographed, using a semiautomatic HPLC system, yielding 512 fractions that were tested for their cytotoxic activity against 2D and 3D models of human colon carcinoma (HCT 116), and non-cancerous cell line hCMEC/D3. Six fractions showed high cytotoxicity against 2D and 3D cell models (group A), and six other fractions were selected by their effects on 3D cells (group B). The metabolome of each group was organized and characterized using the MolNetEnhancer workflow, and its processing with MetaboAnalyst allowed discrimination of the mass features with the highest fold change, and thus the ones that might be bioactive. Of those, mass features without precedented identification were mostly found in group A, indicating seven possible novel bioactive molecules, alongside in silico putative annotation of five cytotoxic compounds. Manual dereplication of group B tentatively identified nine pheophytin and pheophorbide derivatives. Our approach enabled the selection of 7 out of 60 cyanobacterial strains for anticancer drug discovery, providing new data concerning the chemical composition of these cyanobacteria.

Keywords: natural products library; cyanobacteria; cytotoxicity; 3D spheroids; untargeted metabolomics; MetaboAnalyst; GNPS

Citation: Ferreira, L.; Morais, J.; Preto, M.; Silva, R.; Urbatzka, R.; Vasconcelos, V.; Reis, M. Uncovering the Bioactive Potential of a Cyanobacterial Natural Products Library Aided by Untargeted Metabolomics. *Mar. Drugs* **2021**, *19*, 633. https://doi.org/10.3390/md19110633

Academic Editor: Bill J. Baker

Received: 15 October 2021
Accepted: 10 November 2021
Published: 12 November 2021

1. Introduction

Natural products continue to inspire many drug discovery programs; as such, more than sixty percent of the approved drugs comprise natural products, their synthetic derivatives, and their pharmacophore-inspired drugs [1]. Cyanobacteria have been regarded as one of the most promising groups of organisms capable of producing metabolites with pharmaceutical applications [2]. Since the 1970s, more than 1630 unique cyanobacterial compounds have been described [3], mainly belonging to the classes of non-ribosomal peptides (NRPs), ribosomally synthesized and post translationally-modified peptides (RiPPs), polyketides (PKs), and the hybrid NRPs/PKs [3,4]. These hybrid molecules contribute to the diversity of structural motifs found in cyanobacterial compounds. In addition, other classes of secondary metabolites have also been isolated from cyanobacteria as alkaloids, fatty acids, terpenes, and UV-protectant pigments [3,4]. Among the reported bioactivities, a great deal of studies have focused on the characterization of the cytotoxic and anticancer activity of cyanobacterial metabolites; among those, dolastatin 10, a tubulin polymerization inhibitor, is the most well-known [3,5]. Its synthetic derivatives monomethylauristatins yielded four approved antibody drug conjugates: Adcetris (2011) and Polivy (2019), used for the treatment of lymphoma; Padcev (2019), applied for the treatment of urinary tract cancers; and Blenrep (2020), for the treatment of relapsed and refractory multiple myeloma [6].

The Blue Biotechnology and Ecotoxicology Culture Collection (LEGE-CC, http://www.ciimar.up.pt/legecc/), hosted at CIIMAR (Matosinhos, Portugal), is a unique biological resource that hosts more than 700 strains of cyanobacteria, covering a wide range of geographical habitats. These are mainly represented by marine and freshwater water systems, but there are also representative strains from brackish, hypersaline, and terrestrial environments [7]. Regardless this biodiversity, this natural resource is still underexplored in terms of the discovery of new chemical entities. Our bioactivity-guided screening endeavors have delivered compounds such as lactylates of chlorinated fatty acids (chlorosphaerolactylates A–D) with antimicrobial effects [8]; chlorophyll derivatives with lipid reducing activity [9]; and compounds with anticancer activity, such as oxadiazine Nocuolin A [10], alkylresorcinol hierridin B [11], and the NRPs portoamides A–B [12] that also proved to have promising antifouling activity [13]. Despite these successes, our classic approach for cyanobacterial natural products discovery is often time consuming, originates false positives (synergistic effects), and ends frequently in the unsuccessful isolation of the active components due to their low concentrations. To overcome these problems and encompass the growing number of new cyanobacterial strains entering LEGE-CC, a new strategy for bioactivity screening is needed in order to accelerate our drug discovery process. In this study, we describe the generation of a natural products library and its assessment for potential cytotoxic activity. An untargeted metabolomics approach was used to discover and highlight the putative bioactive molecules.

2. Results and Discussion

2.1. *Cyanobacterial Natural Products Library (LEGE-NPL)*

In the last 10 years, LEGE-CC has had a significant increase in the number of deposited strains; nevertheless, its associated drug discovery has not been able to keep the same pace. As a possible solution for this problem, we designed a methodology for a cyanobacterial natural products library (LEGE-NPL). To test this approach, 60 cyanobacterial strains and 4 environmental samples were used (Table S1). The selected strains belong to different cyanobacterial orders following the classification of Komárek et al. [14]: Synechococcales (46%), Oscillatoriales (27%), Nostocales (15%), Chroococcales (10%), and Pleurocapsales (2%), representing the phylogenetic diversity of LEGE-CC (Figure 1). In addition, these orders have been considered to be a good asset for secondary metabolites research due to the richness in biosynthetic gene clusters found in their genomes [3,5,15].

The LEGE-NPL was designed to have a solid inventory (MeOH extracts) and a liquid inventory of fractions. The raw material that supplied the solid inventory was derived from 4 L cultures of cyanobacteria that yielded on average 2.57 g of dry weight (Figure S1). MeOH was chosen as solvent to produce the solid library because of its the ability to extract components with different polarities; previous results using sequential extraction did not show advantage of using different solvents over the single use of MeOH [9]. The average yield of extraction was 15.50% of the lyophilized biomass (Figure S1). The liquid inventory, constituted by eight fractions (denominated from A to H) derived from each MeOH extract, was designed to be fully compatible with a 96-well plate format for bioactivity screening. It was produced in semiautonomous fashion using a HPLC system coupled to an automatic injector, PDA detector, and an automatic fraction collector. Hence, the 64 MeOH extracts were separated on a C8 column using a gradient of H_2O/MeCN, yielding a total of 512 fractions. The total run time, including gradient recovery, was 20 min per strain. These chromatographic conditions were optimized to ensure a good mass separation between all eight fractions that were estimated to have 2.50 mg. These plates were dried using a centrifugal evaporation system, resuspended in DMSO, and stored in 96-deep well plates as mother plates. The choice of the stationary phase considered the recent woks of the National Cancer Institute Program for Natural Products Discovery that indicated C8 as a preferred stationary-phase over the classical C18 or silica due to a better separation between lipophilic and medium polarity compounds [16].

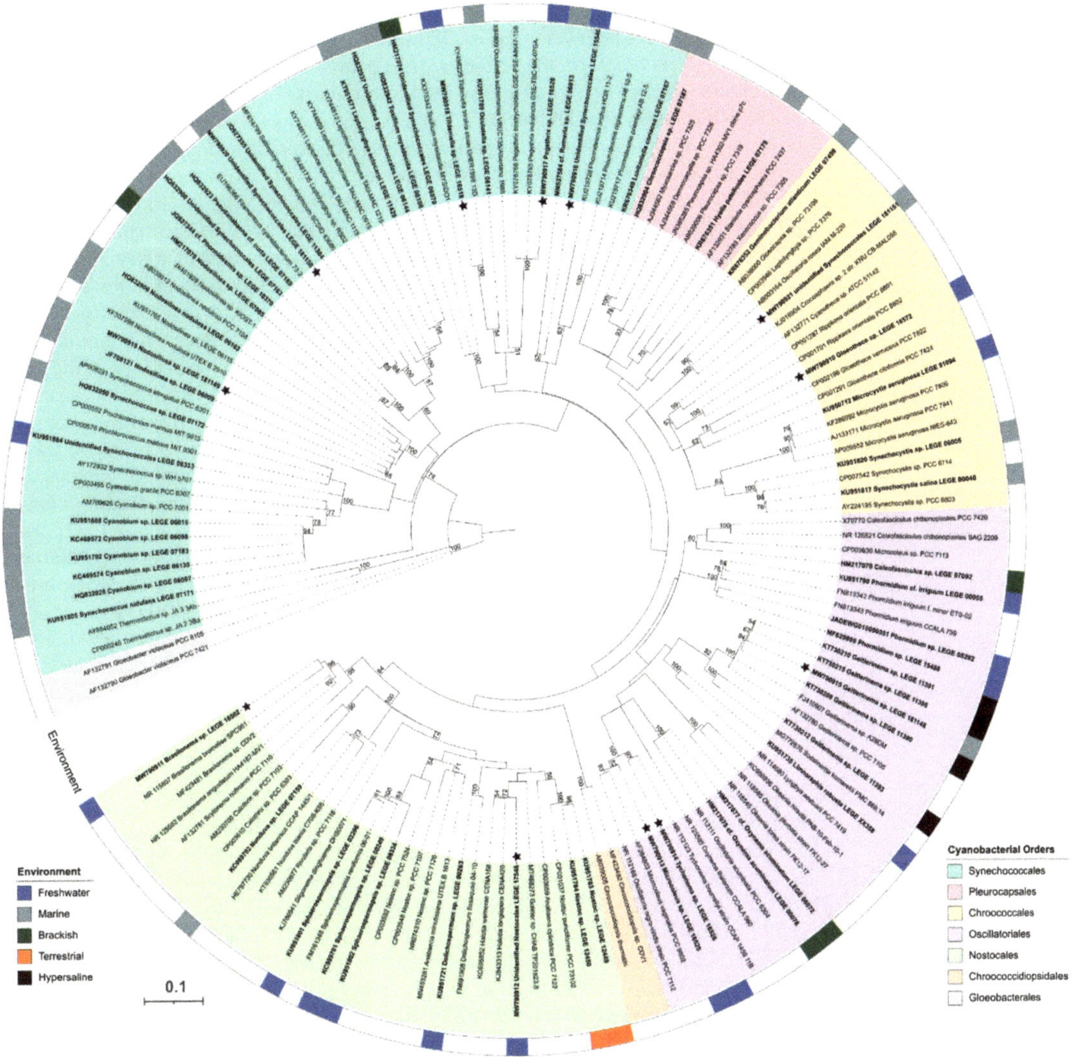

Figure 1. Maximum likelihood phylogenetic tree based on 146 partial 16S rRNA gene sequences of cyanobacteria. *Gloeobacter violaceus* PCC 7421 and *G. violaceus* PCC 8105 were used as outgroup. LEGE-CC strains used in this work are indicated in bold. The different color segments represent strain placement at order level following Komárek et al. [14]. Different colored strips around the tree represent the environment from where strains were isolated. Bootstrap values over 50% are indicated at the nodes. Black stars represent the strains whose sequences were obtained in this work.

2.2. Bioactivity Screening

Another aim of this work was to use cancer spheroids in routine screenings of LEGE-NPL. The cancer spheroids are characterized by a hypoxic core with quiescent cells and a prolific outer shell, and thus, they more accurately simulate the tumor microenvironment than 2D cultures. Due to this complexity, 3D culture systems are considered to be less prone to showing effects of unspecific activities or to overestimate the activity of compounds, increasing the chances of finding potent lead compounds [17].

The colon carcinoma cell line HCT 116 was chosen due to its ability to form uniform spheroids using the liquid-overlay technique, and because it had already been used in confirmation assays for cyanobacterial compounds [10,18]. Moreover, the assays using HCT 116 cells were used to compare the 2D versus 3D hit selection. The endpoints and readout techniques were adjusted accordingly to the nature of the cell culture system. For 2D cell cultures, cell viability was assessed by the standard MTT assay after a 48 h incubation period. This colorimetric assay was not suitable to measure cell viability in spheroids (Figure S2). This was verified mainly due to the poor diffusion of the dye, which can be attributed to the 3D matrices and tight cell–cell junctions present in the multilayer cell spheroids [19], resulting in low differentiation of the metabolic activity of the cells. Thus, for 3D cell cultures, cell viability was measured using the acid phosphatase assay after 96 h (longer exposure times in 3D cell cultures increase the sensitivity of the assay and reduce the false negative hits [19]). Moreover, to test the hypothesis that our methodology would be able to detect active compounds in fractionated extracts, the strain *Phormidium* sp. LEGE 05292 was included in the study set (as a positive control). This strain is known to produce the cytotoxic peptides portoamides A and B in a proportion of 3:1 [12]. This mixture presented IC_{50} values of 3.38 µM and 12.67 µM, respectively, to monolayer cultures and multicellular spheroids of HCT 116 cells. These results indicated that an approximate 4-fold higher concentration is needed to induce cytotoxicity in spheroids [18].

The 512 fractions of LEGE-NPL (25 µg mL^{-1}) were screened for their cytotoxic effect on the colon carcinoma cells (2D HCT 116, 3D HCT 116) and a non-carcinogenic cell line hCMEC/D3 (Figure 2). The non-carcinogenic cell line was not used to select hits; instead it was used to test if the fractions exerted a generalized cytotoxicity or if they had selectivity towards cancer cells. The results were expressed as the percentage of cell viability normalized to the solvent control. To characterize the dynamic range of the assays, the Z′ factor was calculated using the positive (LEGE 05292_C) and solvent control (DMSO) data. The Z′ scores of 0.64–0.83 indicated that the mean and standard deviation of the controls were well separated [20], and thus the criteria to select positive hits was established as the mean viability of LEGE 05292_C plus three times its standard deviation ($\mu_{LEGE\ 05292_C} + 3\sigma_{LEGE\ 05292_C}$). The monolayer assay with HCT 116 cancer cells had a hit rate of 0.4%, selecting the active fractions LEGE 181150_D and LEGE 17548_C (Figure 2). For the 3D HCT 116 cell assay, 11 active fractions were selected (2.1% hit rate) that correspond to one environmental sample and eight cyanobacterial strains (Figure 2). Contrary to what we expected, a higher hit rate was observed for the 3D spheroids than for the monolayer counterpart. Hence, the cell viability data from the three cell models was correlated in a 3D scatter plot to disclose any bioactivity tendency. As such, two bioactive groups could be recognized (Figure 3). Group A contains 5 fractions that present strong cytotoxicity towards the cancer and non-cancer cells (Table 1), whereas group B contains fractions selected for their activity in HCT 116 spheroids despite the moderate activity in the other monolayer assays. In light of these results, the fractions from both groups were selected for metabolomics studies in order to discover the potential cytotoxic compounds.

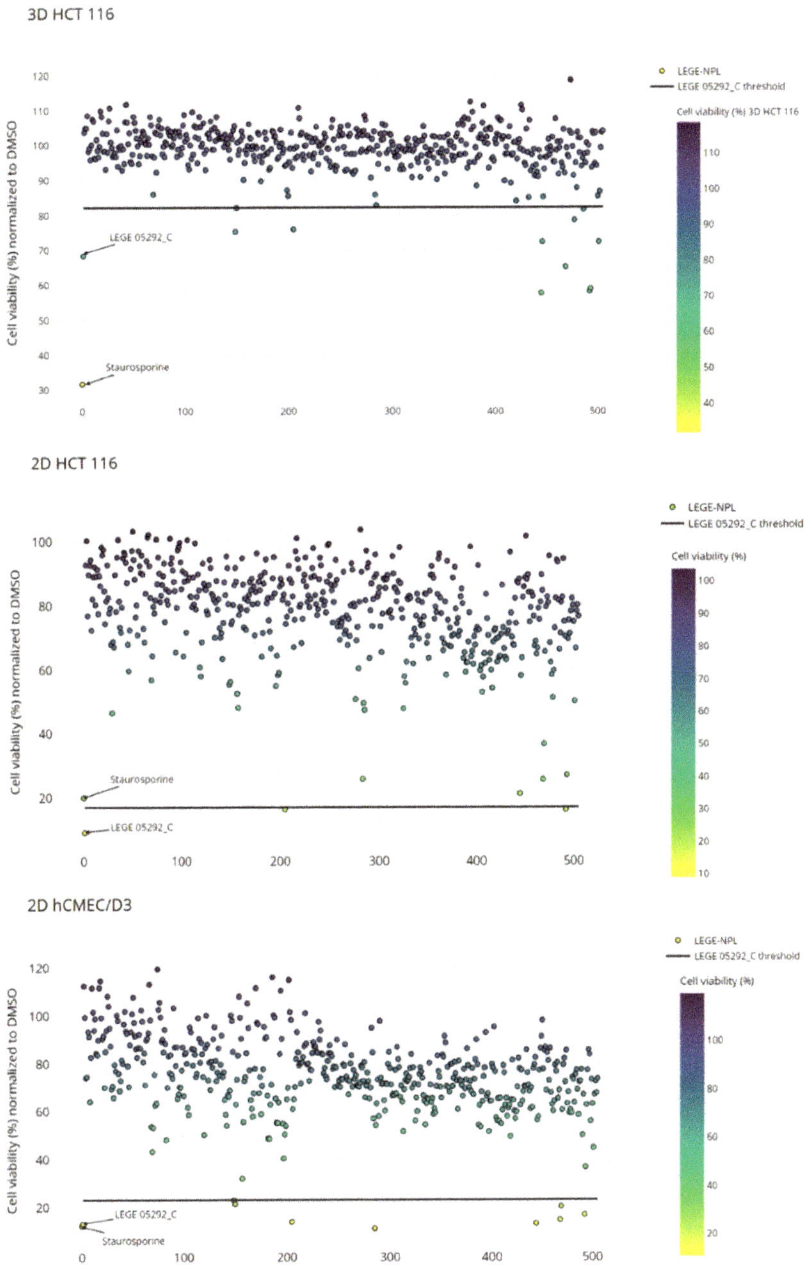

Figure 2. Cytotoxicity screening of 512 fractions of LEGE-NPL (at 25 μg mL^{-1}) against 3D cell spheroids of HCT 116 cells, 2D HCT 116 cells, and hCMEC/D3. The percentage of cell viability was normalized to DMSO. The threshold for selection of positive hits was defined as mean viability of the cytotoxic faction LEGE 05292_C plus three times its standard deviation. All the assays were done in triplicate.

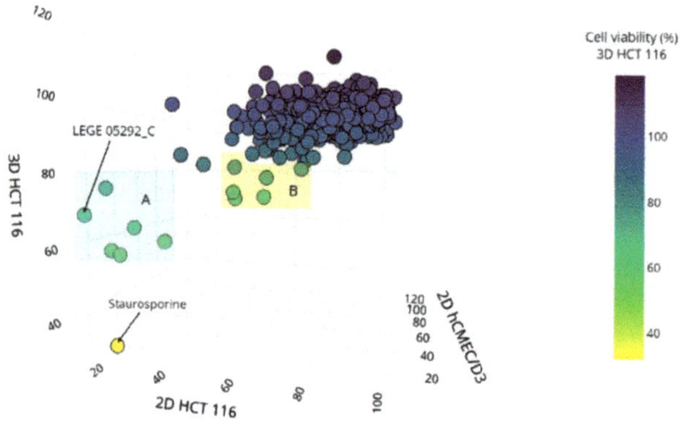

Figure 3. 3D plot correlation of the cytotoxic profile of 512 fractions on the different cell models (3D HCT 116, 2D HCT 116, and hCMEC/D3). The x, y, and z axis represent the percentage of cell viability (normalized to DMSO). Two groups were defined based on the cytotoxic profile: group A and group B.

Table 1. Cytotoxic profile of the selected fractions of group A, B, and C.

	Fractions	Cell Viability (%)		
		3D HCT 116	2D HCT 116	2D hCMEC/D3
Group A	LEGE 16572_C	57.54 ± 20.74	21.30 ± 8.79	12.97 ± 5.14
	LEGE 17548_C	58.05 ± 11.10	16.33 ± 8.50	16.67 ± 11.84
	LEGE 17548_D	58.74 ± 13.40	27.08 ± 17.23	36.52 ± 16.23
	LEGE 15488_C	65.16 ± 10.30	25.69 ± 21.02	14.51 ± 8.65
	LEGE 181150_D	75.95 ± 4.25	16.40 ± 3.26	13.80 ± 3.14
	LEGE 05292_C	68.32 ± 4.60	9.13 ± 2.64	12.83 ± 3.35
Group B	LEGE XX358_D	72.28 ± 16.86	50.11 ± 20.43	44.60 ± 14.66
	LEGE 16572_D	72.34 ± 6.05	58.15 ± 23.40	56.18 ± 19.94
	JM1 Amb_D	75.25 ± 7.14	55.30 ± 3.11	22.77 ± 5.59
	LEGE 15546_D	78.51 ± 7.16	58.44 ± 18.34	59.17 ± 15.65
	LEGE 16502_E	81.53 ± 13.30	71.38 ± 13.24	58.29 ± 7.41
	JM1 Amb_E	82.07 ± 3.02	56.16 ± 12.80	21.15 ± 5.76
Group C	JM5_amb_D	90.07 ± 1.24	52.49 ± 5.34	31.85 ± 4.39
	JM5_amb_E	94.92 ± 5.66	48.11 ± 12.12	55.44 ± 7.66
	LEGE 06078_D	99.29 ± 7.89	46.51 ± 12.42	69.21 ± 15.63
	LEGE 07092_D	94.96 ± 6.94	47.77 ± 3.62	55.86 ± 3.63
	LEGE 07167_C	85.76 ± 2.54	25.86 ± 1.36	56.83 ± 4.00
	LEGE 07167_D	82.74 ± 3.25	49.51 ± 1.90	10.93 ± 2.87
	LEGE 07167_E	99.70 ± 4.71	47.34 ± 1.59	53.96 ± 3.48
	LEGE 08333_D	106.90 ± 5.38	85.02 ± 1.57	80.56 ± 5.12
	LEGE 15488_D	99.09 ± 4.96	36.76 ± 23.26	20.17 ± 15.65
	LEGE 181148_E	93.04 ± 6.94	64.14 ± 14.46	48.58 ± 4.75
	LEGE 181148_F	93.49 ± 6.54	71.52 ± 20.38	48.44 ± 2.02
	LEGE 181149_D	94.01 ± 7.29	64.47 ± 22.29	40.25 ± 2.66
Selection threshold	LEGE 05292_C + 3σ	82.12	17.03	
Staurosporine		31.67 ± 6.84	20.07 ± 4.40	12.05 ± 2.55

2.3. Group A: Metabolomics Analysis and Dereplication of the Putative Active Molecules

In an attempt to discover which metabolites could be responsible for the observed activity, an untargeted metabolomics analysis was performed. The metabolomes of fractions of group A were compared with a group of 12 fractions without activity on cancer spheroids (group C; Table 1). The extracted mass features with MZmine 2 were submitted to fold change (FC) analysis in MetaboAnalyst 5.0, which allowed for the potential differences in the metabolite profiles to be identified, and hence the bioactive compounds could be highlighted.

The chemical space of A/C was then represented as a molecular network constructed using the feature-based molecular networking workflow [21]. The characterization of the molecular families and annotation of compounds were estimated based on the integration of the in silico tools available from the Global Natural Product Social Molecular Networking (GNPS) platform: DEREPLICATOR [22], MS2LDA [23], Network Annotation Propagation (NAP) [24], and MolNetEnhancer [25]. The size of the nodes in the molecular networks was represented relative to the log2(FC) (Figure 4A).

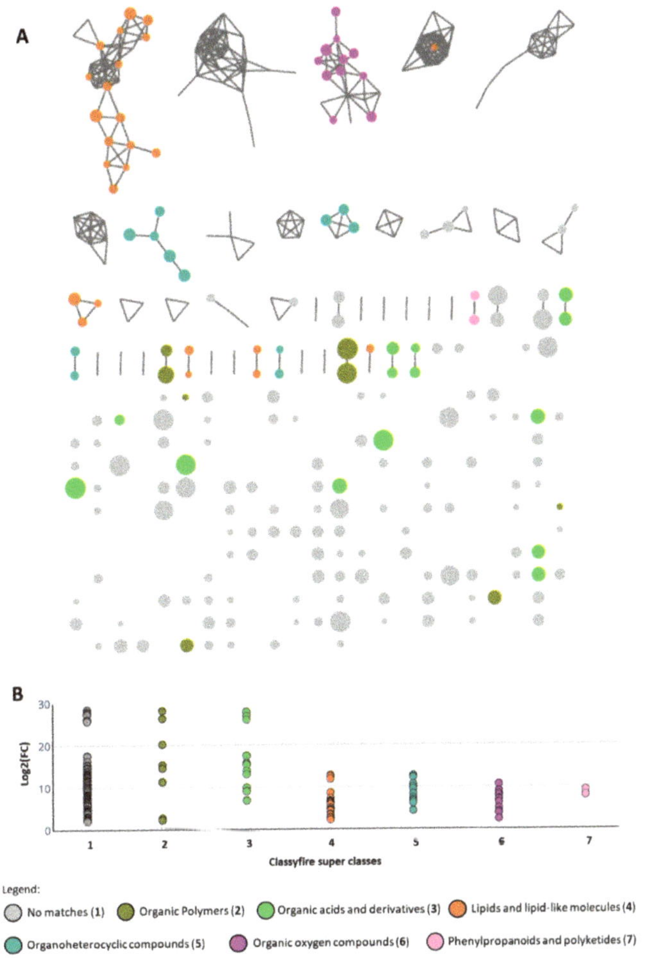

Figure 4. Feature-based molecular network of groups A/C annotated with MolNetEnhancer workflow. The nodes are color-coded accordingly to the ClassyFire super class classification, and their size is related to their fold change log2(FC) value (**A**). Distribution of the nodes with log2(FC) higher than 2 through each ClassyFire super class (**B**).

The analysis of the molecular network revealed 191 nodes with log2(FC) between 2.00 and 28.45, of which 72 nodes were characterized as 13% lipids and lipid-like molecules, 8% organic acids and derivatives, 6% organic oxygen compounds, 6% organoheterocyclic compounds, 4% organic polymers, and 1% phenylpropanoids and polyketides, according to the ClassyFire super class classification [26]. The 17 top features with highest fold change (≥20) were distributed between the super classes' organic polymers, organic acids and derivatives, and the category of no matches (Figure 4B). Such high fold change values reflect the uniqueness of these mass features among the studied metabolomes, which were found for all the active fractions except for LEGE 15488_C (Table 2). Detailed examination of these 17 ions indicated the majority to be related to the cytotoxic compounds portoamides A, B, and C, known to be produced by *Phormidium* sp. LEGE 05292 (Table 2) [27].

Table 2. Characterization and annotation of the putative cytotoxic molecules present in the active fractions of group A.

m/z	Isotope/ Fragments	Rt (min)	Log2(FC)	Super Class	Direct Parent	Molecular Framework	Putative Annotation
			LEGE 05292_C				
1313.6991 [M+H]⁺		7.21	25.71	3	8	9	Portoamide C $C_{62}H_{96}N_{12}O_{19}$ Δ 0.27 ppm
1532.7887 [M+H]⁺		7.51	28.18	2	10	9	Portoamide A $C_{74}H_{109}N_{13}O_{22}$ Δ 0.27 ppm
1502.7780 [M+H]⁺		7.74	26.34	2	10	9	Portoamide B $C_{73}H_{107}N_{13}O_{21}$ Δ 0.18 ppm
			LEGE 17548_C				
1154.6172 [M+Na]⁺		8.73	26.07	-	-	-	[Minutissamide A + CH_3] * $C_{52}H_{85}N_{13}O_{15}$ Δ −1.55 ppm
1118.6187 [M+H]⁺		8.76	26.86	3	8	11	Minutissamide A $C_{51}H_{83}N_{13}O_{15}$ Δ −1.55 ppm
			LEGE 17548_C, LEGE 17548_D and LEGE 16572_C				
762.5468 [M+H]⁺		12.60	27.91	-	-	-	-
			LEGE 16572_C				
703.5092 [M+H]⁺		12.31	27.33	-	-	-	-
			LEGE 181150_D				
895.0778	897.0759 [M+2 isotope]	7.92	25.98	-	-	-	Leptochelin
851.1284	853.1257 [M+2 isotope]	7.81	17.43	-	-	-	Leptochelin-like *
1011.8493		14.57	27.92	-	-	-	-
			LEGE 15488_C				
655.3808 [M+H]⁺		5.73	8.27	-	-	-	-
858.5795 [M+H]⁺		7.29	8.10	-	-	-	-
	331.2010	7.28	8.15	-	-	-	-
	528.3863	7.28	9.05	3	12	11	-
1520.7861 [M+H]⁺		7.87	5.07	2	10	9	Portoamide-like * $C_{73}H_{109}N_{13}O_{22}$ Δ −1.44 ppm

2—Organic polymers; 3—organic acids and derivatives; 8—cyclic peptides; 9—aromatic heteropolycyclic compounds; 10—polypeptides 11—aliphatic heteropolycyclic compounds; 12—Cyclic depsipeptides; * tentative identification.

Moreover, in the fraction C of the unidentified Nostocales LEGE 17548 the cyclic lipopeptide minutissamide A was putatively annotated, together with an ion at *m/z* 1154.6172 $[M+Na]^+$, that could correspond to a methylated minutissamide A (+14.01 Da mass shift). Minutissamide A was previously isolated from cultures of *Anabaena minutissima* (UTEX 1613), and its antiproliferative activity characterized using HT-29 human colon cancer cells (IC_{50} of 2.0 μM) [28], which correlates well with our bioactivity findings. However, *Anabaena minutissima* (UTEX 1613) and the unidentified Nostocales LEGE 17548 fall in different clades according to our phylogenetic study, the latter being more related to strains of the genus *Halotia* (Figure 1).

It is interesting to note that in the case of portoamides or minutissamides, the molecular network was not able to form clusters containing related ions. The absence of clustering led to poor propagation of library annotation as was observed for the sodium or potassium adducts of portoamides and minutissamides that were classified as "no matches".

Furthermore, four mass features, with significant fold change, could not be classified or dereplicated using the GNPS in silico tools or manual search in the databases Dictionary of Natural Products and CyanoMetDB [29], making them potential targets for the isolation of novel active compounds. Of these, the mass feature 897.0759 found in fraction LEGE 181150_D (Table 2) formed a cluster with another ion at *m/z* 853.1257 (7.81 min; log2(FC) = 17.43); analysis of the mass spectrum showed that these masses were in fact M + 2 isotope peaks, thus revealing the presence of halogenated atoms in these molecules. The complexity of the isotopic pattern suggests a combination of chlorine and/or bromine atoms (Figure 5). In addition, the mass difference of 43.94 Da between the compounds might correspond to Cl ↔ Br change. Preliminary GNPS experiments led us to two PhD theses reporting leptochelin (formerly phormidamide) [30,31], a compound with *m/z* 895.0786 and whose mass spectrum and isotopic pattern are very similar to our findings (*m/z* 895.0778; Δ 0.8 mDa). Nevertheless, the structure of this compound seems to not be fully elucidated yet. According to both reports, the compound presented potent cytotoxicity towards mouse neuro-2a neuroblastoma cells (LD_{50} = 1.2 μM) [30] and human NCI-H460 lung cancer cells (IC_{50} = 153 nM) [31], which is in line with the strong reduction of cell viability observed in our assays (Table 1). Leptochelin was isolated from the Red Sea *Leptolyngbya* sp. RS02 and from the Indonesian *Leptolyngbya* sp. HB_3/1/2, which share identical 16S rRNA gene sequences even though they were collected in different geographical locations. Interestingly, our strain, unidentified Synechococcales LEGE 181150, was collected from a marine environment in the Cape Verde archipelago and falls in a subclade apart from the *Leptolyngbya* strains (Figure 1), suggesting the compound to be produced by a different genus of cyanobacteria. Nevertheless, all these locations fall in the tropical region, which might suggest an ecological role subjacent to the production of this compound.

For fraction C of *Phormidium* sp. LEGE 15488, there were no mass features with striking values of fold change. This fact could be explained by the similarity in composition to fraction LEGE 15488_D that was included in group C (Figure S3). Thus, for the fraction LEGE 15488_C, the ions with the highest fold change will most probably be the ones responsible for the cytotoxic activity. As such, three protonated molecules were cherry-picked (Table 2). For these molecules, we could not retrieve any dereplication results either using the GNPS tools or manual search in the databases (Dictionary of Natural Products and CyanoMetDB). For the protonated molecule at *m/z* 1520.7861, the ClassyFire categories Direct Parent (descriptor for the largest structural feature that defines a compound) and Molecular Framework (descriptor for overall aliphaticity/aromaticity and number of cycles) suggested this compound to have a scaffold of the cyclic peptide-type containing aromatic amino acids. In addition to this in silico prediction, the presence of the doubly charged ion at *m/z* 760.8961 $[M+2H]^{2+}$ also reinforces the possible large structure of this compound. Considering these observations and given the taxonomic position of *Phormidium* sp. LEGE 15488 and *Phormidium* sp. LEGE 05292 (Figure 1), we hypothesize that this mass could correspond to an undescribed portoamide-type compound with a proposed molecular formula of $C_{73}H_{109}N_{13}O_{22}$ (calculated for 1519.7810). As for the parent mass 858.5795 $[M+H]^+$, it was found to be associated with the ESI in-source fragments at m/z 331.2010 and 528.3863. For the latter, the in silico annotation can give insights into the nature of this molecule, as it was categorized as a possible cyclic depsipeptide without aromatic amino acids (Table 2).

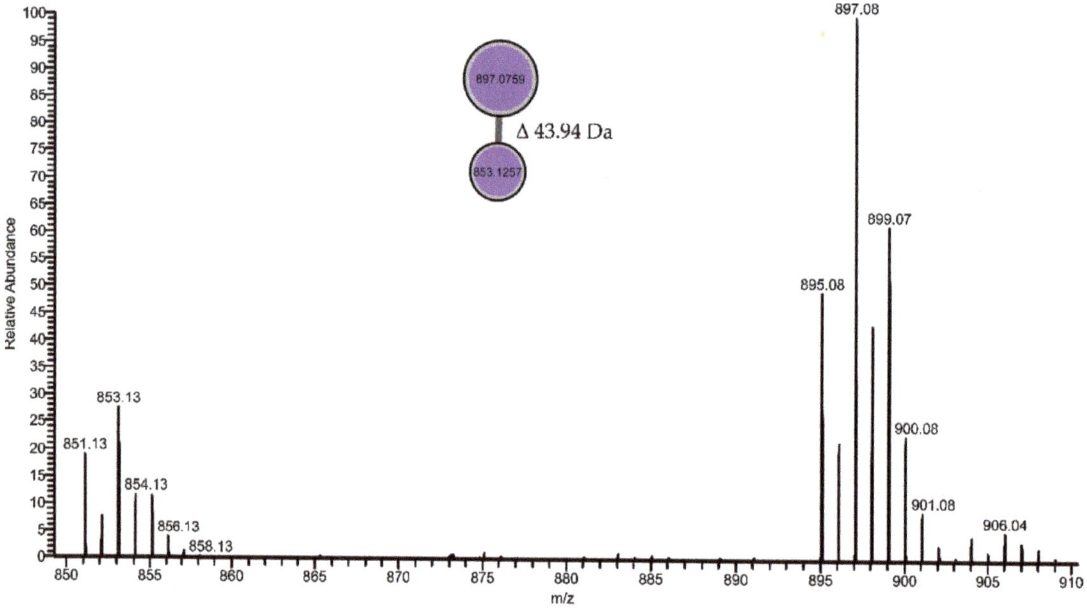

Figure 5. Mass spectrum and the respective cluster of two halogenated compounds present in fraction D of the unidentified Synechococcales LEGE 181150. The nodes are color-coded accordingly to the identity of the fraction. These mass features were exclusively found in the unidentified Synechococcales LEGE 181150.

In this group of cytotoxic fractions, it is worth noting the following aspects: the group is mainly constituted by polar fractions (fraction C); the in silico chemical classification predicted the significant mass features to have a peptide-type scaffold (Figure 4B, Table 2); and the in silico dereplication lead to the putative annotation/identification of known peptides whose cytotoxic activity towards cancer cells had been previously described. Given that these predictions worked correctly with *Phormidium* sp. LEGE 05292 (strain producer of portoamides), we hypothesize that the strains *Phormidium* sp. LEGE 15488 (Amazon River, Brazil; Table S1) and the unidentified Nostocales LEGE 17548 (Mira lagoon, Beira Litoral, Portugal; Table S1) might be potential producers of cytotoxic peptide-type compounds. Furthermore, the strains *Gloeothece* sp. LEGE 16572 (isolated from a fountain, Monchique, Portugal; Table S1) and unidentified Synechococcales LEGE 181150 have potential for the discovery of totally unknown structures.

2.4. Group B: Metabolomics Analysis and Dereplication of the Putative Active Molecules

The same untargeted metabolomics approach described above was applied for group B. The fold change analysis highlighted 34 mass features with log2(FC) between 2.14 and 17.13. Fifteen nodes were characterized, according to ClassyFire superclass, as organoheterocyclic compounds all belonging to the tetrapyrroles and derivatives class (23%) and phenylpropanoids and polyketides (21%) (Figure 6). Contrary to group A, in group B there were no mass features with high fold change values. In fact, the only three mass features that presented log2(FC) higher than 10 were 636.4814, 1245.5650, and 1267.5473. The m/z 636.4814 (12.9 min; log2(FC) = 17.14) was found in samples LEGE 16502_E and

LEGE 15546_D, being characterized as a potential macrolide-type compound. However, its manual query on the mass databases did not retrieve any identification.

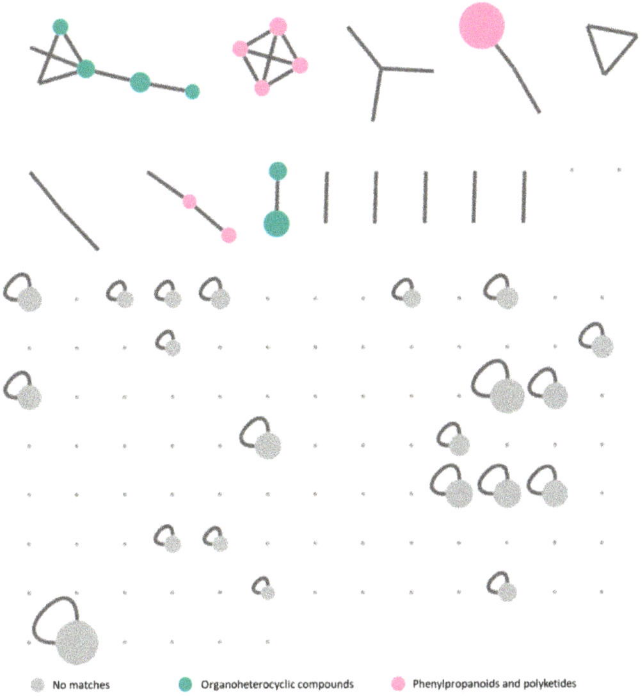

Figure 6. Feature-based molecular network of groups B/C annotated with MolNetEnhancer workflow. The nodes are color-coded accordingly to the ClassyFire super class classification, and their size is related to their fold change log2(FC) value.

The mass features 1245.5650 and 1267.5473, respectively, with log2(FC) of 15.85 and 11.59, were found to be the $[2M+H]^+$ and $[2M+Na]^+$ ions of the protonated molecule at m/z 623.2865 (11.68 min; log2(FC) = 7.54), predicted as a tetrapyrrole-type molecule. Despite this classification, the putative annotation via GNPS tools was not successful. Thus, 13^2-hydroxy-phaeophorbide a methyl ester, was tentatively identified by manual search in the Dictionary of Natural Products and study of its MS2 fragmentation pattern (Table 3, Figure S4). This compound was found to be one of the main components of the samples LEGE 16572_D, LEGE 15546_D, and LEGE xx358_D (Figure 6, Table 3). This putative pheophorbide appeared clustered with a protonated molecule at m/z 609.2706 (11.30 min; log2(FC) = 3.90). The difference of 14.01 Da between the molecules suggested the loss of a methyl group, and thus was tentatively identified as 13^2-hydroxy-pheophorbide a. This molecule was found in the environmental sample of a cyanobacterial mat (JM1_amb_E) and in the strain *Brasilonema* sp. LEGE 16502 (LEGE 16502_E). Moreover, further manual dereplication led to the tentative identification of other pheophytins and pheophorbides (Table 3). The lack of GNPS annotation for these compounds might be due to the fact that the masses deposited in the GNPS database were acquired in low resolution mass spectrometers, and thus, did not match with our search criteria.

Table 3. Characterization and annotation of the putative cytotoxic molecules present in the active fractions of group B.

m/z	Rt (min)	Log2(FC)	Super Class	Precursor Intensity	Tentative Identification
LEGE 16572_D, LEGE 15546_D and LEGE xx358_D					
653.2971 $[M+H]^+$	12.12	7.72	1	1.19×10^{10}	15^1-hydroxy-lactone-pheophorbide a ethyl ester $C_{37}H_{40}N_4O_7$ Δ 0.19 ppm
623.2865 $[M+H]^+$	11.68	7.54	1	2.55×10^{10}	13^2-hydroxy-phaeophorbide a methyl ester $C_{36}H_{38}N_4O_6$ Δ 0.14 ppm
639.2813 $[M+H]^+$	11.88	5.99	2	2.44×10^9	15^1-hydroxy-lactone-pheophorbide a methyl ester $C_{36}H_{38}N_4O_7\Delta$ −0.04 ppm
LEGE 16502_E, JM1_amb_E					
593.2759 $[M+H]^+$	11.77	6.99	2	2.97×10^{10}	pheophorbide a $C_{35}H_{36}N_4O_5$ Δ 0.09 ppm
535.2704 $[M+H]^+$	12.24	4.18	2	3.85×10^9	pyrophaeophorbide a $C_{33}H_{34}N_4O_3\Delta$ 0.06 ppm
609.2706 $[M+H]^+$	11.29	3.90	1	5.22×10^8	13^2-hydroxy-phaeophorbide a $C_{35}H_{36}N_4O_6$ Δ −0.26 ppm
All samples					
903.5618 $[M+H]^+$	14.41	4.58	2	1.47×10^{10}	15^1-hydroxy-lactone-phaeophytin a $C_{55}H_{74}N_4O_7\Delta$ −1.36 ppm
887.5664 $[M+H]^+$	14.30	3.67		4.80×10^{10}	13^2-hydroxy-pheophytin a $C_{55}H_{74}N_4O_6\Delta$ −1.93 ppm
JM1_amb_D, JM1_amb_E, LEGE 16502_E					
917.5777 $[M+H]^+$	14.70	2.16	2	2.02×10^9	13-methyldioxy-phaeophytin a/ ficusmicrochlorin B C56H76N4O7 Δ −1.07 ppm

1—No Matches, 2—Organic polymers.

These pheophytins and pheophorbides are products of the degradation pathway of chlorophyll a, and their anticancer activity has been widely reported [32] Such molecules are commonly found in photosynthetic organisms, which suggests that the bioactivity results obtained for group B could be related to a higher content of these compounds in the fractions. Future studies will help to elucidate this observation and address possible ecological relationships.

3. Materials and Methods

3.1. *Cyanobacteria Culture Conditions*

The 60 cyanobacterial strains were obtained from the Blue Biotechnology and Ecotoxicology Culture Collection (LEGE-CC) (Table S1). To establish the natural products library, these microorganisms were cultured up to 4 L, in the appropriate growth media, and maintained under standard laboratory conditions: 25 °C with light/dark cycle of 14/10 h at a light intensity of 10–30 µmol photons m^{-2} s^{-1}. The freshwater strains were cultured using Z8 medium, while the marine strains were grown using Z8 medium supplemented with 25‰ of synthetic sea salts (Tropic marin, Berlin, Germany) and 1‰ of vitamin B_{12} (Table S1). Depending on the strain, after 30 to 160 days of growth, the biomass was harvested either by centrifugation for unicellular strains, or by filtration for filamentous strains, through an appropriately sized mesh. All biomasses were freeze-dried (LyoQuest, Telstar, Terrassa, Spain) before organic extraction.

3.2. DNA Extraction, Amplification (PCR) and Sequencing

Twelve strains of cyanobacteria were characterized for the first time in this work (Figure 1). For taxonomic studies, these strains were grown in 50 mL culture flasks and cells were harvested after 15–20 days of cultivation. Genomic DNA was extracted using the Genomic DNA Mini Kit (Invitrogen, Waltham, MA, USA), according to the manufacturer's instructions for Gram-negative bacteria. To obtain the complete sequence of 16S rRNA gene, PCR amplification was performed using the oligonucleotide primers set 27F [33] and 23S30R [34]. PCR reactions were performed in a final volume of 20 μL containing 1× Green GoTaq Flexi Buffer, 2.5 mM of $MgCl_2$, 125.0 mM of each deoxynucleotide triphosphate, 1.0 μM of each primer, 0.5 U of GoTaq Flexi DNA Polymerase (Promega, Madison, WI, USA), 10 mg mL^{-1} of bovine serum albumin (BSA), and 10–30 ng of template DNA, on a TProfessional Standard thermal cycler (Biometra, Göttingen, Germany). The PCR conditions were as follows: initial denaturation at 94 °C for 5 min, followed by 10 cycles of denaturation at 94 °C for 45 s, annealing at 57 °C for 45 s, and extension at 72 °C for 2 min, followed by 25 cycles of denaturation at 92 °C for 45 s, annealing at 54 °C for 45 s, and extension at 72 °C for 2 min with a final elongation step at 72 °C for 7 min. The PCR reactions were performed in duplicate. PCR products were separated by 1.5% agarose gel stained with SYBR® safe (Invitrogen, Waltham, MA, USA) and DNA fragments with the expected size were excised and purified using NZYGelpure (NzyTech, Genes and Enzymes, Lisbon, Portugal) according to the manufacturer's instructions. Since the sequences were obtained by direct sequencing of purified amplicons, internal primers CYA359F, CYA781R [35], and 1494R [33] were used to improve the quality of the sequences. The sequencing was performed at GATC Biotech (Ebersberg, Germany) and the nucleotide sequences obtained were manually inspected for quality and assembled using the Geneious 11.1.5 software (Biomatters Ltd., Auckland, New Zealand). Possible chimera formation during the sequences was checked using the software DECIPHER [36] before any phylogenetic analysis. Sequences obtained were inserted in the BLASTn (Basic Local Alignment and Search Tool for Nucleotides) database and the results were analyzed. The sequences associated with this study were deposited in the GenBank database under the accession numbers MW790910 to MW790921 (Table S1).

3.3. Phylogenetic Analysis

A total of 146 sequences were used in the final analysis, including 2 strains of *Gloeobacter violaceus* as outgroup, 85 sequences of cyanobacteria including type and reference strains retrieved from GenBank (National Center for Biotechnology Information, NCBI, Bethesda, MD, USA), and 59 sequences of LEGE-CC strains from which 12 were obtained in this work. Multiple sequence alignment was constructed using ClustalW in MEGA7 [37,38], and sequences were manually proofread and edited. Maximum likelihood (ML) analysis was carried out using substitution model GTR+G+I according to the Bayesian information criterion (BIC) and Akaike information criterion (AIC) scores with 1000 bootstrap resampling replicates using the MEGA7 software [38]. The final phylogenetic tree was edited on iTOL (Interactive Tree of Life) [39].

3.4. Cyanobacterial Natural Products Library

The LEGE-NPL (natural products library) solid inventory is composed of crude extracts. Thus, freeze-dried biomass was extracted three times with MeOH, with a sonication step of 5 min in between extractions, and was filtered and concentrated at 30 °C, using a rotary evaporator. The yields of extraction are described in the Supplementary Material (Figure S1). The extracts were then fractionated by reverse-phase HPLC in a Waters Alliance e2695 Separations Module instrument, coupled to a photodiode array detector (Waters 2998 PDA) and an automatic Waters Fraction Collector III (Waters, Mildford, MA, USA). Each crude was injected at 40 mg mL^{-1} (500 μL; 1 mL loop) and separated on an ACE 10 C8 column (50 ×10 mm, ACE, Reading, UK), using a H_2O:MeCN gradient (Table 4). Hence, each cyanobacterial extract was chromatographed into eight fractions (4 mL final volume, named A–H) into 48-deep well plates (Riplate, Ritter, Schwabmünchen, Germany), which were then dried on a CentriVap Concentrator (LabConco, Kansas City, MO, USA). These fractions were solubilized in 500 μL of DMSO and transferred to 96-deep well microplates (Nest Scientific, Woodbridge Township, NJ, USA) and stored at −80 °C, thus forming the LEGE-NPL liquid library (mother plates).

Table 4. HPLC chromatographic and collection program for generating the fractions for LEGE-NPL liquid inventory.

Time (min)	Flow ($mL \cdot min^{-1}$)	MeCN (%)	H_2O (%)	Collection Time (min)	Fraction
0.0	3.0	10	90	1.00–2.30	A
2.0	3.0	80	20	2.30–3.60	B
3.0	3.0	80	20	3.60–4.90	C
4.0	3.0	100	0	4.90–6.20	D
8.9	3.0	100	0	6.20–7.50	E
9.2	3.5	100	0	7.50–8.80	F
12.0	3.5	100	0	8.80–10.36	G
12.3	3.0	100	0	10.36–11.50	H
14.0	3.0	100	0		
15.0	3.0	10	90		
18.0	3.0	10	90		

3.5. Cell Culture

The human colon carcinoma cell line HCT 116 was obtained from Sigma-Aldrich (St. Louis, MO, USA) and the human brain endothelial cell line hCMEC/D3 was kindly donated by Dr. P. O. Courad (INSERM, Paris, France). HCT 116 was cultured with McCoy's 5A medium (CarlRoth, Kasruw, Germany) and hCMEC/D3 with Dulbecco's modified Eagle medium (DMEM) (Gibco, Thermo Fisher Scientific, Waltham, MA, USA), both supplemented with 10% of fetal bovine serum (Biochrom, Berlin, Germany), 1% of penicillin/streptomycin (Biochrom, Berlin, Germany), and 0.1% of amphotericin (GE Healthcare, Little Chafont, Buckinghamshire, UK). Both cell lines were grown at 37 °C with 5% CO_2 atmosphere.

3.6. Bioactivity Screening Using 2D Cell Models

The HCT 116 and hCMEC/D3 cells were seeded on 96-well plates, at a density of 3.3×10^4 cells mL^{-1} for 24 h. Then, the cells were incubated with 25 μg mL^{-1} of LEGE-NPL fractions (0.5% DMSO final concentration) and 1.25 μM of staurosporine (positive control) for 48 h. After this period of exposure, cell viability was evaluated by the MTT colorimetric assay (3-(4,5-dimethylthiazol-2-yl)-2,5-diphenyltetrazolium bromide). Thus, the cells were incubated with 20 μL of MTT reagent, at a final concentration of 200 μg mL^{-1} over 3–4 h, and afterwards 100 μL of DMSO was used to dissolve formazan crystals. Absorbance was read at 550 nm on a multi-detection microplate reader (Synergy HT, Biotek, Bart Frederick Shahr, Germany). All assays were repeated three times. Cell viability was calculated using the following formula:

$$\%\ cell\ viability\ (to\ negative\ control) = \frac{\overline{x}\ (Absorbance_{sample})}{\overline{x}\ (Absorbance_{negative\ control})} \times 100$$

3.7. Bioactivity Screening Using 3D Cell Models

The cancer spheroids were produced using the scaffold-free liquid-overlay technique [40]. Briefly, 200 μL of McCoy's medium with a HCT 116 cell density of 5×10^4 cells mL^{-1} was added to ultra-low attachment round-bottom 96-well plates (Costar, Corning, New York, NY, USA). Cells were allowed to settle for 30 min, at room temperature, and then incubated for 5 days, at 37 °C under 5% CO_2 atmosphere, until the spheroids were properly formed. After renewal of the culture medium, the spheroids were incubated with 25 μg mL^{-1} of

LEGE-NPL fractions (0.5% DMSO final concentration) and 1.25 μM staurosporine (positive control) for 96 h. Cell viability was evaluated using the acid phosphatase assay. Hence, media was removed, the wells were carefully washed with PBS, and the spheroids were incubated for 2 h in 100 μL of p-nitrophenyl phosphate (2 mg mL^{-1}) in sodium acetate buffer (0.1 M). To stop the reaction, 10 μL of NaOH (1 N) was added to each well and the absorbance was read at 405 nm on a multi-detection microplate reader (Synergy HT, Biotek, Bart Frederick Shahr, Germany). All assays were performed in triplicate and cell viability was calculated according to the formula above. Graphics were designed using Plotly Chart Studio [41].

3.8. Untargeted Metabolomics Analysis

To identify the putative cytotoxic compounds, an untargeted metabolomics approach was performed. Groups A and B were constituted by the active fractions of the study (Table 1, Figure 4). Group C was constituted by 12 fractions that were not considered active: JM5_amb_D, JM5_amb_E, LEGE 06078_D, LEGE 07092_D, LEGE 07167_C, LEGE 07167_D, LEGE 07167_E, LEGE 08333_D, LEGE 15488_D, LEGE 181148_E, LEGE 181148_F, and LEGE 181149_D. The liquid chromatography-high resolution electrospray ionization tandem mass spectrometry (LC-HRESIMS/MS) data were acquired on a system composed of a Dionex UltiMate 3000 HPLC with a MWD-3000RS UV/VIS detector, coupled to a Q Exactive Focus mass spectrometer controlled by Xcalibur 4.1 software (Thermo Fisher Scientific, Waltham, MA, USA). Then, 5 μL (1 mg mL^{-1} in MeOH) was separated on an ACE UltraCore 2.5 SuperC18 column (75 × 2.1 mm, ACE, Reading, UK), at 40 °C, using a gradient from 99.5 to 10% H_2O/MeOH/formic acid (95:5:0.1, v/v) to 0.5 to 90% iso-propanol/MeOH/formic acid (95:5:0.1, v/v) for 9.5 min, maintaining the last mixture until 15.5 min before returning to the initial conditions, with a flow rate of 0.35 mL min^{-1} [42]. The UV absorbance was monitored at 254 nm. HRESIMS-MS was obtained in positive mode using a capillary temperature of 262.5 °C, spray voltage of 3.5 kV, full MS scan at the resolution of 70,000 FWHM (m/z range of 150–2000), and data dependent MS^2 ($ddMS^2$, Discovery mode) at the resolution of 17,500 FWHM (isolation window used was 3.0 amu and normalized collision energy was 35). Raw data files were converted to the mzML format with MSConvert, using the parameters recommended for the Global Natural Product Social Molecular Networking (GNPS) [43]. MZmine 2 v.2.53 (http://mzmine.github.io/) was used to generate the quantification file used in the fold change analysis of MetaboAnalyst 5.0 (https://www.metaboanalyst.ca/), and to generate the MS^2 spectral summary file and quantification file for feature-based molecular networking (parameters used in MZmine 2 for mass feature detection, chromatogram building, and alignment can be found in Table S2). The appropriate files were uploaded to the GNPS web platform, and the feature-based molecular networking (FBMN) was constructed using the default settings. This molecular network was analyzed with the integrated GNPS tools DEREPLICATOR [22], MS2LDA [23], and Network Annotation Propagation (NAP) [24], which were all combined via the MolNetEnhancer [25] workflow. The web links that gave origin to the results are provided in Table S3 and the structure database used for NAP can be found as Supplementary Material. For the fold change analysis with MetaboAnalyst 5.0, the data was uploaded in comma separated values (.csv) format, with 18 unpaired samples (fractions) in columns and mass features in rows (474 mass features for group A/C and 137 mass features for group B/C; PCA and fold change charts are shown in Figure S5). No data filtering or data normalization was performed, and missing values were replaced by 1. Cytoscape 3.8.2 was used to combine the GNPS and MetaboAnalyst results and visualize the resulting molecular network. Manual dereplication was done by using the Dictionary of Natural Products 30.1 Chemical Search (https://dnp.chemnetbase.com) and CyanoMetDB [29].

4. Conclusions

Cyanobacteria have acquired an indisputable role in natural products drug discovery. Our in-house culture collection of cyanobacteria (LEGE-CC) harbors a great potential to explore for biotechnological applications, but in prior works, this was often very laborious and unsuccessful. Therefore, there was a need to develop a new strategy to access the chemical richness of LEGE-CC in a more expedited way. In summary, the semiautomated HPLC fractionation of 64 crudes generated 512 fractions that were tested for their cytotoxic potential using different cell models. The conjugation of monolayer assays and 3D cancer spheroids lead to the selection of 11 active fractions, whose chemical space was studied using an untargeted metabolomics approach. The putative annotation and identification of several cytotoxic compounds contributed to expanding the knowledge of the biochemical composition of 7 LEGE-CC strains that were characterized herein for the first time. This study was relevant to prioritize the strains with potential to discover compounds of unknown structure, work that will be addressed in the near future.

Supplementary Materials: The following are available online at https://www.mdpi.com/article/10.3390/md19110633/s1, Table S1: List of LEGE-CC strains and environmental samples used in this work. Asterisks (*) represent sequences that were obtained for this work. Table S2: Parameters used in MZmine 2 for mass feature detection, chromatogram building and feature alignment for comparison of group A with C and group B with C. Table S3: GNPS jobs used for the construction of the molecular networks. Figure S1: Boxplot representing the max, min, median and mean amounts of lyophilized biomass (A), MeOH extract (B) and final yield (C). Figure S2: IC50 graphs from the optimization of the MTT and acid phosphatase assays on 3D spheroids of the HCT 116 human colon carcinoma cell line. A range of concentrations, from 0.1 nM to 10 μM, of the anticancer drug staurosporine was used to determine the most sensitive method for evaluating cytotoxicity in cell spheroids. Figure S3: Total ion chromatograms of fractions LEGE 15488_C (upper) and LEGE 15488_D (lower). Figure S4: MS/MS spectrum of the protonated molecule at m/z 623.2865. The MS2 fragments and molecular formula were consistent with the tentative identification of 13^2-hydroxy-phaeophorbide a methyl ester. Figure S5: Principal component analysis (PCA) and fold change plots of the untargeted metabolic analysis of group A/C (A) and group B/C (B).

Author Contributions: Conceptualization, M.R.; methodology, L.F., M.P., R.U., and M.R.; investigation, L.F. (creation of library, bioactivity assays, untargeted metabolomics), J.M., R.S. (DNA extraction, amplification (PCR), sequencing, and phylogenetic analysis), and M.R. (untargeted metabolomics); resources, V.V. and M.R.; data curation, M.R.; writing—original draft preparation, L.F. and M.R.; writing—review and editing, all authors. All authors have read and agreed to the published version of the manuscript.

Funding: This research was developed under CYANCAN project PTDC/MED-QUI/30944/2017-NORTE-01-0145-FEDER-030944, co-financed by NORTE 2020, Portugal 2020, and the European Union through the ERDF, and by FCT through national funds and was additionally supported by the FCT and strategic funds UIDB/04423/2020 and UIDP/04423/2020 andby the project ATLANTIDA (ref. NORTE-01-0145-FEDER-000040), supported by the Norte Portugal Regional Operational Program (NORTE 2020), under the PORTUGAL 2020 Partnership Agreement and through the European Regional Development Fund (ERDF).

Institutional Review Board Statement: Not applicable.

Informed Consent Statement: Not applicable.

Data Availability Statement: The data presented in this study are available in the Supplementary Materials.

Acknowledgments: We deeply thank Pedro Leão and the Cyanobacterial Natural Products team at CIIMAR for all the help with the mass spectrometry data acquisition.

Conflicts of Interest: The authors declare no conflict of interest.

References

1. Newman, D.J.; Cragg, G.M. Natural Products as Sources of New Drugs over the Nearly Four Decades from 01/1981 to 09/2019. *J. Nat. Prod.* **2020**, *83*, 770–803. [CrossRef]
2. Khalifa, S.A.M.; Shedid, E.S.; Saied, E.M.; Jassbi, A.R.; Jamebozorgi, F.H.; Rateb, M.E.; Du, M.; Abdel-Daim, M.M.; Kai, G.Y.; Al-Hammady, M.A.M.; et al. Cyanobacteria—from the Oceans to the Potential Biotechnological and Biomedical Applications. *Mar. Drugs* **2021**, *19*, 320. [CrossRef]

3. Demay, J.; Bernard, C.; Reinhardt, A.; Marie, B. Natural Products from Cyanobacteria: Focus on Beneficial Activities. *Mar. Drugs* **2019**, *17*, 320. [CrossRef] [PubMed]
4. Nandagopal, P.; Steven, A.N.; Chan, L.-W.; Rahmat, Z.; Jamaluddin, H.; Mohd Noh, N.I. Bioactive Metabolites Produced by Cyanobacteria for Growth Adaptation and Their Pharmacological Properties. *Biology* **2021**, *10*, 1061. [CrossRef] [PubMed]
5. Tan, L.T.; Phyo, M.Y. Marine Cyanobacteria: A Source of Lead Compounds and Their Clinically-Relevant Molecular Targets. *Molecules* **2020**, *25*, 2197. [CrossRef]
6. Dyshlovoy, S.A.; Honecker, F. Marine Compounds and Cancer: Updates 2020. *Mar. Drugs* **2020**, *18*, 643. [CrossRef]
7. Ramos, V.; Morais, J.; Castelo-Branco, R.; Pinheiro, Â.; Martins, J.; Regueiras, A.; Pereira, A.L.; Lopes, V.R.; Frazão, B.; Gomes, D.; et al. Cyanobacterial Diversity Held in Microbial Biological Resource Centers as a Biotechnological Asset: The Case Study of the Newly Established LEGE Culture Collection. *J. Appl. Phycol.* **2018**, *30*, 1437–1451. [CrossRef] [PubMed]
8. Gutiérrez-del-Río, I.; Brugerolle de Fraissinette, N.; Castelo-Branco, R.; Oliveira, F.; Morais, J.; Redondo-Blanco, S.; Villar, C.J.; Iglesias, M.J.; Soengas, R.; Cepas, V.; et al. Chlorosphaerolactylates A–D: Natural Lactylates of Chlorinated Fatty Acids Isolated from the Cyanobacterium *Sphaerospermopsis* sp. LEGE 00249. *J. Nat. Prod.* **2020**, *83*, 1885–1890. [CrossRef]
9. Freitas, S.; Silva, N.G.; Sousa, M.L.; Ribeiro, T.; Rosa, F.; Leão, P.N.; Vasconcelos, V.; Reis, M.A.; Urbatzka, R. Chlorophyll Derivatives from Marine Cyanobacteria with Lipid-Reducing Activities. *Mar. Drugs* **2019**, *17*, 229. [CrossRef]
10. Sousa, M.L.; Preto, M.; Vasconcelos, V.; Linder, S.; Urbatzka, R. Antiproliferative Effects of the Natural Oxadiazine Nocuolin a Are Associated with Impairment of Mitochondrial Oxidative Phosphorylation. *Front. Oncol.* **2019**, *9*, 224. [CrossRef]
11. Freitas, S.; Martins, R.; Costa, M.; Leão, P.; Vitorino, R.; Vasconcelos, V.; Urbatzka, R. Hierridin B Isolated from a Marine Cyanobacterium Alters VDAC1, Mitochondrial Activity, and Cell Cycle Genes on HT-29 Colon Adenocarcinoma Cells. *Mar. Drugs* **2016**, *14*, 158. [CrossRef] [PubMed]
12. Ribeiro, T.; Lemos, F.; Preto, M.; Azevedo, J.; Sousa, M.L.; Leão, P.N.; Campos, A.; Linder, S.; Vitorino, R.; Vasconcelos, V.; et al. Cytotoxicity of Portoamides in Human Cancer Cells and Analysis of the Molecular Mechanisms of Action. *PLoS ONE* **2017**, *12*, e0188817. [CrossRef] [PubMed]
13. Antunes, J.; Pereira, S.; Ribeiro, T.; Plowman, J.E.; Thomas, A.; Clerens, S.; Campos, A.; Vasconcelos, V.; Almeida, J.R. A Multi-Bioassay Integrated Approach to Assess the Antifouling Potential of the Cyanobacterial Metabolites Portoamides. *Mar. Drugs* **2019**, *17*, 111. [CrossRef]
14. Komárek, J. A Polyphasic Approach for the Taxonomy of Cyanobacteria: Principles and Applications. *Eur. J. Phycol.* **2016**, *51*, 346–353. [CrossRef]
15. Gerwick, W.H.; Coates, R.C.; Engene, N.; Gerwick, L.; Grindberg, R.v.; Jones, A.C.; Sorrels, C.M. Giant Marine Cyanobacteria Produce Exciting Potential Pharmaceuticals. *Microbe* **2008**, *3*, 277–284. [CrossRef]
16. Thornburg, C.C.; Britt, J.R.; Evans, J.R.; Akee, R.K.; Whitt, J.A.; Trinh, S.K.; Harris, M.J.; Thompson, J.R.; Ewing, T.L.; Shipley, S.M.; et al. NCI Program for Natural Product Discovery: A Publicly-Accessible Library of Natural Product Fractions for High-Throughput Screening. *ACS Chem. Biol.* **2018**, *13*, 2484–2497. [CrossRef] [PubMed]
17. Belfiore, L.; Aghaei, B.; Law, A.M.K.; Dobrowolski, J.C.; Raftery, L.J.; Tjandra, A.D.; Yee, C.; Piloni, A.; Volkerling, A.; Ferris, C.J.; et al. Generation and Analysis of 3D Cell Culture Models for Drug Discovery. *Eur. J. Pharm. Sci.* **2021**, *163*, 105876. [CrossRef]
18. Sousa, M.L.; Ribeiro, T.; Vasconcelos, V.; Linder, S.; Urbatzka, R. Portoamides A and B Are Mitochondrial Toxins and Induce Cytotoxicity on the Proliferative Cell Layer of in Vitro Microtumours. *Toxicon* **2020**, *175*, 49–56. [CrossRef] [PubMed]
19. Kijanska, M.; Kelm, J. In Vitro 3D Spheroids and Microtissues: ATP-Based Cell Viability and Toxicity Assays. In *Assay Guidance Manual [Internet]*; Eli Lilly& Company and the National Center for Advancing Translational Sciences: Bethesda, MD, USA, 2016; pp. 1–13.
20. Zhang, J.H.; Chung, T.D.Y.; Oldenburg, K.R. A Simple Statistical Parameter for Use in Evaluation and Validation of High Throughput Screening Assays. *J. Biomol. Screen.* **1999**, *4*, 67–73. [CrossRef]
21. Nothias, L.F.; Petras, D.; Schmid, R.; Dührkop, K.; Rainer, J.; Sarvepalli, A.; Protsyuk, I.; Ernst, M.; Tsugawa, H.; Fleischauer, M.; et al. Feature-Based Molecular Networking in the GNPS Analysis Environment. *Nat. Methods* **2020**, *17*, 905–908. [CrossRef]
22. Mohimani, H.; Gurevich, A.; Shlemov, A.; Mikheenko, A.; Korobeynikov, A.; Cao, L.; Shcherbin, E.; Nothias, L.F.; Dorrestein, P.C.; Pevzner, P.A. Dereplication of Microbial Metabolites through Database Search of Mass Spectra. *Nat. Commun.* **2018**, *9*, 4035. [CrossRef] [PubMed]
23. Wandy, J.; Zhu, Y.; van der Hooft, J.J.J.; Daly, R.; Barrett, M.P.; Rogers, S. Ms2lda.Org: Web-Based Topic Modelling for Substructure Discovery in Mass Spectrometry. *Bioinformatics* **2018**, *34*, 317–318. [CrossRef]
24. Da Silva, R.R.; Wang, M.; Nothias, L.F.; van der Hooft, J.J.J.; Caraballo-Rodríguez, A.M.; Fox, E.; Balunas, M.J.; Klassen, J.L.; Lopes, N.P.; Dorrestein, P.C. Propagating Annotations of Molecular Networks Using in Silico Fragmentation. *PLoS Comput. Biol.* **2018**, *14*, e1006089. [CrossRef] [PubMed]
25. Ernst, M.; Kang, K.B.; Caraballo-Rodríguez, A.M.; Nothias, L.F.; Wandy, J.; Chen, C.; Wang, M.; Rogers, S.; Medema, M.H.; Dorrestein, P.C.; et al. Molnetenhancer: Enhanced Molecular Networks by Integrating Metabolome Mining and Annotation Tools. *Metabolites* **2019**, *9*, 144. [CrossRef]
26. Djoumbou Feunang, Y.; Eisner, R.; Knox, C.; Chepelev, L.; Hastings, J.; Owen, G.; Fahy, E.; Steinbeck, C.; Subramanian, S.; Bolton, E.; et al. ClassyFire: Automated Chemical Classification with a Comprehensive, Computable Taxonomy. *J. Cheminform.* **2016**, *8*, 61. [CrossRef] [PubMed]

27. Leao, P.N.; Pereira, A.R.; Liu, W.-T.; Ng, J.; Pevzner, P.a.; Dorrestein, P.C.; Konig, G.M.; Vasconcelos, V.M.; Gerwick, W.H. Synergistic Allelochemicals from a Freshwater Cyanobacterium. *Proc. Natl. Acad. Sci. USA* **2010**, *107*, 11183–11188. [CrossRef]
28. Kang, H.S.; Krunic, A.; Shen, Q.; Swanson, S.M.; Orjala, J. Minutissamides A-D, Antiproliferative Cyclic Decapeptides from the Cultured Cyanobacterium Anabaena Minutissima. *J. Nat. Prod.* **2011**, *74*, 1597–1605. [CrossRef]
29. Jones, M.R.; Pinto, E.; Torres, M.A.; Dörr, F.; Mazur-Marzec, H.; Szubert, K.; Tartaglione, L.; Dell'Aversano, C.; Miles, C.O.; Beach, D.G.; et al. CyanoMetDB, a Comprehensive Public Database of Secondary Metabolites from Cyanobacteria. *Water Res.* **2021**, *196*, 117017. [CrossRef]
30. Vulpanovici, F.A. Biosynthesis, Production and Structural Studies of Secondary Metabolites in Cultured Marine Cyanobacteria. Ph.D. Thesis, Oregon State University, Corvallis, OR, USA, 2004.
31. Thornburg, C.C. Investigation of Unique Marine Environments for Microbial Natural Products. Ph.D. Thesis, Oregon State University, Corvallis, OR, USA, 2013; pp. 1–276.
32. Saide, A.; Lauritano, C.; Ianora, A. Pheophorbide A: State of the Art. *Mar. Drugs* **2020**, *18*, 257. [CrossRef]
33. Lane, D.J. 16S/23S rRNA sequencing. In *Nucleic Acid Techniques in Bacterial Systematics*; John Wiley and Sons: Chichester, UK, 1991; pp. 115–175.
34. Lepère, C.; Wilmotte, A.; Meyer, B. Molecular Diversity of Microcystis Strains (Cyanophyceae, Chroococcales) Based on 16S RDNA Sequences. *Syst. Geogr. Plants* **2000**, *70*, 275–283. [CrossRef]
35. Nübel, U.; Garcia-Pichel, F.; Muyzer, G. PCR Primers to Amplify 16S RRNA Genes from Cyanobacteria. *Appl. Environ. Microbiol.* **1997**, *63*, 3327–3332. [CrossRef]
36. Wright, E.S.; Yilmaz, L.S.; Noguera, D.R. DECIPHER, a Search-Based Approach to Chimera Identification for 16S RRNA Sequences. *Appl. Environ. Microbiol.* **2012**, *78*, 717–725. [CrossRef] [PubMed]
37. Thompson, J.D.; Higgins, D.G.; Gibson, T.J. CLUSTAL W: Improving the Sensitivity of Progressive Multiple Sequence Alignment through Sequence Weighting, Position-Specific Gap Penalties and Weight Matrix Choice. *Nucleic Acids Res.* **1994**, *22*, 4673–4680. [CrossRef] [PubMed]
38. Kumar, S.; Stecher, G.; Tamura, K. MEGA7: Molecular Evolutionary Genetics Analysis Version 7.0 for Bigger Datasets. *Mol. Biol. Evol.* **2016**, *33*, 1870–1874. [CrossRef] [PubMed]
39. Letunic, I.; Bork, P. Interactive Tree of Life (ITOL): An Online Tool for Phylogenetic Tree Display and Annotation. *Bioinformatics* **2007**, *23*, W293–W296. [CrossRef] [PubMed]
40. Carlsson, J.; Yuhas, J.M. Liquid-Overlay Culture of Cellular Spheroids. In *Spheroids in Cancer Research*; Springer: Berlin/Heidelberg, Germany, 1984; Volume 95, pp. 1–23.
41. Plotly Technologies Inc. Collaborative Data Science. Available online: https://Chart-Studio.Plotly.Com/ (accessed on 18 March 2021).
42. Girão, M.; Ribeiro, I.; Ribeiro, T.; Azevedo, I.C.; Pereira, F.; Urbatzka, R.; Leão, P.N.; Carvalho, M.F. Actinobacteria Isolated from Laminaria Ochroleuca: A Source of New Bioactive Compounds. *Front. Microbiol.* **2019**, *10*, 683. [CrossRef]
43. Aron, A.T.; Gentry, E.C.; McPhail, K.L.; Nothias, L.F.; Nothias-Esposito, M.; Bouslimani, A.; Petras, D.; Gauglitz, J.M.; Sikora, N.; Vargas, F.; et al. Reproducible Molecular Networking of Untargeted Mass Spectrometry Data Using GNPS. *Nat. Protoc.* **2020**, *15*, 1954–1991. [CrossRef]

marine drugs

MDPI

Article

Application of Networking Approaches to Assess the Chemical Diversity, Biogeography, and Pharmaceutical Potential of Verongiida Natural Products

James Lever [1], Robert Brkljača [2], Colin Rix [1] and Sylvia Urban [1,*]

[1] School of Science (Applied Chemistry and Environmental Sciences), RMIT University, GPO Box 2476, Melbourne, VIC 3001, Australia; james.lever@rmit.edu.au (J.L.); colin.rix@rmit.edu.au (C.R.)

[2] Monash Biomedical Imaging, Monash University, Clayton, VIC 3168, Australia; Robert.brkljaca@monash.edu

* Correspondence: sylvia.urban@rmit.edu.au

Abstract: This study provides a review of all isolated natural products (NPs) reported for sponges within the order Verongiida (1960 to May 2020) and includes a comprehensive compilation of their geographic and physico-chemical parameters. Physico-chemical parameters were used in this study to infer pharmacokinetic properties as well as the potential pharmaceutical potential of NPs from this order of marine sponge. In addition, a network analysis for the NPs produced by the Verongiida sponges was applied to systematically explore the chemical space relationships between taxonomy, secondary metabolite and drug score variables, allowing for the identification of differences and correlations within a dataset. The use of scaffold networks as well as bipartite relationship networks provided a platform to explore chemical diversity as well as the use of chemical similarity networks to link pharmacokinetic properties with structural similarity. This study paves the way for future applications of network analysis procedures in the field of natural products for any order or family.

Keywords: network analysis; cheminformatics; verongiida sponges; natural products; in silico mapping

Citation: Lever, J.; Brkljača, R.; Rix, C.; Urban, S. Application of Networking Approaches to Assess the Chemical Diversity, Biogeography, and Pharmaceutical Potential of Verongiida Natural Products. *Mar. Drugs* **2021**, *19*, 582. https://doi.org/10.3390/md19100582

Academic Editors: Susana P. Gaudencio and Florbela Pereira

Received: 23 September 2021
Accepted: 14 October 2021
Published: 18 October 2021

1. Introduction

Marine sponges (phylum Porifera, Grant 1836 [1]) are benthic invertebrates that play host to a rich and diverse number of microbial symbionts. Marine sponge holobionts or their symbionts have been the source of an extraordinary number of biologically important chemical compounds, termed natural products (NPs). The compounds isolated have generally been of high chemical diversity and are often unique, not only in the structures that they exhibit, but also in the broad range of biological activities that they display [2]. This array of bioactivity has sustained great interest in marine sponges as a source of compounds with pharmaceutical potential.

Contemporary NP research is centred around the hypothesis that targeting organisms or sampling sites with high biodiversity will lead to more chemically diverse compounds, and thus a larger variety of bioactivities [3–5]. The understanding of biogeographical and ecological diversity, and the distribution trends of organisms that produce NPs, can be informative for future isolation efforts [6,7].

To date, the study of biogeographical trends which influence sponge NP production has been hindered by the dynamic nature of sponge taxonomy, particularly those within Verongiida Bergquist, 1978 [8], because the primary diagnostic tool is the structure and architecture of the laminated fibres. This, together with both the tendency of these organisms to occur in different forms under different environmental pressures, due to natural morphological plasticity, and the presence of diverse microbial symbionts, can create difficulty when deciding on the origin of compounds that are isolated from marine sponges. With more widespread and accurate data having been accumulated regarding taxonomy and the distribution of NPs across many families, the task of describing NP diversity and distribution is becoming a more achievable one.

A large body of work exists in the literature documenting and reviewing NPs isolated from specific genera within the order Verongiida [9–13]. This distinct marine sponge order is differentiated both phylogenetically and morphologically from other sponge orders [14]. The Verongiid sponges lack a mineral skeleton, displaying instead a heavily collagenous mesohyl which obtains shape and structure from spongin fibres that exhibit a granulated "pith" interior, together with a laminated "bark" exterior [14,15]. This marine sponge order has seen particular interest from the NP community over the past 50 years, due in part to the large number of bioactive bromotyrosine alkaloids (BTAs) that they produce [12]. BTAs from Verongiida show significant chemical diversity as a class, and provide effective chemical defence for these sessile invertebrates against predation [16,17] and fouling organisms [18,19].

Whilst these compounds are not exclusive to Verongiida [20], they do occur in greater quantities and present more structural variants within this order than any other. Given the taxonomic spread and geographic ubiquity of BTAs across this order, it is clear why they are considered by many as a significant taxonomic marker for Verongiida sponges [21–23].

BTAs represent a compound class of interest due to their chemical diversity as well as their propensity for wide ranging bioactivity [9–12]. Notable examples include the disulphide-linked psammaplins, first isolated from an unidentified specimen of *Psammaplysilla* Keller, 1889 (= *Pseudoceratina* Carter, 1885), in 1987 [24]. These compounds have inspired further studies of Verongiid sponges as well as the design of synthetically targeted anti-cancer drug libraries [25–27]. The BTA compounds from the Verongiid sponges show enormous pharmaceutical potential, with many viewed as being promising targets within the preclinical pipeline. Preclinical assays on BTAs have highlighted many candidates for antimalarial [28,29], antibacterial [30–33], antiprotozoal [30,34], anticoagulant [28,35,36] as well as potential central nervous system drugs [30,31,37,38]. This significant and broad-spectrum activity has provided much impetus to further study this order of sponge and its associated NPs.

Much debate has ensued regarding the origin of these NPs, with putative evidence suggesting contradicting theories of host vs. symbiont origins from Verongiid sponges [39–42]. It has even been suggested that the biogenetic origins of these compounds begin within sponge cells, followed by the translocation of intermediates for further biosynthetic transformation performed by symbiont microbes [43]. Whichever the case, it is a process that is poorly understood. Multi-omic related work on Verongiid sponges has shown a correlation between the microbial and metabolic architectures of a range of species sampled from differing locations [39]. This assessment implies that despite the differing core microbiomes of varying taxa of Verongiid sponges, there is chemical consistency when comparing species from different locations. Moreover, this aligns with the current understanding of the core microbiome as being highly species-dependent across differing geospatial and temperature gradients [44–48]. However, species specificity has not brought us any closer to understanding the origin of NPs from the Verongiid sponges; instead, it has highlighted that these organisms exist in a complex mutualistic ecosystem.

The geospatial and taxonomic conservation of microbiome architectures provides an opportunity to better understand the biogeographic and chemotaxonomic distribution of Verongiida NPs. With approximately 633 NPs reported from over 43 different species in the literature, there appears to be a suitable number of compounds with a wide enough taxonomic spread of species to provide a solid foundation on which to base an understanding of any trends in the distribution of NPs.

The goal of this data mining exercise was to characterise the geographical distribution of all NPs produced by sponges within the order Verongiida, highlighting key trends that may assist NP isolation efforts in the future. The work also addresses the distribution of NPs across different genera within the order Verongiida to identify possible chemotaxonomic or biosynthetic trends. Finally, the predicted structural similarities and pharmaceutical activity of these NPs is discussed, utilising network analysis methodologies.

2. Results and Discussion

In total, 215 papers were surveyed, which reported NPs that had been isolated from four families (43 species) of Verongiid sponges across approximately 126 geographical locations (see Supporting Information S1 for full reference list). Prior to this current study, reviews had been published on the genus *Aplysina* Nardo, 1834 [49], and its associated NPs in 2011 [10] and 2015 [11]. These reviews focused primarily on the listing and reporting of ^{13}C NMR data and biological activity, as well as providing some insight into the proposed biosynthesis of some BTA compounds. In 2019, a review was also published on the genus *Suberea* Bergquist, 1995 [50], including compound lists as well as bioactivity and proposed biosynthesis [9]. A 2005 review documented the bioactivity and biosynthesis of the marine BTA derivatives as a compound class [12].

To date, there remains no review that encompasses the entire order of Verongiida. The present work rectifies this situation and focusses on NPs reported between the period of 1960 to May 2020. Compound types that have been described from this order of marine sponges are largely comprised of BTAs, including spiroisoxazolines (SIA) existing in both mono- and bis-configurations (mSIA and bSIA), spirooxepinisoxazolines, brominated phenolics, dibromocyclohexadienes, verongiabenzenoids, verongiaquinols, brominated oximes, oxime disulfides, bromotyramines (BT), bromotyramine oximes (BTOx), bastadins and hemibastadins. Further compounds that are not associated with the BTA biosynthetic route which are also found in the order, include hydroquinones, pyrroles, quinolines, guanidine alkaloids, indole alkaloids, benzonaphthyridines, benzofurans isoprenoids, sesterterpenoids, sesquiterpenoids, merosesquiterpenoids and macrolides.

2.1. Biosynthesis and Distribution of BTAs

The SIA and BT classes form the basis of many sub classes of BTA including a large array of mono- and bis- spiro isomers. In addition, both SIAs and BTs are incorporated to create some of the higher molecular weight compound classes (Figure 1). Mono- and bis-SIA compounds are also observed together with BTs that form end groups using cyclised guanidine (Gdn) expressed as either imidazole, amino imidazole or imidazoline. These three classes, SIA, BT and BTOx, represent approximately 48% of all the NPs reported for Verongiida sponges and appear to be the major biosynthetic outcomes for these organisms. The SIA, BT and BTOx units are then utilised as the building blocks to create many more diverse structures, somewhat reminiscent of combinatorial chemistry (Figure 1 and Table 1). Approximately 18% of SIAs, BTs and BTOxs incorporate Gdn into their structures, resulting in either imidazole, imidazoline, imidazole amine or non-cyclic Gdn functionalities. Biosynthetically, these groups are often found as chain-terminating entities, except in the rare situations when Gdn can be found to reside between two SIA head groups. In this situation, the NH group of an imidazole ring provides an attachment point for another SIA head group.

SIAs appear to be the only spiro class of NP created by Verongiid sponges expressed with bis configurations. A bis spirooxepinisoxazoline has yet to be observed, despite the two classes supposedly originating from the same arene oxide intermediate. The formation of bis compounds would appear to be exclusive to the spirocyclohexadiene structure shown by SIAs. Conversion of the epoxide intermediate to either an SIA or a spirooxepinisoxazoline has been postulated to be enantioselective, rather than enantiospecific, as both (+) and (−) SIAs have been reported in differing quantities, suggesting enantiodivergence from the intermediate epoxide [51,52].

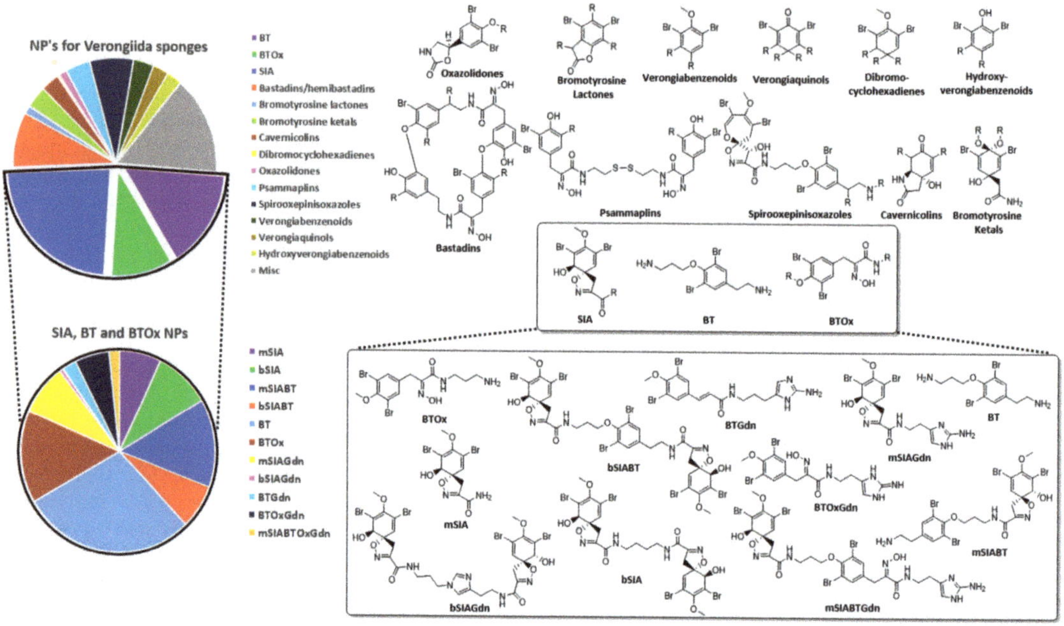

Figure 1. Classes of SIA, BT and BTOx. Mono spiroisoxazolines (mSIA), bis spiroisoxazolines (bSIA), bis spiroisoxazoline bromotyramine (bSIABT), mono spiroisoxazoline bromotyramine (mSIABT), mono spiroisoxazoline guanidine (mSIAGdn), bromotyramine (BT), bromotyramine oxime (BTOx), bis spiroisoxazoline guanidine (bSIAGdn), mono spiroisoxazoline bromotyrmamine oxime guanidine (mSIABTOxGdn), bromotyramine guanidine (BTGdn), bromotyramine oxime guanidine.

The distribution of these NPs (Table 1) across the order of Verongiida reflects that the two most studied genera, *Aplysina* and *Pseudoceratina* Carter, 1885 [53], have a wide variety of compound classes. Both genera have many species with reported bSIA and mSIA compounds, which are indicative of the presence of compounds such as aerothionin, homoaerothionin and purealidin R or purpuroacetic acid, respectively. *Aplysina* differs from *Pseudoceratina* in the production of compounds that possess Gdn derived moieties. *Aplysina* species appear to always express mSIAGdns, often in the form of aerophobin compounds, but only *A. archeri* (Higgin, 1875) [54] and *A. lacunosa* (Lamarck, 1814) [55] have been reported with other Gdn compounds. Comparatively, species of *Pseudoceratina* sponges show more complex chemistry with a wider variety of SIA/BT/Gdn combinations. The absence of Gdn also extends to the genus *Ianthella* Gray, 1869 [56], which has also displayed an apparent absence of the BTOx class of NP. This probably arises from the apparent tendency for *Ianthella* sponges to produce hemibastadins from their oxime bromotyramines prior to any O-methylation, which then acts as the precursor for the macrocyclic bastadins. This absence of BTOx compounds (other than hemibastadins) is informative, as they seem to produce the required BT precursors for the BTOx compounds that are largely absent, suggesting that the hemibastadins are the preferential biosynthetic route for *Ianthella*. The scarcity of SIAs reported for *Ianthella* indicates significant biogenetic divergence of this genus from the remainder of the Verongiid sponges, which is supported by its unique mesohyl biology and differentiation within Verongiida in the family Ianthellidae Hyatt, 1875 [57].

Table 1. Distribution of SIA and BT compound classes amongst Verongiida sponges (see Supporting Information S1 for references).

Species	mSIA	bSIA	mSIA BT	bSIA BT	BT	BTOx	mSIA Gdn	bSIA Gdn	BTGdn	BTOx Gdn	mSIA BTOxGdn
Aiolochroia crassa (Hyatt, 1875)	+		+	+	+		+				
Anomoianthella popeae (Bergquist, 1980)					+						
Aplysina aerophoba (Nardo, 1833)		+		+			+				
Aplysina archeri (Higgin, 1875)		+		+				+			
Aplysina caissara (Pinheiro and Hajdu, 2001)		+					+				
Alplysina cauliformis (Carter, 1882)	+	+	+				+				
Aplysina cavernicola (Vacelet, 1959)		+		+			+				
Aplysina fistularis (Pallas, 1766)		+		+	+	+	+				
Aplysina fulva (Pallas, 1766)	+	+	+	+			+				
Aplysina gerardogreeni (Gomez and Bakus, 1992)		+									
Aplysina insularis (Duchassaing and Michelotti, 1864)	+	+		+			+				
Aplysina lactuca (Pinheiro, Hajdu and Custodio, 2007)		+		+							
Aplysina lacunosa (Lamarck, 1814)	+	+	+	+			+		+	+	+
Aplysina laevis (=*Pseudoceratina durissima* Carter, 1885)											
Aplysina solongeae (Pinheiro, Hajdu and Custodio, 2007)		+		+							
Aplysina sp. (Nardo, 1834)	+	+	+	+	+	+					
Aplysina thiona (=*Aiolochroia thiona* Laubenfels, 1930)		+									
Aplysinella rhax (de Laubenfels, 1954)											
Aplysinella sp. (Bergquist, 1980)		+	+		+					+	
Aplysinella strongylata (Bergquist, 1980)											
Hexadella dedritifera (Topsent, 1913)						+					
Hexadella indica (Dendy, 1905)					+						
Hexadella sp. (Topsent, 1896)			+		+						
Ianthella basta (Pallas, 1766)					+						
Ianthella flabelliformis (Linnaeus, 1759)			+								
Ianthella quadrangulata (Bergquist and Kelly-Borges, 1995)					+						
Ianthella reticulata (Bergquist and Kelly-Borges, 1995)											
Ianthella sp. (Gray, 1869)			+	+	+						
Pseudoceratina arabica (Keller, 1889)					+						
Pseudoceratina crassa (=*Aiolochroia crassa* Hyatt, 1875)	+	+	+	+	+					+	
Pseudoceratina durissima (Carter, 1885)		+		+							
Pseudoceratina purea (=*P. purpurea* Carter, 1880)	+		+		+	+	+			+	+
Pseudoceratina purpurea (Carter, 1880)	+		+	+	+	+	+			+	+
Pseudoceratina sp. (Carter, 1885)	+	+	+	+	+	+	+	+		+	+
Pseudoceratina verrucosa (Bergquist, 1995)	+		+	+	+	+	+		+	+	+
Suberea clavata (Pulitzer-Finali, 1982)							+		+	+	
Suberea creba (Bergquist, 1995)	+	+		+							
Suberea ianthelliformis (Lendenfeld, 1888)			+		+						
Suberea mollis (Row, 1911)		+			+		+		+		
Suberea praetensa (Row, 1911)				+							
Suberea sp. (Bergquist, 1995)	+				+	+					
Verongula gigantea (Hyatt, 1875)	+	+		+			+			+	
Verongula rigida (Esper, 1794)	+	+	+	+			+		+		
Verongula sp. (Verrill, 1907)	+	+		+							

The current literature also shows an apparent absence of low molecular weight verongiabenzenoids, dibromocyclohexadienes and verongiaquinols within species of *Ianthella*. This evidence tends to contradict a postulate that no SIAs are observed due to biotransformation of these higher molecular weight compounds to lower molecular weight derivatives via the hypothesised wound induced chemical defence process.

This same observation could be made for both *Hexadella* Topsent, 1896 [58] and *Aplysinella* Bergquist, 1980 [59]; however, these two genera are far less well-studied than *Aplysina*, *Pseudoceratina* and *Ianthella*. Despite this lack of SIAs for *Aplysinella* and *Hexadella*, it is still significant to note that only *Hexadella* sp. and *Aplysinella* sp. produced SIA compounds, while the remaining species either produced BTs or BTOx type compounds (Table 1). *Aplysinella rhax* (de Laubenfels, 1954) [60] and *A. strongylata* (Bergquist, 1980) [59] showed the presence of only psammaplin and spirooxepinisoxazolines, respectively, providing many derivatives of the psammaplin and psammaplysin classes of compounds and clearly displaying high biosynthetic preference toward these over SIAs.

Verongula Verill, 1907 [61] demonstrated the same trends as *Pseudoceratina*, with many mSIA and bSIA compounds documented across all species. The major difference is the lack of BT and BTOx compounds reported, which suggests that this genus efficiently converts these classes into bSIABTs, mSIABTs, BTGdns or BTOxGdns.

The biosynthesis of BTAs has yet to be completely elucidated, but it is thought to begin with the catalysed hydroxylation of phenylalanine to form tyrosine, followed by bromination through flavin-dependent halogenases. Brominated tyrosine is thought to be the source of psammaplin compounds arising through reaction with, in the case of psammaplin A, pre-psammaplin, which is derived from cysteine. Alternatively, the production of methoxylated nitriles or oxidation of the amine group can produce an oxime intermediate which provides the basis for a cascade of phenolic nitriles and amides created through decarboxylation and dehydrogenation. The oxime intermediate can also combine with bromotyramine to form, via the hemibastadin precursor, the bastadin series of compounds. Epoxidation of the oxime intermediate can also yield the SIA ring system as well as the spirooxepinisoxazolines and dibromocyclohexadienes. It has been suggested that dibromocyclohexadienes might also be generated through the degradation of SIAs to ultimately produce a highly bioactive dienone which provides part of a wound-induced chemical defence against predation [11,62,63]. In addition, the oxime intermediate can also combine with BT compounds to produce the class BTOx (Figure 2).

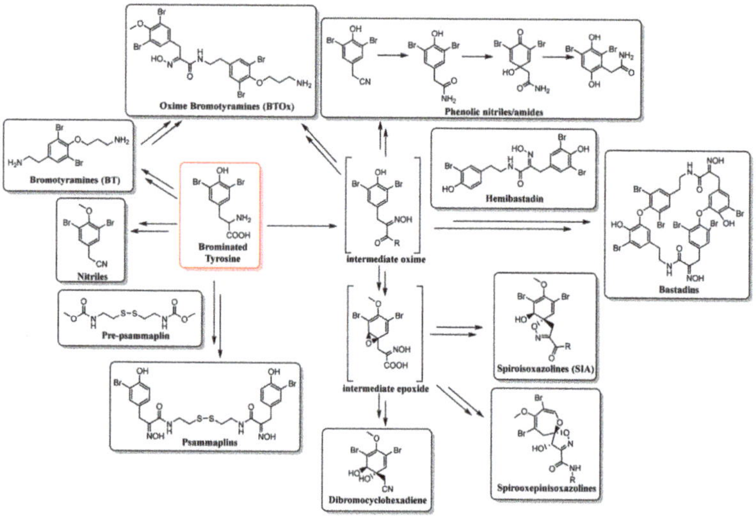

Figure 2. Proposed biosynthesis of BTAs from brominated tyrosine [9,11,12,64].

2.2. *Biogeography and Hotspots for Verongiida NPs*

Sponges of the order Verongiida are known to predominately inhabit tropical and temperate regions of the world, being present in the Central Indo-Pacific, Tropical Western Atlantic and Temperate Australasian realms (Figure 3). These sponges are found to dominate deeper reefs in the Caribbean region and New Caledonian waters, as well as the southern and eastern coasts of Australia, including the Great Barrier Reef (GBR).

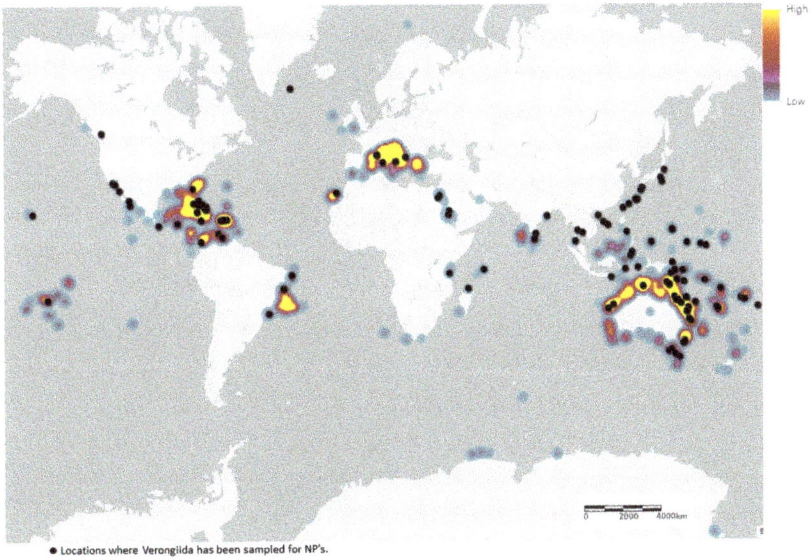

Figure 3. Known distribution of Verongiida sponges globally, data from Ocean Biodiversity Information System (OBIS) (heat map) [65,66]. Locations where Verongiida sponges have been sampled, yielding natural products (black dot).

Despite being relatively well-distributed throughout temperate and tropical environments, NP studies have been focused on specimens collected from the Central Indo-Pacific and Tropical Atlantic regions. This is understandable, as these regions provide exceptional biodiversity and are thus prime sampling locations for providing chemical diversity. However, this leaves several regions considerably understudied, including the western coast of Brazil (within the Tropical Atlantic realm) as well as Temperate Northern Atlantic waters, especially the Mediterranean and Adriatic Seas. These regions offer potentially untapped NP resources that should be investigated in more detail.

Regions in Japan, north of the Okinawa prefecture, have been a rich source of sponges from the genus *Pseudoceratina*, as have Hachijo-jima Island [67–69] and Oshima-shinsone [70], and have all yielded NPs from *Pseudoceratina* sponges, despite not being listed as regions of frequent habitation for Verongiida sponges by the OBIS. This has also been true for regions in China, such as Hainan Island [71,72] and Yong Xing Island [73], as well as Tonga [24,74] and the Gulf of Thailand, near Kho Chang Island [75]. This same trend was also observed for *Hexadella* sponge samples sourced in Jervis Inlet, British Columbia, Canada [76,77] and the *Aplysinella* sponges sampled from Pingelap Atoll, Micronesia [78]. These occurrences draw attention to the large body of biodiversity and geographical distribution data that are still undescribed for the phylum Porifera [79].

Variation in distribution and sampling was observed across all families of Verongiida. In some cases, geographical variation was linked to chemical differences even at the species level. While this dataset cannot allow for a full description of metabolomic differences between each species, it can still be instructive to explore the more apparent cases of metabolomic divergence observed between NPs reported in the literature. The Central-Indo Pacific realm, including the GBR, is an area that has shown the largest number of sampled and studied Verongiida sponges across nearly all genera (Figure 4). The sheer number of diverse NPs attests to this region's biodiversity.

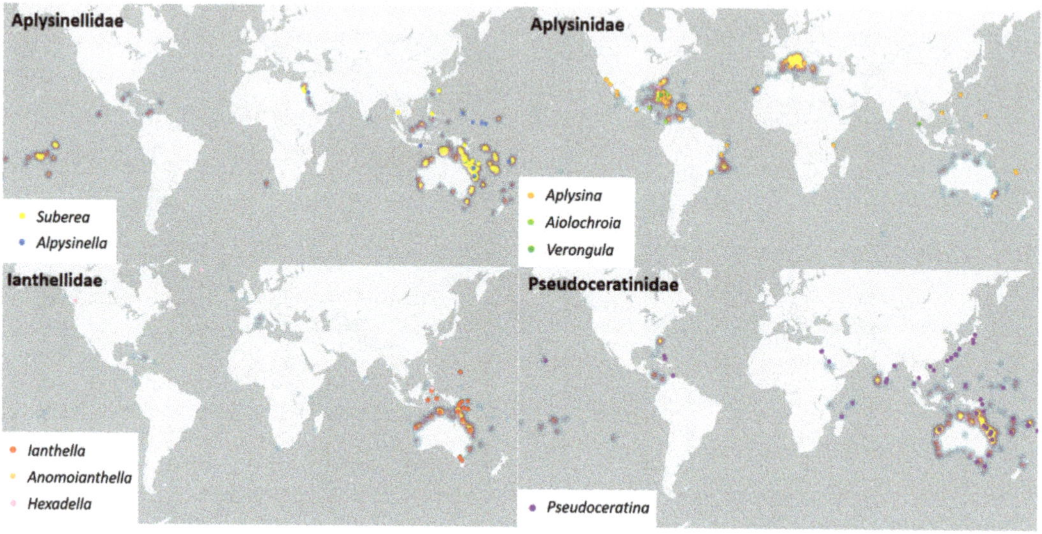

Figure 4. OBIS distribution of Verongiida sponge families (heat map). Locations of Verongiida sponges that have been sampled yielding NPs (coloured dots).

The genus *Pseudoceratina*, belonging to the family Pseudoceratinidae Carter, 1885 [53], has been one of the major genera sampled and studied in this region, with the most highly represented species being *P. purpurea* (Carter, 1880) [80] and *Pseudoceratina.* sp., although sampling was not limited to these species, with *P. durissima* (Carter, 1885) [53,81] and *P. verrucossa* (Bergquist, 1995) [50,82,83] also being studied from the GBR and New Caledonian regions (Figure 4). The Tropical Atlantic realm, including the Bahamas, has yielded exclusive species, including *P. crassa* Hyatt, 1875 (= *Aiolochroia crassa* Hyatt, 1875) [57,84–86], and no other Pseudoceratinidae species. *P. crassa* displayed the presence of several verongiabenzenoids, as well as SIAs and BT compounds, together with cyclitol glycolipids, which is unique to this species within the Verongiida order.

The Red Sea, in the Western Indo-Pacific, was another realm that showed species specificity, proving to be the only location outside of Madagascar [87] where *P. arabica* (Keller, 1889) [88] was sampled and studied for NPs [89–91]. This species yielded BTs, verongiabenzenoids and spirooxepinisoxazoline compounds, with some exhibiting a rare 2-(methyl)cyclopent-4-ene-1,3-dione moiety as well as incorporating BTs into their structure [91]. However, no related mSIABT compounds were reported from this species despite having the necessary BT precursors. Pseudoceratinidae sponges have been sampled and studied from many of the regions that show high levels of distribution, except for the South Pacific Ocean near the French Polynesian shelf.

Ianthellidae displays far more localised distribution, with much of the sampling occurring within the Central-Indo Pacific realm surrounding the GBR and Papua New Guinea (PNG) regions [92], although some species, such as *I. flabelliformis* (Linnaeus, 1759), can be found at more southerly latitudes, such as the Port Phillip Bay region in Victoria, Australia. Comparisons of the NPs reported for *I. flabelliformis* sampled within the southerly region of Port Phillip Bay [93], and its two North Australian counterparts in Shelburne Bay, Queensland [94] and Darwin Harbour, Northern Territory [95], yielded quite different chemistry. The Port Phillip Bay sample showed an interesting array of lactam sesquiterpenes, as well as some more common indole alkaloids, two classes unrelated to the BTA biosynthetic pathway, whereas the two northern locations displayed SIAs as well as bastadins. Bastadins represented the more common biosynthetic outcome for *Ianthella*, but SIAs proved to be a more significant find, as products of the isooxazoline biosynthetic route are far more rare from *Ianthella* sponges [96]. Macrocyclic bastadin isomers where also isolated from *I. flabelliformis* sampled from PNG [97].

The species *I. basta* (Pallas, 1766) [98] is the most studied sponge of the family Ianthellidae, and has been sampled across a number of localities, including Guam [99,100], PNG [97,101–103], Indonesia [104–109], GBR [110–112], and the Exmouth Gulf, Western Australia [113,114]. All samples across all localities yielded a very similar chemistry, proving *I. basta* to be a large producer of bastadins and their precursor, the hemi-bastadins. The only notable difference was that sponges sampled from both Guam and the Exmouth Gulf both exhibited sulfated monoesters of the bastadins and hemibastadins.

Ianthella quadrangulata (Bergquist, 1995) [92] was collected from three locations across the GBR. The Heron Island collection, which was the most southerly of the three, produced the most interesting chemistry [115,116]. This sample provided many bastadin congeners, but more significantly several novel dimeric brominated benzofurans were discovered, all of which were shown to have incorporated *O*-sulfate esters into their structures. This indicated that perhaps this is a biosynthetic trend that persists throughout the genus *Ianthella* and is not specific to a single species. Collections from Orpheus Island [37] and Sykes Reef [117], which were more northerly locations, appeared to mostly yield bastadin congeners, as well as an octopamine derivative. Interestingly, a number of sponges were sampled from the GBR region that were only identified at the genus level, *Ianthella.* sp. Additionally observed from this collection was a series of benzofuran compounds very similar to those produced by *I. quadrangulata* [118,119]. Unfortunately, sample details only reported GBR as the region of collection so it could not be confirmed if benzofurans are more likely to be found in Heron Island *Ianthella* sponges. Collections of *Ianthella.* sp. from the Bass Strait region of Australia yielded the most unique chemistry for the genus *Ianthella*, including pyrrolidones, lamellerins, a new class of furanones and a rare class of pyrrolidone–lamellerin hybrids called the dictyodendrins, all of which are highly unusual for *Ianthella* [120,121]. This is significant, as it appears that *Ianthella* sponges sampled from more southerly locations such as the Bass Strait and Port Phillip Bay appear to display more chemistry which is independent of the brominated tyrosine biosynthetic pathway.

Aplysinidae Carter, 1875 [122], sponges are almost as extensively studied as Pseudoceratinidae sponges. The genus *Aplysina* accounts for a great deal of this, especially in the Tropical Atlantic realm, where the biodiversity hotspots of the Bahamas, Puerto Rico and Cuba have yielded large numbers of NPs, as well as those from the Temperate Northern Atlantic within the Mediterranean region. A great deal of knowledge has been accumulated regarding the distribution of BTAs within this genus, allowing *Aplysina* to be used as an effective model in understanding the relationships between production of BTAs and biogeographical trends involving the study of depth, spatial differences, and seasonal variation on quantities of key BTAs.

The species *A. aerophoba* (Nardo, 1833) [123] and *A. cavernicola* (Vacelet, 1959) [124] are found in large quantities in the Mediterranean region and show somewhat similar chemistry, with both exhibiting SIAs as well as some characteristic pigments. Comparative studies have been performed on *A. aerophoba* and *A. cavernicola,* illustrating specific differences in the secondary metabolomes of these two species, despite both inhabiting similar regions of the Mediterranean. Differences were found between the two species in the relative concentrations of the key SIAs: aerothionin, aerophobin-2, isofistularin-3, and aplysinamisin-1, indicating these to be appropriate markers to differentiate the two species. During transplantation experiments, depth was found to play little or no role in the variability of the production of key secondary metabolites [125]. Depth was also shown to play little to no role in the chemical variability of *A. aerophoba* in a quantitative analysis of key BTAs, with the largest amount of chemical variability being explained by spatial scale between sampling sites. Interestingly, large variations were observed for sponges that were sampled in close proximity as well as those that were sampled with larger distances between sites, seeming to indicate that while proximity plays a role in secondary metabolism, there are also other factors contributing to this variability [126]. This became evident in a follow up study confirming the effect of seasonal variation on the quantitative variation of metabolites within *A. aerophoba* [127]. Seasonal and water temperature effects were also shown to be the major influences contributing to increased production of NPs for *A. cavernicola* [128]. In the case of *A. fulva* (Pallas, 1766) [98], sampled from locations in the Caribbean, USA (South Atlantic Bight, Georgia and Key Largo, Florida) as well as the Brazilian coastline, it was observed that while both locations consistently yielded SIA derivatives, only samples from the South Atlantic Bight location produced compounds such as aerophobin-1 with an imidazole functional group [21,129–132].

The genus *Verongula*, family Aplysinidae, has been sampled in many of the same Caribbean locations as *Aplysina*, as well as once from the Kho Ha Islets on the coast of Thailand. The *Verongula* sponges exhibited the same plethora of SIAs and verongiabenzenoids [133–136] that could be found across much of the rest of the order Verongiida; however, a unique array of brominated tryptamine-derived alkaloids, merosesquiterpenoids and a benzonaphthyridine were also reported. As well as being new to the family Aplysinidae, these compounds were also previously unreported within the order Verongiida, and thus have no biosynthetic precedents within this order, making *Verongula* unique amongst its Verongiida counterparts [137–141].

Aplysinella and *Suberea*, both within the family Aplysinellidae Bergquist, 1980 [59], were sampled mainly from the Central Indo-Pacific realm and accounted for the majority of NPs reported for this family. *A. rhax* was sampled from the GBR [142,143], Fiji [144], Palau [145], Guam [16,145] and Micronesia [145]. The production of psammaplin type compounds was conserved across all five locations with several derivatives of this class being reported. These studies also confirmed that despite different sample locations, the production of the pharmaceutically significant NP psammaplin A was conserved in *A. rhax*. Within this genus, *A. strongylata* was also studied and appeared to exhibit a different class of BTAs to *A. rhax*, and has yet to have any psammaplin type compounds isolated from its crude extracts. *A. strongylata* was only sampled from Tulamben beach, Bali, Indonesia, and produced large quantities of the spirooxepinisoxazoline compounds, psammaplysins [146–148]. Unlike *A. rhax*, which produced the disulfide psammplins, *A. strongylata* produced no BTAs that incorporated sulfur into their structure.

Aplysinella sp. specimens from Micronesia were reported with both spirooxepinisoxazolines and SIAs representing both the spirocycloheptadiene and spirocyclohexadiene ring structures [78,149–151]. This is of particular interest, as both spiro systems are thought to be biosynthetically derived from the same arene oxide intermediate [9,12]. This suggests that *Aplysinella* sponges possess the ability to produce NPs using both biosynthetic pathways. A separate *Aplysinella* sp. yielded BT compounds that were also found to be present in several *Aplysina* and *Pseudoceratina* sponges across many biogeographical realms [38,151]. Another *Aplysinella* sp. was also sampled from the Red Sea, yielding a very similar set of secondary metabolites to that of *A. strongylata*, with both producing psammaplysin derivatives showing very little biosynthetic divergence in the secondary metabolites isolated [152].

The genus *Suberea* showed similar geographic distribution to *Aplysinella* but displayed quite different chemistry. *S. ianthelliformis* (Lendenfeld, 1888) [153] sourced from the GBR [32] and Solomon Islands [34] was reported to have BTs that contained higher-molecular weight compounds than those of other genera, with many of the BTs appearing to have incorporated putrescine into their structures, reminiscent of aerothionin. However, *S. ianthelliformis* sampled from French Polynesia [154] was reported to produce unsaturated BTs as well as some quinoline derivatives. Quinoline derivatives were also identified in a study performed on a sample of *S. creba* (Bergquist, 1995) [50], sampled from the Coral Sea, but were confirmed to be produced by the isolated symbiont *Pseudomonas* sp. [9]. Curiously, other samples of *S. creba* obtained from the Coral Sea showed the presence of an array of common small molecular weight amides and nitriles such as subereaphenols, dibromoverongiaquinols and aeroplysinins, making these two *S. creba* samples quite distinct from each other [9]. The sponge *S. clavata* (Pulitzer-Finali, 1982) [155] was only sampled from the GBR and produced some species-specific clavatadines as well as some SIA derivatives, all of which incorporated Gdn as a functionality [35,36].

Marine ecoregions were used to display the frequency of isolated NPs from Verongiida sponges (Figure 5) and appear to suggest that the frequencies are highly location-dependent, with regions such as the Caribbean, GBR, the Red Sea and the Okinawan coast producing the largest numbers of NPs. Aside from the Okinawan coast, all these regions are known to have sponges that yield NPs from all four families, making them both significant Verongiida habitats as well as being diverse. However, this result may be misleading, as the regions studied are likely to have been targeted because they are readily accessible and are known to be rich sources of many tropical marine species, including sponges. Hence, the lack of study may simply reflect a lack of opportunity, or a reduced interest in other regions.

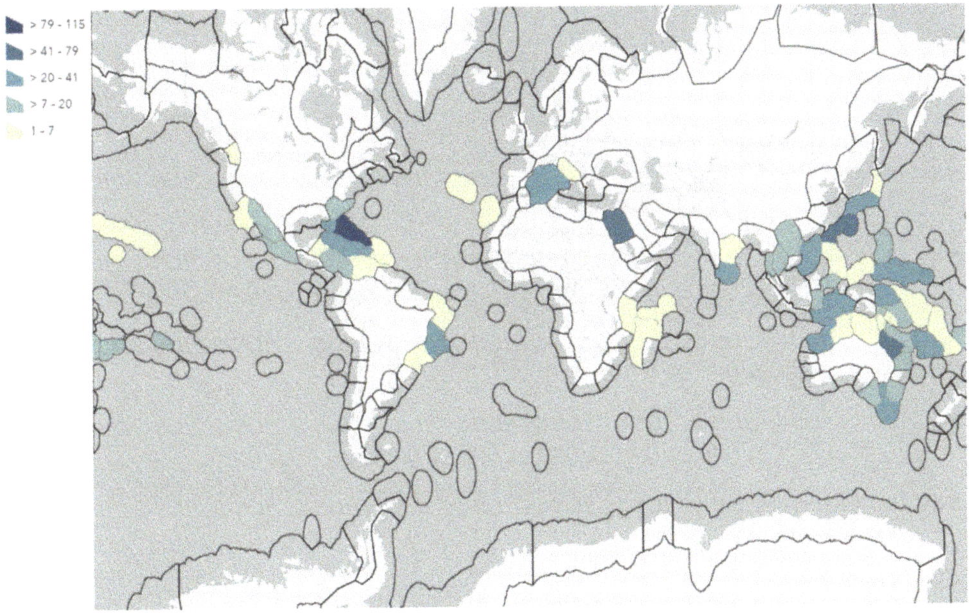

Figure 5. Marine ecoregions of the world (MEOWs) (Black borders) [156] displaying the total number of NPs isolated from Verongiida sponges in each region.

2.3. *Natural Product Diversity across Genera of Verongiida—A Network Analysis Investigation*

Many of the Verongiida species that have been studied possess NPs derived from closely related biosynthetic pathways, and this raises the following questions:

1. To what degree do these genera differ with regard to their secondary metabolites?
2. What compound classes contribute to the largest amount of variance between the genera studied?
3. Which sponges offer biosynthetic outcomes that are the most exploitable in terms of drug discovery?

Answers to these questions were sought using bipartite networks and chemical scaffolding methods to explore NP inter-relationships and diversity. Initially, a direct comparison of shared metabolites was created using a bipartite network consisting of two distinct classes of nodes. The first are nodes that represent every compound reported for the order Verongiida. The second type of node represents species that have had compounds reported in the literature. The network displays edges between compounds and species when a compound has been reported in the literature for that species. In this situation, no edges are created for species–species or compound–compound. To aid with analysis, node size was organised such that nodes with a higher degree (number of edge attachments) are larger than those with a lower node degree. This approach highlights the species or compounds that have the greatest interconnection, as illustrated in Figure 6.

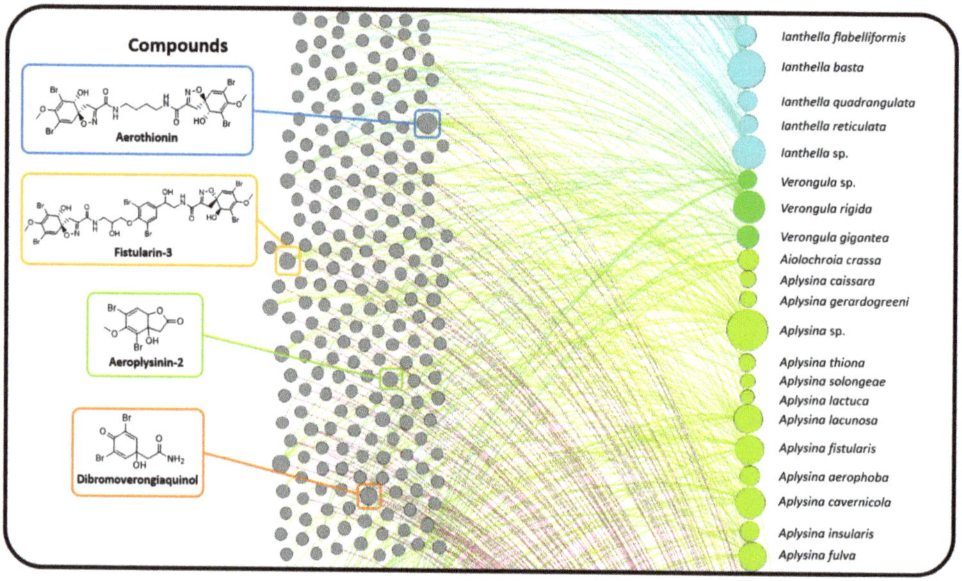

Figure 6. Bipartite network representation of species (nodes, right) and compounds (nodes, left) that exist within species (edges = curved lines) for the sponges in the order Verongiida.

Monopartite projection of this bipartite network with respect to the species nodes gives the species network (Figure 7). In this projection, edges (curved lines) are drawn between species that share at least one compound, with a thicker edge width (weight), indicating the sharing of multiple compounds between species. The monopartite projection (Figure 7) provides a valuable visualisation, clearly indicating which species share compounds with each other. The sharing of a common compound between two species provides some evidence of shared biosynthetic pathways between the two species, thereby supporting taxonomic relationships [157]. As with the bipartite network, the node size is ordered to represent node degree, and thus indicates which species share compounds with the largest number of species within this order of sponges. Species from the genus *Aplysina* are the most interconnected in this network representation, both within the genus *Aplysina* and to external genera. This is largely due to the high numbers of common BTs and SIA compounds that these species possess, which are shared by other prominently studied species, such as the sponges from the genus *Pseudoceratina*.

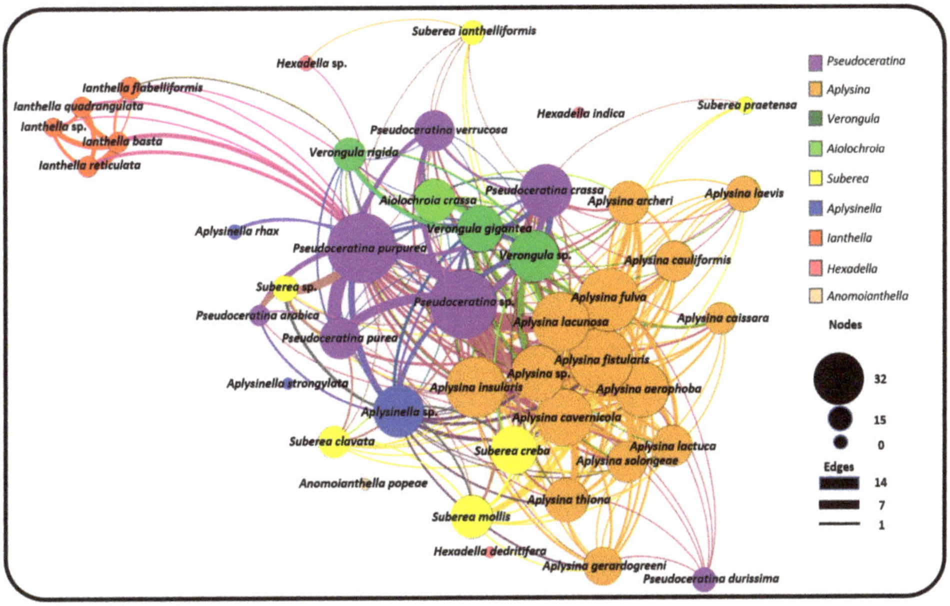

Figure 7. Monopartite projection of the bipartite network with respect to species (visualised using the Force Atlas layout algorithm in Gephi).

The relatively central positioning of the *Pseudoceratina* nodes illustrates the commonalities this genus displays with many other species from different families, including the *Ianthella* genus. *Ianthella* forms a unique cluster, in the large part due to the high numbers of shared bastadins that they all possess. While *Ianthella* is observed with many intra-genus edges, nearly all inter-genus linkages observed for the entire genus *Ianthella* are with the sponge species *P. purpurea*. The positional isolation of Ianthellidae sponges in Figure 7 seems to be conserved for other genera of this family, such as *Anomoianthella* Bergquist, 1980 [59] and *Hexadella*, which also exhibit very small node degrees, together with a tendency to only form edge relationships within their respective genera or not at all. Figure 8A shows the cross section of the Verongiida sponges by family, where Ianthellidae sponges are shown to have the lowest number of inter-family compounds. Interestingly, sponges of the genus *Suberea* display sharing of compounds with a higher number of inter-genera species, whilst almost no intra-genera connections are observed. This can also be seen with the genus *Aplysinella*, where *Aplysinella.* sp. shows wide ranging connections across several species outside the *Aplysinella* genus.

Initially, it was thought that the amount of interconnection amongst other species in the monopartite projection could simply be explained by the fact that species with a higher total number of compounds reported in the literature would be more likely to have a high node degree, or rather, a higher number of species with shared compounds. However, this was shown to be false, as Figure 8C shows the distribution of node degree from the monopartite graph with respect to the total number of compounds reported for each species. Except for the two *Pseudoceratina* species that have higher than usual numbers of reported compounds, there appears to be little or no correlation between the total number of compounds reported and the number of species with shared compounds. Whilst it is true that some *Aplysina* species have both high numbers of compounds and high node degrees, it can also be concluded that some *Ianthella* species have a high total number of compounds reported but a low node degree. This type of variance can also be seen within the genus *Suberea*, where both situations can be observed.

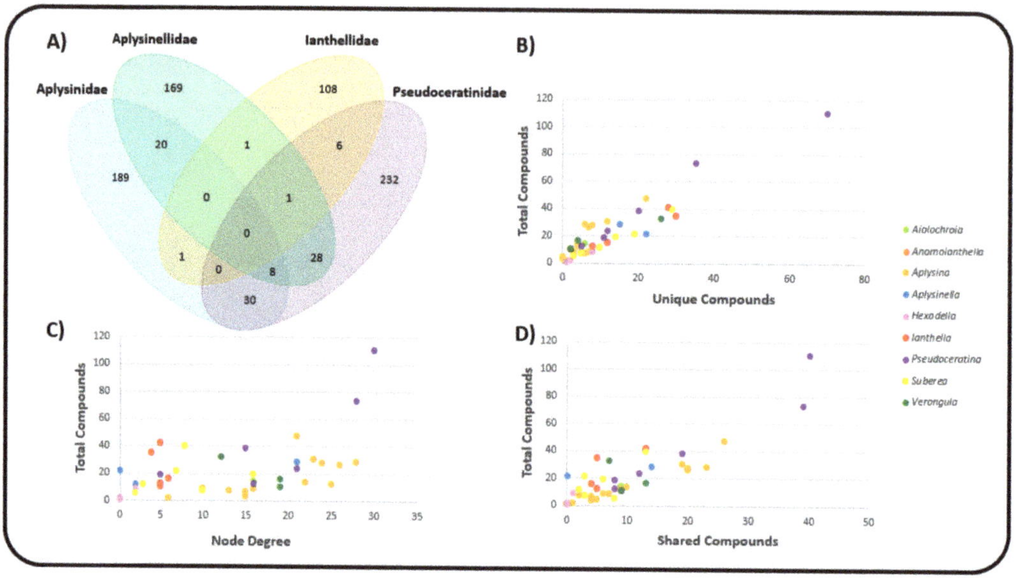

Figure 8. (**A**) Venn diagram for compounds distributed across families of Verongiida. (**B**) Total number of unique compounds for each species. (**C**) Node degree for each species in monopartite projection. (**D**) Number of compounds that are shared with at least one other species.

The distribution of the total compounds reported was mapped against both the number of unique compounds (Figure 8B) and the number of shared compounds (Figure 8D). In both situations, a positive correlation was observed across all Verongiida sponges. In Figure 8B,D, it is apparent that many of the *Aplysina* species exhibit far more common chemistry than the other genera in Verongiida, as they display a lower number of unique compounds per total reported compounds, as well as many shared compounds per total reported compounds. Compounds from the genera *Ianthella, Suberea* and *Aplysinella* exhibit greater uniqueness and a lower amount of relative sharing. *Pseudoceratina* shares many compounds with a large number of species, as well as having many unique compounds

While Figure 8D shows a trend of shared compounds from one species to another, it is not clear if the compounds are being shared according to any predictable pattern. Keeping taxonomical distance in mind, one would expect species within the same genera to share many compounds, as they have closer genetic ties, and their biosynthetic processes are expected to be similar. As a way of investigating this 'shared compound hypothesis', the total compounds reported were mapped against both the intra-genera sharing of compounds and the inter-genera sharing of compounds, and the results are presented in Figure 9A,B, respectively.

The data in Figure 9A support the earlier conclusion from the monopartite projection graph, namely that the *Suberea* sponges appear to show minimal intra-genus compound sharing, and that *Aplysina* sponges display both large intra- and inter-genus sharing of compounds.

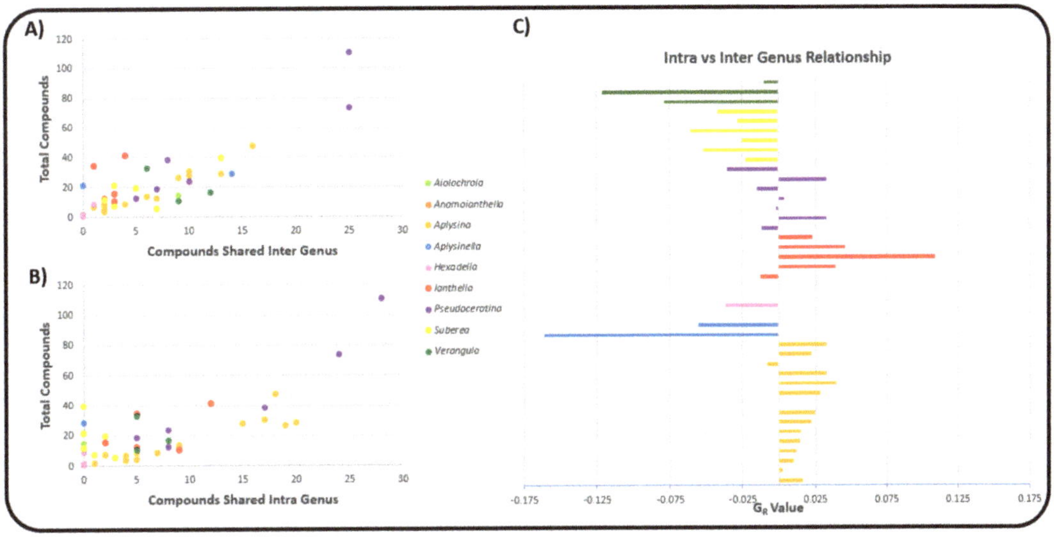

Figure 9. (**A**) G_R Value assessing overall intra- vs. inter-genera sharing of compounds. (**B**) Number of compounds shared with species of the same genus. (**C**) Number of compounds shared with species of different genera.

To quantify this difference between intra- vs. inter-genus sharing of compounds, the genus relationship (G_R) value was calculated for each species according to Equation (1). In this instance, species are compared via their number of intra-genus shared compounds (C_{intra}) and their number of inter-genus shared compounds (C_{inter}). The genus relationship value was then calculated with respect to total reported compounds (T_C) and the total number of species for a particular genus (G_S), so comparisons are possible between species across differing genera.

$$G_R = \frac{(C_{intra} - C_{inter})}{T_C} \div G_S \quad (1)$$

The results of the G_R score for each species are illustrated in Figure 9C. Values that are positive show a tendency for that species to share a larger proportion of compounds with species in the same genus. Negative values show a higher propensity to share compounds with inter-genera species. Figure 8C, derived from the monopartite projection, indicates that species within the *Aplysina* genus of sponge appeared to share compounds with many species of sponge within the order Verongiida. However, reference to Figure 9C and the associated G_R values of the *Aplysina* sponges indicates that much of the compound sharing for the *Aplysina* sponges occurs within the genus *Aplysina*. This suggests that *Aplysina* sponges are largely insular with regard to sharing compounds between species of sponges. However, because the G_R value focusses on the relationship between intra- and inter-sharing, it misses an interesting cross section of *Aplysina* species that share the same compounds both with intra-genus species and inter-genus species. The monopartite projection (Figure 7) shows the most intra-shared compounds for each major genus, together with the compounds that are most shared between inter-genera species. In this instance, it is evident that a large proportion of the most shared compounds within the *Aplysina* genus are also shared with species from other genera, such as *Pseudoceratina* and *Suberea*.

Sponges within the genus *Ianthella* show similar trends to *Aplysina*, with largely positive G_R values; however, when considering Figure 8C, *Ianthella* sponges show lower numbers of species that have shared compounds. Figure 8B also shows that *Ianthella* sponges, as a genus, exhibit many more unique compounds compared to those of the *Aplysina* sponges.

Figure 8D shows that the *Suberea* sponges have a variety of species that contain shared compounds, but only have negative G_R values. This is noteworthy, because while *Suberea* shows extensive inter-genus sharing of compounds, these species also have a significantly larger number of unique compounds, as is the case for the *Ianthella* species.

It has been made clear from investigating the most shared compounds from both intra- and inter-genera species that, with the possible exception of the bastadins found in *Ianthella* sponges, there is no class of compounds that is shared almost exclusively in an intra-genera manner specific to one genus and no other. Rather, there appears to be a subset of compounds that are common to all, or nearly all, species across multiple genera. There are also compounds that are specific to species in each genus, but this may also be found outside that genus. This creates uniqueness for that species within its genus, but this does not mean it is unique when considering the entire order.

Scaffold analysis was performed on compounds that were reported for each genus, with the aim of investigating the frequency of each chemical scaffold for each genera, together with assessing the diversity and novelty of the chemistry in each genera. Murcko scaffolds (N) were created from NPs (M) and used to calculate genera diversity (N/M), where the frequency of each Murcko scaffold indicated importance to the genera. Scaffolds that existed in only one genus were termed scaffold singletons (N_{sing}) and used to calculate genera novelty (N_{sing}/M) (Table 2) [158,159].

Table 2. Murcko scaffold analysis for NPs of all genera within the order Verongiida.

Genus	Natural Products (M)	Murcko Scaffolds (N)	Singleton Scaffolds (N_{sing})	Diversity (N/M)	Novelty (N_{sing}/M)
Aiolochroia	15	8	0	0.533	0
Anomoianthella	1	1	0	1	0
Aplysina	140	44	20	0.314	0.143
Aplysinella	63	19	8	0.301	0.127
Hexadella	12	9	0	0.75	0
Ianthella	95	29	20	0.305	0.211
Pseudoceratina	232	67	35	0.289	0.151
Suberea	115	47	24	0.409	0.209
Verongula	51	28	13	0.549	0.255

A high diversity of scaffolds was reported for *Verongula* and *Suberea*, with diversity scores of 0.549 and 0.409, respectively. These were significantly higher than other genera such as *Pseudoceratina* and *Aplysina*, which appear to have a larger number of compounds that are represented by a relatively low number of scaffold classes. Furthermore, they also displayed low novelty scores and there were many shared scaffolds between the two genera (Figure 10). While novelty and diversity are advantageous for drug discovery efforts, a lack of these properties combined with many shared scaffolds could suggest similarities in terms of the biosynthetic origins of the compounds produced by two genera, thereby also providing chemotaxonomic value. It should be noted that although *Aiolochroia* Wiedenmayer, 1977 [160], *Anomoianthella* and *Hexadella* also achieved much higher diversity scores as well, it is likely that this is simply a result of the low number of NPs reported in the literature for these genera. Cumulative scaffold frequency graphs of each genus show *Pseudoceratina* to have the highest number of compounds represented by the lowest number of scaffolds. Interestingly, the genus *Aplysinella* shows a similar trend, with a sharp rise at the beginning of the curve indicating an upper end of scaffolds that dominate its dataset.

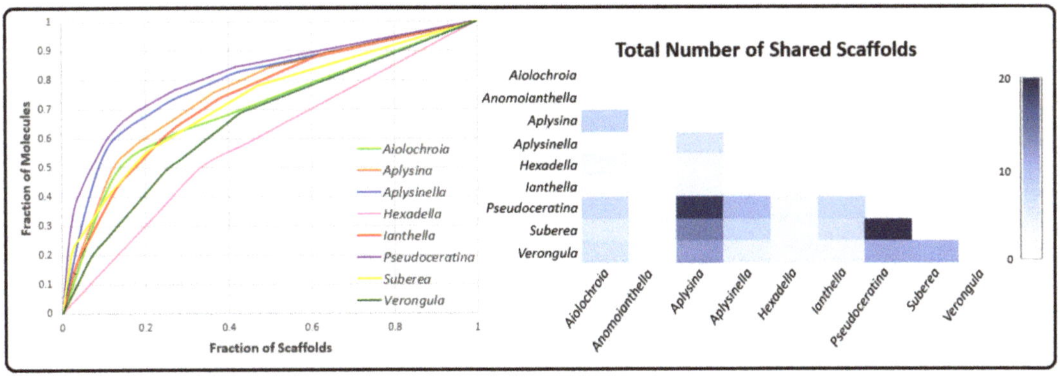

Figure 10. Cumulative scaffold frequency by genus (**left**). Number of shared scaffolds by genus (**right**).

Pseudoceratina has approximately 23.6% of its compounds represented by the benzene Murcko scaffold (representative of phenolic nitriles, amides and BTs), as well as SIA (4.5%) and BTOx (5.4% and 4.5%) scaffolds (Figure 11). *Aplysinella*, on the other hand, has many more scaffolds created through the alternate biosynthetic route of spirooxepinisoxazolines. *Hexadella* and *Verongula* both display curves representing a low ratio of molecules per scaffolds, indicating the presence of only a small number of derivatives present in their listed NPs. This type of data analysis can inform future isolations and could provide evidence of two situations: (i) that the organism only produces single derivatives of the same scaffold, or (ii) that there simply has not been many of these derivatives discovered. Either way, the combination of high scaffold diversity and novelty that *Verongula* displays, together with the low ratio of molecules to scaffolds, make this genus an ideal target for drug discovery, with the potential to provide novel scaffolds as well as derivatives of known scaffolds.

The number of shared scaffolds between *Pseudoceratina* and *Aplysina*, the two genera with the highest number of reported NPs, implies a strong biosynthetic connection. *Aplysina* and *Pseudoceratina* have many compounds represented by the SIA scaffold with 7.9% and 4.5% for each, respectively. This, together with the high frequency of benzene, demonstrates the utilisation of a number of common biosynthetic routes to achieve these scaffolds. However, *Aplysina* appears to produce more compounds that have lower MW Murcko scaffolds such as BTs, cavernicolins, bromotyrosineketals and verongiaquinols, whereas *Pseudoceratina* has higher MW scaffolds that are created from the NP classes of BTOx, SIABTs or BTOxGdns. *Suberea* sponges exhibit a variety of scaffolds from *Aplysinella*, *Pseudoceratina* and *Aplysina*, with a mixture of SIAs and spirooxepinisoxazolines. This subset of common scaffolds, which are shared between the more widely studied genera within the Verongiida order, suggests that all biosynthetic outcomes of the BTA class of compounds are available to each genus, but variance is created at the species level. Considering this, it would be useful to understand if species share more in common with their intra-genus counterparts than with inter-genera species.

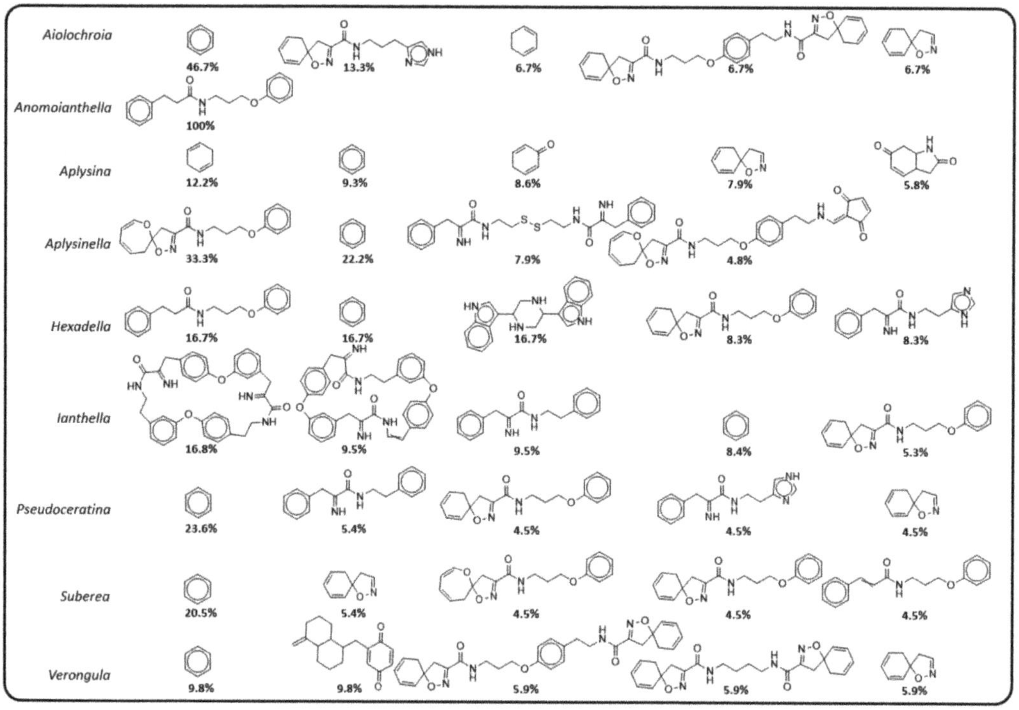

Figure 11. Most frequently occurring Murcko scaffolds for each genus.

To this end, scaffold trees were created using the RDKit scaffolding package [161] and were arranged to create a scaffold network (SN) as presented in Figure 12A. These networks include nodes representing individual species, whole compounds (initialised compounds), as well as common scaffolds created from whole compounds. Edges (links) between species nodes (coloured) and initialised compounds (dark grey) represent a compound that has been reported for that species. Each compound is iteratively fragmented into its substituent scaffolds, and edges (links) are placed between the initialised compounds and the scaffolds (light grey). This provides a chemical space where species are placed based on the structural features of their associated secondary metabolites. Scaffolds exist between two species that would have otherwise not been connected in a bipartite network projection due to them not having a single metabolite in common. As species are distributed according to their metabolites, it is possible to assess their likeness to each other with respect to their local environments within the network. Environmental similarity was assessed using the python networking tool SimRank [162], where a domain-specific view of each species was taken. In this way, species were compared to each other based on their respective environments where two objects are similar to each other if they are both connected to similar objects.

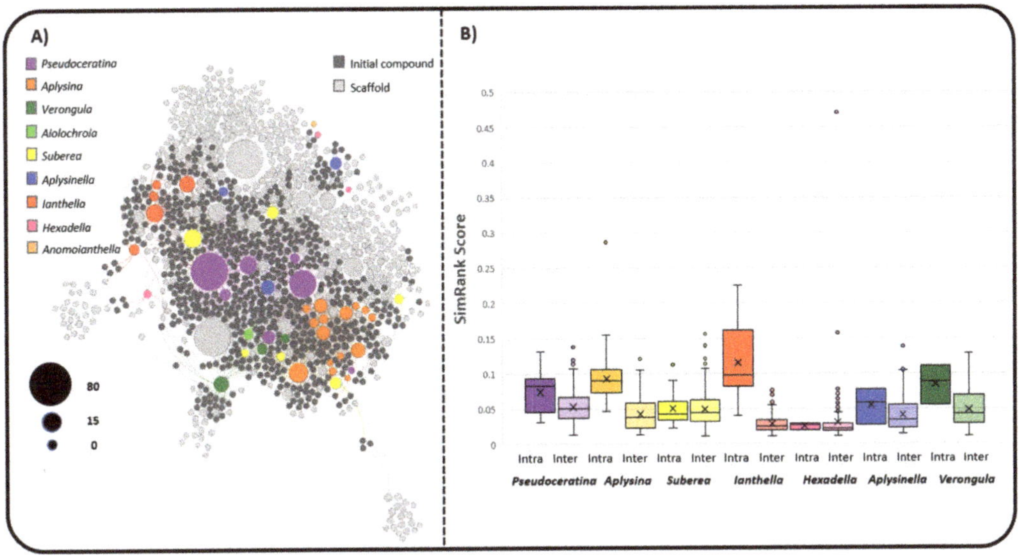

Figure 12. (**A**) Scaffold network (SN) created using HierS type scaffolds that displays species (coloured), initialised compounds (dark grey) and scaffolds (light grey). (**B**) SimRank score data calculated for each species comparison in the SN, organised via genera comparing intra/inter genera relationships.

Figure 12B presents the box plot results of SimRank scores between all species nodes in the SN created by considering intra-genera versus inter-genera similarity comparisons. SimRank scores show similar trends to the G_R score method of comparison when considering *Ianthella* and *Aplysina*, where there is a strong tendency towards similar chemistry within their respective genera, as opposed to species from other genera. This trend is due to the large number of unique bastadin compounds that are found in the genus *Ianthella*, and the high density of common SIA compounds that are found in *Aplysina*, which are extensively shared within the genus, whilst also exhibiting very similar scaffolding.

Suberea show very low numbers of shared compounds within the genus, but it appears that there is a very similar number of common scaffolds both intra- and inter- genera when considering the SimRank results for this genus. *Suberea* shares a large proportion of SIAs with other genera, such as *Aplysina* and *Pseudoceratina*, but also displays many compounds that are species-specific to *Suberea* and have similar scaffolds and overall chemical structures.

The genera *Aplysinella* and *Verongula* appear to have more inter-genera shared compounds when considering G_R score, but when considering chemical features and common scaffolds in the SN, there is a larger proportion of similar scaffolds in their intra-genera species as opposed to inter-genera species. This is likely to be reflective of the fact that the G_R score, while useful for direct comparisons of shared compounds across species, does not accurately depict the relative chemistry of species that have only very low numbers of connections in the monopartite projection of shared compounds. If a species is present with only a very low number of shared compounds for both inter- and intra-genus comparison, there is little that can be concluded without further information regarding the chemical classes present. *A. rhax* and *A. strongylata* have very limited interconnection with both inter- and intra-genera species (Figure 7), leaving the trend for the genus *Aplysinella* to be dictated entirely by *Aplysinella*. sp. This results in a misconception when comparing genera via shared compounds, because it is entirely likely that species within a genus will produce compounds that are structural variants and thus will not be reflected in sharing, but rather in shared or common scaffolds. This means that while shared compounds can provide a useful insight into shared biosynthesis, it needs to be considered together with shared common scaffolds to provide context to the compounds that are not shared frequently, and the compounds that are potentially missing from the data. This is most important, as not all datasets are complete, especially in NPs research, where datasets are subject to how rigorously each species has been investigated and by what methodologies.

2.4. Verongiida NP Drug Score and Drug-Likeness Assessment

The compounds produced by Verongiida sponges were assessed for their pharmaceutical potential using both the Lipinski/Veber rules and the drug score metric calculated on the OSIRIS property explorer [163]. Chemical space was first represented using principal component analysis (PCA) with chemical descriptors derived from the Lipinski/Veber rules, such as molecular weight (MW), topological polar surface area (TPSA), number of rotatable bonds (nRotB), total number of hydrogen bond donors and acceptors (nHBDon/Acc) and the octanol water partition coefficient (cLogP), forming the basis of compound features, with the results illustrated in Figure 13. Descriptive statistics of the PCA plots in Table 3 show that 93.5% of the cumulative variance of this data is described by the first three principal components. Table 4 shows that PC1 has a strong positive correlation with the descriptors MW, TPSA, nHBDon as well as nHBAcc; PC2 has a large positive correlation with the cLogP coefficient and nRotB; while PC3, which contributes to only 8.4% of variance, has a positive correlation with the nRotB descriptor and a negative correlation with cLogP.

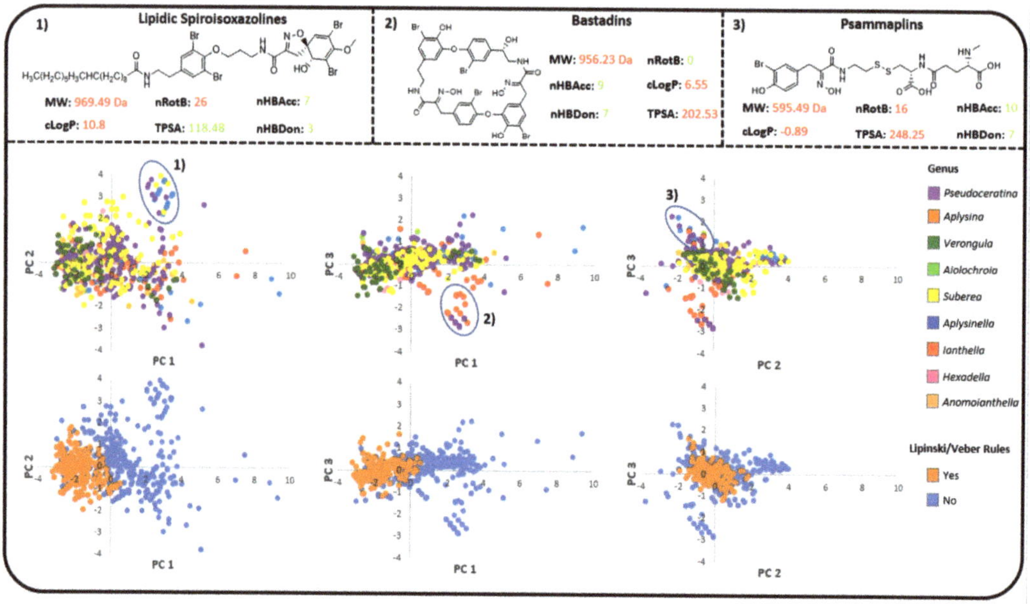

Figure 13. PCA analysis of chemical descriptors MW, TPSA, nRotB, nHBDon, nHBAcc and cLogP.

Most outliers in these PCA plots are accounted for by variance in PC1, with a few associated with variance in PC2. Some small cluster groupings can be observed where compounds from *Suberea*, *Pseudoceratina* and *Aplysinella* form a cluster of spiroisoxazoline compounds that have long lipidic tails. This cluster is formed due to the compounds displaying unusually large cLogP and nRotB values, which corresponds to the two descriptors showing large positive correlations with PC2 in Table 4. Some clustering was also observed along the PC3 axes, which can be accounted for by the bastadin compounds, which are found primarily in the genera *Pseudoceratina* and *Ianthella* and are unique, as they are the only macrocyclic compounds found in this order of sponge. This often results in high MW compounds that have very low numbers of nRotB. The psammaplins were also observed to form a small cluster when comparing PC2 and PC3. These compounds exhibit the only disulfide functionality across the entire order, and are found in *Aplysinella, Ianthella* and *Pseudoceratina* sponges. Outliers in this analysis were found to be highly lipophilic compounds that exhibited large cLogP values, MW and TPSA values.

Table 3. PCA descriptive statistics.

	PC1	PC2	PC3	PC4	PC5
Eigenvalues	3.8916	1.2130	0.5068	0.2505	0.0841
Proportion of variance	0.649	0.202	0.084	0.014	0.009
Cumulative proportion	0.649	0.851	0.935	0.991	1.000

Table 4. PCA loadings for all compound descriptors.

	PC1	PC2	PC3	PC4	PC5
MW	0.472	0.147	−0.133	−0.476	−0.636
TPSA	0.458	−0.338	0.020	0.049	0.538
nHBAcc	0.471	−0.199	0.122	−0.453	0.277
nHBDon	0.420	−0.374	−0.153	0.681	−0.374
nRotB	0.307	0.522	0.748	0.270	−0.002
cLogP	0.273	0.642	−0.619	0.172	0.299

The Euclidean distance between each genus, which correlates with their degree of relatedness, was studied and the results are summarised in Figure 14. Euclidean distance measurements were performed using the PUMA cheminformatics server [164,165]. This measurement of similarity between genera appeared to display similar trends to the SimRank score plot, despite using pharmacokinetic features to describe molecular structure rather than chemical scaffolds.

The genus *Ianthella* showed a smaller Euclidean distance of 3.21 when compared to itself, whereas the inter-genus scores against all other genera were found to be larger in magnitude. *Aplysina* had a short Euclidean distance value of 2.63; however, it showed smaller distances when compared to *Aiolochroia* and *Hexadella,* which both scored distances of 2.53. *Pseudoceratina* appeared to have higher inter-genus distances, compared to the intra-genus value of 2.82, than *Suberea, Verongula* and *Aplysinella,* which showed values of 2.9, 2.94 and 3.52, respectively.

This contrasted with the values observed with other genera, which were all much lower. *Ianthella, Aplysinella* and *Verongula* are suggested to have the most unique chemistry based on the descriptors, and these provided the highest Euclidean distances. This tends to agree with the SN results and the PCA plots. *Aplysinella* shows the greatest amount of variance along PC2, due primarily to its compounds that have a large range of cLogP values. It also has a single species in the SN that displays highly unique scaffolding and a very large distance to other genera. The entire genus *Ianthella* shows unique scaffolding in the SN and also relatively large data variance across all three principal components, as shown in Table 3. *Verongula* appears to derive most of its uniqueness from the variance along principal component 1 and the fact that, as with *Aplysinella,* it has a single species that produces unique scaffolds in the SN.

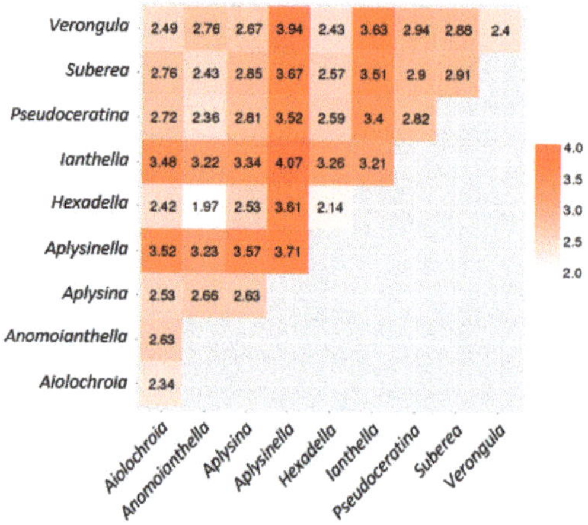

Figure 14. Euclidean distance of genera based on pharmacokinetic properties of compounds.

PCA analysis showed large numbers of compounds from *Pseudoceratina*, *Verongula*, *Suberea*, *Aplysina* and *Aplysinella* occupying the chemical space of Lipinski/Veber-abiding compounds. Many of the compounds that do not abide by these rules were discounted due to excessively high MW, cLogP and/or nRotB values.

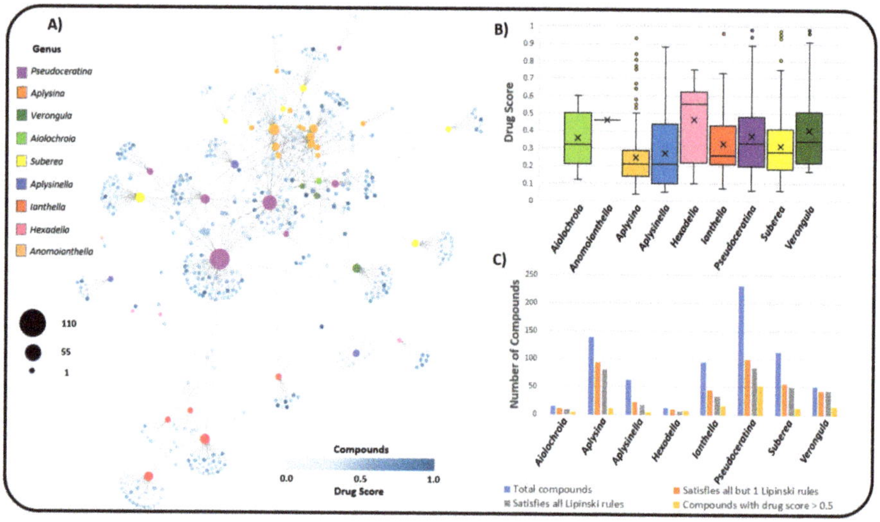

Figure 15. (**A**) Species drug score network. (**B**) Drug score distribution by genus. (**C**) Lipinski statistics by genus.

Figure 15A shows a network where the distribution of compounds amongst genera can be observed as well as the compound's associated drug score, as calculated by the OSIRIS property explorer [163]. The drug score of a compound is used to assess its potential pharmaceutical value, based on parameters such as cLogP, solubility, molecular weight, drug likeness and any associated toxicity risks, on a scale between 0 and 1 (where 1 indicates a high potential to qualify as a drug). The drug score is a powerful value that encapsulates core druglike descriptors and is particularly useful for providing a snapshot of the compound's drug feasibility, whilst also considering its predicted toxicity.

The genera that exhibit the highest mean drug score for compounds are *Hexadella*, *Verongula*, *Pseudoceratina* and *Aiolochroia*. The genera *Aplysina* has a relatively low drug score profile for its compounds, as seen in Figure 15B, but it does display a number of compounds with particularly high drug scores as outliers. In Figure 15A, it can be observed that many of the high drug score compounds for *Aplysina* are found only within *Aplysina* sponges. This contrasts with *Pseudoceratina*, where many of the high druglike compounds are found to be shared amongst other genera such as *Aplysinella*, together with many high drug score compounds that are exclusive to *Pseudoceratina*. Many other genera, especially *Ianthella*, show the same trend as *Aplysina*, where the high drug score compounds are not shared with inter-genus species. Despite having many compounds reported for both *Aplysina* and *Pseudoceratina*, of which a relatively large percentage conform to all Lipinski and Veber's rules for druglikeness, (57.5% and 36.2%, respectively), Figure 15C shows that an incredibly small percentage of these compounds possess appropriate properties to achieve a drug score higher than 0.5, and this is attributed to the predicted toxicity and mutagenic properties of these compounds being too high to allow for an effective drug score.

To further explore the relationship between drug score and chemotype in this order of sponges, chemical space networks (CSNs) [166] were used to create a chemical space for compounds based on chemical similarity, as illustrated in Figure 16. Network analysis, based on chemical similarity, provides a direct connection of cluster analysis with chemotype without loss of information due to dimensionality reduction, as would be observed in PCA.

This type of network connects compounds (nodes) to other compounds based on structural similarity as expressed via the Tanimoto score between two compounds. A network threshold value of 0.5 was used to maximise the assortativity degree and average clustering coefficient, whilst also minimising the number of singletons and providing an appropriate network density. The Louvain clustering algorithm (default Gephi clustering algorithm) was used to cluster the compounds in this network. This resulted in 20 clusters having three or more nodes. Major clusters represent the major chemotypes present in this order of sponge, as can be seen in Figure 16A. Chemical assessment of the major clusters in this network showed that the predominant chemotypes present are SIAs (Cluster 1), BTOx (Cluster 2), BT's (Cluster 3), spirooxepinisoxazolines (Cluster 4), bastadins (Cluster 5), bromotyrasineketals and verongiaquinols (Cluster 6), as well as cavernicolins and bromotyrosine lactone derivatives (Cluster 7).

The Lipinski/Veber rules and drug score ranking were then applied to this network, as illustrated in Figure 16C,D, respectively. Figure 16C shows darker nodes for compounds that comply with all the Lipinski/Veber rules. It should be noted that when comparing Figure 16C,D, compliance with the Lipinski/Veber rules does not necessarily guarantee a high drug score. This is likely due to the compounds having lower druglikeness values and/or also having high predicted toxicity values for either mutagenic or irritant properties. Upon comparing Figure 16D with Figure 16A, it was observed that the cluster of compound classes that achieve the highest drug score ranking includes the BTOx compounds (Cluster 2) and the simple BT compounds (Cluster 3). These two classes of compounds are found widely across the order Verongiida and contribute to the mean drug score of most genera.

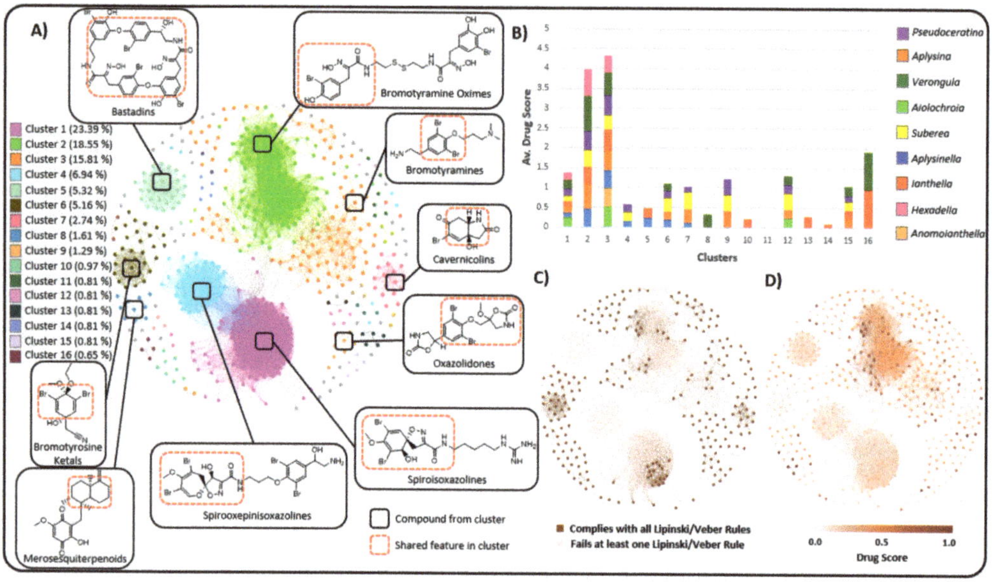

Figure 16. (**A**) Similarity network with Louvain clustering applied. (**B**) Average drug score for each cluster arranged by genera. (**C**) Similarity network highlighting compounds that conform to the Lipinski/Veber rules. (**D**) Similarity network ranking compounds based on their drug score.

For example, *Verongula* gains much of its high mean drug score in Figure 16B due to the presence of high drug score compounds from cluster 2, achieving a mean drug score from this cluster of 0.89, and from cluster 16, where compounds from this genus achieve a mean drug score of 0.94. For genera such as *Ianthella,* which achieve a relatively low mean drug score of 0.33 for its compounds, it can be inferred from Figure 16D that much of this can be attributed to the high prevalence of bastadin-type compounds. The macrocyclic bastadins exhibit high molecular weights, large numbers of nHBAcc and high cLogP values, all contributing to low drug scores for the *Ianthella* genera set of compounds. While these compounds lower the mean drug score for *Ianthella,* there are other clusters, such as cluster 16, where *Ianthella* shows a considerably higher mean drug score of 0.96 (see Figure 16B). This seems to suggest that *Ianthella* sponges do produce compounds with a drug potential that is higher than that of their most frequently occurring compound class, which are the bastadins (cluster 5). Information such as this is important when considering future isolation strategies and investigations for these species of sponges, as it would be wise to use an approach that avoids the isolation of bastadins, and that preferentially aims to isolate compounds such as those found in clusters achieving high mean drug scores, such as components in clusters 2 (BTOx), 3 (BT) and 16 (Aplysinopsins). This does not mean that the isolation of bastadins should be ignored, since as macrolides they may possess useful membrane disrupting properties, but rather that they should not be the primary targets for small molecule isolation.

This type of network analysis could conceivably be utilised to prioritise isolation strategies for compounds with high drug scores, although it would not provide insight into predicting which organisms would produce novel chemicals that are highly bioactive. Nevertheless, it may still be of use in designing isolation strategies that target specific chemotypes that are assessed as being likely drug candidates with higher drug scores. This type of structure-based similarity network that relies on thresholds is useful for identifying the major types of compounds present across a dataset and can provide insight into structure–activity relationships in compounds. Compounds can be compared to each other within a single network with a threshold value, but it is relatively difficult to compare those across multiple networks due to different network statistics. This, however, does not invalidate this type of network analysis in terms of understanding chemotype–drug viability relationships across chemical space.

Recent studies of BTA compounds have shown this class of compounds as being promising candidates within the preclinical pipeline [25–38]. Despite this, the large majority of BTAs from Verongiida sponges have been understudied when it comes to biological activity and function, leaving a potentially untapped resource for drug development.

Figure 17 shows the compounds that have achieved a drug score of 0.75 or higher, with all molecular descriptors displayed in Table 5. Many of the compounds that achieve high drug scores are from clusters 2 (BTOx) and 3 (BT) of the CSN. In addition, a large proportion of these compounds are from miscellaneous clusters that are either singletons or simply have three nodes or fewer contributing to their cluster information. This suggests that this type of network analysis is useful for observing activity trends only when the dataset contains large numbers of compounds with high similarity, as can be observed in clusters 2 and 3.

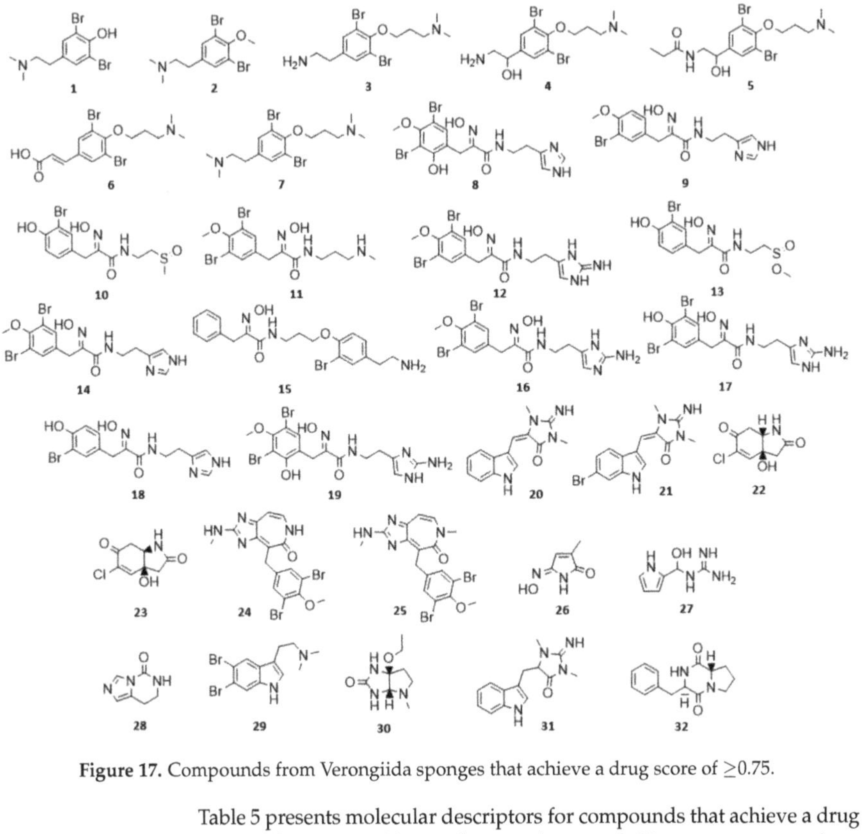

Figure 17. Compounds from Verongiida sponges that achieve a drug score of ≥0.75.

Table 5 presents molecular descriptors for compounds that achieve a drug score higher than 0.75. Aplysamine-1 (**7**) was shown to be a weak H_3 receptor antagonist compared to a standard of conessine achieving an IC_{50} value of 0.34 μg/mL (0.83 μM) [167]. Compounds **24** and **25** (ceratamine A and B, respectively) are cytotoxic and antimitotic in a variety of assays covering a number of human and rat cell lines [168–170]. Compound **28** was assessed as being a potent antifungal agent against the fungus *Geotrichum candidum* [171]. Compound **29** showed some antidepressant activity during a rodent forced swim test [138,172]. Compound **32** has been reported to be antibacterial, antimycobacterial and an effective inhibitor of human ETA receptors as well as neuropeptide Y1 receptors [173–175]. It is noteworthy that none of the other listed compounds have had any form of bioassay undertaken despite being ideal drug candidates that achieve high drug scores and generally conform to the Lipinski/Veber rules. This clearly presents an opportunity for further work to evaluate the therapeutic potential of these compounds.

Table 5. Molecular descriptors for compounds that achieve a drug score ≥ 0.75.

Compound	Cluster	Drug Score	Genus	MW	TPSA	nHBAcc	nHBDon	nRotB	cLogP
1	3	0.81	*Aplysina, Suberea*	323.03	23.47	2	1	3	2.82
2	3	0.84	*Aplysina*	337.05	12.47	2	0	4	3.09
3	3	0.79	*Pseudoceratina*	380.12	38.49	3	1	7	2.63
4	3	0.81	*Pseudoceratina*	396.12	58.72	4	2	7	1.56
5	3	0.79	*Pseudoceratina*	452.19	61.8	4	2	9	2.42
6	3	0.78	*Pseudoceratina*	407.1	49.77	4	1	7	1.89
7	3	0.75	*Aplysina, Suberea, Pseudoceratina*	408.18	15.71	3	0	8	3.25
8	2	0.77	*Aplysina, Pseudoceratina*	460.13	99.6	6	4	7	2.56
9	2	0.88	*Aplysinella, Pseudoceratina, Verongula*	381.23	99.6	5	3	7	1.84
10	2	0.81	*Aplysinella*	323.23	118.2	5	3	6	0.14
11	2	0.8	*Pseudoceratina*	437.13	82.95	5	3	8	2.39
12	2	0.77	*Pseudoceratina*	475.14	118.83	7	5	7	1.84
13	2	0.77	*Aplysinella*	379.23	127.43	5	3	7	1.19
14	2	0.77	*Pseudoceratina*	460.13	99.6	5	3	7	2.56
15	2	0.77	*Pseudoceratina*	434.33	96.94	5	3	10	3.16
16	2	0.75	*Hexadella*	475.14	125.62	6	4	7	2.25
17	2	0.77	*Pseudoceratina*	461.11	136.62	6	5	6	1.98
18	2	0.89	*Pseudoceratina*	367.2	110.6	5	4	6	1.56
19	2	0.75	*Pseudoceratina*	475.14	125.62	7	5	7	2.25
20	16	0.96	*Ianthella*	254.29	63.19	3	2	1	1.01
21	16	0.91	*Verongula*	333.19	63.19	3	2	1	1.74
22	7	0.93	*Suberea*	201.61	66.4	3	2	0	−0.57
23	7	0.93	*Aplysina*	201.61	66.4	3	2	0	−0.57
24	21	0.79	*Pseudoceratina*	454.12	75.08	5	2	3	1.94
25	21	0.77	*Pseudoceratina*	468.15	66.29	5	1	3	2.19
26	42	0.94	*Pseudoceratina*	126.11	61.69	3	2	0	0.06
27	50	0.95	*Suberea*	154.17	97.92	4	5	2	−1.28
28	39	0.98	*Pseudoceratina, Verongula*	137.14	46.92	2	1	0	0.38
29	19	0.81	*Verongula*	346.07	19.03	1	1	3	3.2
30	43	0.79	*Pseudoceratina*	185.23	53.6	3	2	2	0.02
31	66	0.97	*Ianthella*	256.31	63.19	3	2	2	0.8
32	57	0.97	*Suberea*	244.29	49.41	2	1	2	0.85

MW = molecular weight, TPSA = total polar surface Area, nHBAcc = number of hydrogen bond acceptors, nHBDon = number of hydrogen bond donors, nRotB = number of rotatable bonds, cLogP = octanol/water partition coefficient.

3. Methodology

3.1. Collection of Chemical Compound Data

All compound data were manually curated from the literature and 'data-mined' from the SciFinder database using keyword search phrases. Keyword searches were performed on all genera that make up the order Verongiida. This process was assisted by using reviews that focus on specific genera within this order [9,10]. Curation of the literature data resulted in a library of 633 NPs that were reported from species within the order Verongiida. This represents a comprehensive list of all secondary metabolites isolated from Verongiida sponges within the period from 1960 to May 2020. It is important to note that since May 2020 to August 2021, a further 7 papers have been published concerning secondary metabolites from this order that were not included in this analysis [176–182]. A full reference list can be found in Supporting Information S1.

This library contains compounds isolated from 43 separate species from across 9 different genera. Of the 5 families that are contained within the order Verongiida, compounds were reported from only 4 families (Aplysinellidae, Aplysinidae, Ianthellidae and Pseudoceratinidae), as listed in Table 6.

Table 6. Taxonomy of sponges in the order Verongiida.

Order	Family	Genera (Total NPs)
Verongiida	Aplysinellidae	*Aplysinella* (63) *Patriciaplysina* (0) *Suberea* (115)
	Aplysinidae	*Aiolochroia* (15) *Aplysina* (140) *Verongula* (51)
	Ernstillidae	*Ernstilla* (0)
	Ianthellidae	*Anomoianthella* (1) *Hexadella* (12) *Ianthella* (95) *Vansoestia* (0)
	Pseudoceratinidae	*Pseudoceratina* (232)

3.2. Network Considerations

Graphical presentations, or networks, are a useful tool when representing chemical space that can otherwise seem inaccessible due to the sheer number of organic molecules that exist within a dataset. This is especially true when considering the number of NPs that have been documented. Networks are created by relationships observed between pairs of data points. Vertices or nodes (V) are connected by edges (E) which can be expressed by the relationship, G(Graph) = (V, E). Network distribution and topology can be defined by several metrics, including degree, density, assortativity, modularity and clustering coefficient (see Supporting Information S2).

Edges can represent either a one-way or two-way relationship between nodes, termed either directed or undirected. Undirected networks display edges that are bidirectional, meaning that the relationship between two nodes is equal in both directions. On the other hand, a directed network displays only connections that exist in one direction. In this study, the NP similarity data were calculated using the Tanimoto value which considers the global similarity of the compound structures; hence, the networks in this study were made with undirected edges.

Edges, whilst representing a relationship between nodes, can also have an associated value or weight. Networks that incorporate edge weights are termed weighted networks. In this situation, a nominal value dictates the significance of the relationship between two nodes, thereby creating certain node relationships that are more significant than others within the structure of a network. Furthermore, some networks can be both weighted and directed. In this instance, networks display edges as arrows rather than lines and will often display edge weight visually by increasing the physical thickness of edges in a network that have higher weightings. All networks in this study were undirected, with some relying on weighting values (monopartite projection network) and others being unweighted (scaffold network).

Networks can also be defined as being either bipartite or monopartite. Monopartite graphs are usually created by considering data that are of a similar kind to be represented by nodes. The network is created to investigate the relationships of objects, as is the case of graphs designed around investigating academic citation patterns, where nodes are the academics and the edges represent a single citation of one author by a second author [183]. In this situation, all nodes are the same type of data (academic authors). However, nodes within networks do not always have to be the same type of object, such as in the case when networking host–microbiota relationships in nature [184]. In this situation, it can be appropriate to use bipartite networks where two distinct groups of nodes are identified (predators and prey) and relationships, or edges, are defined between the two groups but not within each group. The work described in this current study presents the exploration of both types of networks within the scope of chemotaxonomy and in the assessment of drug viability.

Network layout is another important factor when considering how to visualise a network, as it can often have a significant influence over the utility and interpretation of the created network. The layout of a network refers to the relative topology of the nodes that comprise the network. Many layout designs exist, but the Fruchtermann Reingold algorithm [185] is the most widely used in networking chemical space, with the force atlas algorithm offered by the Gephi software [186] also being a popular choice, both of which have been used in this study.

3.3. *Molecular Fingerprints, Similarity and Scaffolding*

Chemical similarity, as a concept, is relative and highly dependent on the methods used to assign it. Considerations need to be made regarding how to view molecules when comparing them, whether it be using global molecular topology (the molecule as a whole) or whether sub-structure methodologies are employed to provide a more focused outlook on important structural motifs (see Supporting Information S3).

Similarity is calculated by considering the features of molecules and comparing the common features that two compounds share. A common method used to ascribe similarity to molecules is the Tanimoto coefficient, sometimes referred to as the Jaccard index. For molecules A and B, let T_c equal the Tanimoto coefficient, where the common features of both A and B are divided by the total number of remaining features for both molecules, as defined by Equation (2).

$$T_c(A,B) = \frac{|A \cap B|}{|A \cup B|} \tag{2}$$

Features that are compared by the Tanimoto coefficient are usually binary bit vectors called structural keys. The structure key used in this study was the Morgan fingerprint from the RDKit package, which is similar to the more common extended connectivity fingerprint (ECFP).

The optimisation of networks requires the use of appropriate 'threshold parameters' to prepare a network that achieves desirable aesthetic qualities without missing key information (see Supporting Information S4).

3.4. *Creation and Visualisation of Networks as Applied to Data for the Verongiida Sponge Order*

3.4.1. Bipartite Networks

Bipartite networks were created from two different types of nodes: (i) NPs in the form of Simplified Molecular Line-Entry System (SMILES) codes and (ii) species from the order Verongiida. This network was created from the n x m matrix between all compounds and all species. The matrix entries are either 0, where a compound is not found in that species, or 1, where that compound has been reported.

The monopartite projections of this network show the relationship between species based on their shared compounds. In these monopartite projections, two species are joined by an edge if they each share a compound in the original bipartite network. Monopartite projections of bipartite networks also exhibit edges that are weighted based on the number of shared compounds between species. That is to say, the more compounds two species share together, the thicker the edge will be in a monopartite projection. Bipartite graphs and monopartite projections were created using the networkx library in Python. These were subsequently visualised using the Gephi networking software package version 0.9.2 (Supporting Information S5).

3.4.2. Scaffold Networks (SNs)

SNs are undirected non-weighted networks that consist of three distinct types of node: (i) species nodes, which are nodes that are exclusively linked to initialising compound nodes (only the compounds that are reported in the literature to be found in those species);(ii) initialising compound nodes, which represent the full structure of a compound found within one or many species and must be linked to at least one species node directly, but are also linked to at least one scaffold node or possibly many; (iii) scaffold nodes, which represent the scaffolds derived from the initialising compounds. The scaffolding of compounds was performed using the RDKit scaffolds package, which follows the HierS method of scaffolding [161,187]. The subsequent SNs were prepared using in-house python applications and visualised using Gephi ver 0.9.2.

3.4.3. Chemical Similarity Networks (CSNs)

All compound similarity values that were used to create networks were calculated on the basis of the Tanimoto coefficient and prepared in a similar fashion to the CSNs created by Maggiora and Bajorath [166]. Compound similarity was calculated using the Morgan fingerprint derived from the RDKit library in python. The compound library that was curated from the literature was processed prior to fingerprint creation using in-house python code to create both node and edge lists that displayed all associated attributes of each compound. Network statistics were calculated using the networkx library in python. The data curation and network creation process are summarised by the schematic in Figure 18.

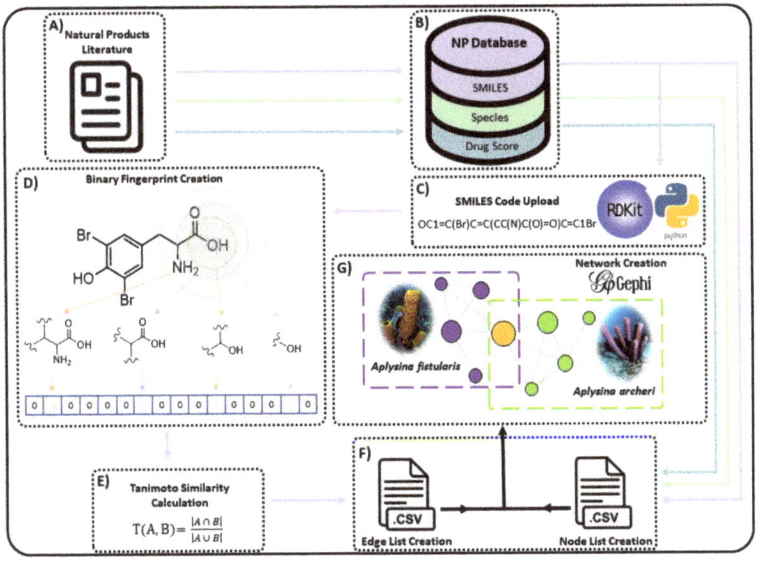

Figure 18. Conceptual scheme for networking NP compound libraries. (**A**) Collecting the NP literature obtained from SciFinder database with an emphasis on keyword searches such as genus and species name. (**B**) Curating the literature to form a database including all pertinent attributes of compounds such as species and sample location. (**C**) Reading and canonising SMILES codes from the NP database using in house python code and RDKit library. (**D**) Creation of a unique binary fingerprint for all molecules. (**E**) Calculating the Tanimoto similarity value for all possible compound comparisons. (**F**) Combining similarity calculations into an edge list describing all edge information for networks and creation of a node list including all nodes that will feature in the network and their attribute information from the NP database. (**G**) Using the Gephi software package to input node and edge list information to visualise the network.

3.5. PCA and Drug Score Assessment

Principal component analysis (PCA) was performed on compounds for each dataset using common chemical descriptors (Lipinski/Veber parameters) that include: molecular weight (MW), topological polar surface area (TPSA), number of rotatable bonds (nRotB), total number of hydrogen bond donors and acceptors (nHBDon/Acc) and the octanol water partition coefficient (cLogP) (Supporting Information S6). This, together with Euclidean distance calculations, was performed using the Platform for Unified Molecular Analysis (PUMA) and Minitab version 19.2 [164,165]. Druglikeness and the drug score for all compounds were assessed using the OSIRIS Property explorer [163]. The drug score is a value that incorporates the pharmacokinetic properties of each compound together with predicted druglikeness and the associated toxicity risk for each compound.

3.6. Limitations

Once the collection and collation of the scientific literature related to this current study were completed, some bias trends were noted in studies related to the extraction and isolation of NPs. Whilst the recognition in these bias trends means that improvements are being noted in more recent natural products publications, there is a need for these biases to be further addressed in order to improve the validity of cheminformatic work seeking to explore biogeographical NP trends as well as for further exploring secondary metabolite distribution amongst specific taxa. The biggest issue concerning some of these publications is related the missing or lacking taxonomic identification and geographical sampling information. This problem could be addressed with the inclusion of appropriate DNA identification of organisms for future NP studies, a suggestion made previously amongst the chemosystematics community [188]. Given this limitation, it is possible that some of the Verongiida sponge taxonomic classifications used in this current study may have been incorrectly classified in the literature, or that they have recently been re-classified as other species. Taxonomic reclassifications can occur many years after the initial studies and many of these reclassifications have been noted herein. In this current study, the taxonomic information obtained from the literature was taken on face value and in good faith. The authors have not attempted to authenticate or to challenge the taxonomic assignments reported in the research, as such a task was beyond the remit of the present work. Such an undertaking would also not be straightforward, as many publications give little, or no, details of how the taxonomy of the sponge was assigned.

Furthermore, many of the trends observed in this work may be subject to researcher bias such as geographical trends, which may simply highlight the focus of researchers on a certain area or species. For example, many data exist for the two genera *Aplysina* and *Pseudoceratina*, more so than any other genus, which is primarily due to the focus of specific NP research groups during the past 20 years. These sponges were also sampled from specific areas in the Caribbean and the Indo-Pacific, resulting in many NPs being reported from these genera and geographic locations, once again reflecting the bias of research focus.

This dataset is also subject to the bias inherent in the extraction and isolation procedures used by the respective research groups investigating each species. The extraction solvent plays a large role in the pool of secondary metabolites that become available for investigation, providing bias across studies as well as in experimental design. Here, the focus on the isolation strategy can affect the outcome of secondary metabolites identified. This is also apparent when comparing the general strategies of isolation seeking a chemical novelty, with targeted approaches seeking a specific pharmaceutically relevant chemotype using for instance, bioassay guided fractionation. Each method of extraction and isolation can potentially miss important secondary metabolites that could be used for cheminformatic style studies.

Data analysis provided its own set of limiting factors on top of data collection which centred around the reduction in complexity when attempting to describe chemical compounds using chemical fingerprints. The relative performance of these fingerprints is discussed frequently amongst the cheminformatics community [189,190]. As much of the similarity and also fingerprint calculations did not amount to quantitative work, but rather relative comparisons, this was deemed not pertinent to the outcomes in this current study.

4. Conclusions

This work has provided valuable insights into the use of network strategies to investigate the distribution and drug potential of natural products within the order Verongiida. Regardless of the true origin of BTA compounds, the review and subsequent networking data investigation conducted herein have made it clear that many diverse NPs isolated from this order require further investigation.

By using bipartite network analysis together with SNs, it has been demonstrated that a variety of approaches can be utilised to display the chemical space of a set of NPs for the purpose of genera group comparison. These methods have shown that species of sponges within this order, overall and not unexpectedly, appear to follow a trend of having more similar NP chemistry with their intra-genera counterparts as opposed to their inter-genera counterparts. The comparison of secondary metabolites across the order Verongiida using networking methodology supports the current systematics of the Verongiid sponges at the family and the genus level.

The construction of similarity networks provided the basis for discussing the chemical space and bioactivity assessment of the BTA derivatives produced by Verongiida sponges. This was also investigated using PCA analysis of pharmacokinetic chemical descriptors followed by Euclidean distance measurements. Each genus of sponge was assessed as a set of secondary metabolites as well as via cluster analysis and the drug score, showing differences across each genus in the predicted drug score. Differences in drug score were discussed via apparent chemotype and assessed using cluster analysis of the similarity networks. This showed that the genus *Verongula* is the most prolific at producing the most chemotypes with the highest mean drug score. In addition, it was shown that the BTA derivatives that contained an oxime moiety (Cluster 2) and the simple BT derivatives (Cluster 3) had the highest mean drug scores.

A noteworthy outcome of this study has been the realisation that targeted isolation strategies can be inferred from a consideration of the mean drug scores derived from an ensemble of compounds of interest. Another significant outcome of this work is the realisation that in the search for new pharmaceuticals among NP libraries, data mining, using the network analyses described herein, can provide a rational approach to the identification of likely lead candidates. While molecular networking schemes have seen more frequent use in both the cheminformatics field and the NP drug discovery field, it is apparent that the full utility of the tools provided by graph theory have yet to be fully realised.

Supplementary Materials: The following are available online at https://www.mdpi.com/article/10.3390/md19100582/s1: Supporting Information S1: Genus Reference List, Supporting Information S2: Network Considerations, Supporting Information S3: Molecular Fingerprints, Similarity and Scaffolding, Supporting Information S4: Network Optimisation and Visualisation, Supporting Information S5: Bipartite Network Compounds vs. Species (Full Size), Supporting Information S6: Physicochemical Properties of Compounds and PCA Analysis, Supporting Information S7: References.

Author Contributions: Conceptualisation, J.L.; methodology, J.L.; software, J.L.; validation, C.R., S.U. and J.L.; formal analysis, J.L.; investigation, J.L.; resources, J.L.; data curation, J.L.; writing—original draft preparation, J.L.; writing—review and editing, C.R., S.U., R.B. and J.L.; visualisation, J.L.; supervision, R.B. and S.U.; project administration, J.L.; funding acquisition, S.U. All authors have read and agreed to the published version of the manuscript.

Funding: This research was funded by RMIT University in the form of a postgraduate scholarship.

Institutional Review Board Statement: Not applicable.

Informed Consent Statement: Not applicable.

Data Availability Statement: The data presented in this study is available in the manuscript and in the Supporting Information File.

Acknowledgments: The authors would like to acknowledge the advice provided by Arathi Arakala, School of Science (Mathematics), RMIT University and the valuable discussions and contributions of Stewart Lever and Oli Moraes (Centre for Urban Research), RMIT University.

Conflicts of Interest: The authors declare no conflict of interest.

References

1. Grant, R.E. Animal Kingdom. In *The Cyclopaedia of Anatomy and Physiology*; Sherwood, Gilber and Piper: London, UK, 1836; pp. 107–118.
2. Carroll, A.R.; Copp, B.R.; Davis, R.A.; Keyzers, R.A.; Prinsep, M.R. Marine natural products. *Nat. Prod. Rep.* **2019**, *36*, 122–173. [CrossRef] [PubMed]
3. De Vries, D.J.; Hall, M.R. Marine biodiversity as a source of chemical diversity. *Drug. Dev. Res.* **1994**, *33*, 161–173. [CrossRef]
4. Wiese, J.; Imhoff, J.F. Marine bacteria and fungi as promising source for new antibiotics. *Drug Dev. Res.* **2019**, *80*, 24–27. [CrossRef]
5. Sigwart, J.D.; Blasiak, R.; Jaspars, M.; Jouffray, J.-B.; Tasdemir, D. Unlocking the potential of marine biodiscovery. *Nat. Prod. Rep.* **2021**, *38*, 1235–1242. [CrossRef] [PubMed]
6. Leal, M.C.; Munro, M.H.; Blunt, J.W.; Puga, J.; Jesus, B.; Calado, R.; Rosa, R.; Madeira, C. Biogeography and biodiscovery hotspots of macroalgal marine natural products. *Nat. Prod. Rep.* **2013**, *30*, 1380–1390. [CrossRef]
7. Leal, M.C.; Puga, J.; Serodio, J.; Gomes, N.C.; Calado, R. Trends in the discovery of new marine natural products from invertebrates over the last two decades—Where and what are we bioprospecting? *PLoS ONE* **2012**, *7*, e30580.
8. Bergquist, P.R. *Sponges*; Hutchinson; University of California Press: Berkeley, CA, USA; London, UK; Los Angeles, CA, USA, 1978; pp. 1–268.
9. El-Demerdash, A.; Atanasov, A.G.; Horbanczuk, O.K.; Tammam, M.A.; Abdel-Mogib, M.; Hooper, J.N.A.; Sekeroglu, N.; Al-Mourabit, A.; Kijjoa, A. Chemical Diversity and Biological Activities of Marine Sponges of the Genus Suberea: A Systematic Review. *Mar. Drugs* **2019**, *17*, 115. [CrossRef]
10. Lira, N.S.; Montes, R.C.; Tavares, J.F.; da Silva, M.S.; da Cunha, E.V.; de Athayde-Filho, P.F.; Rodrigues, L.C.; da Silva Dias, C.; Barbosa-Filho, J.M. Brominated compounds from marine sponges of the genus *Aplysina* and a compilation of their ^{13}C NMR spectral data. *Mar. Drugs* **2011**, *9*, 2316–2368. [CrossRef]
11. Niemann, H.; Marmann, A.; Lin, W.; Proksch, P. Sponge derived bromotyrosines: Structural diversity through natural combinatorial chemistry. *Nat. Prod. Comm.* **2015**, *10*, 219–231. [CrossRef]
12. Peng, J.; Li, J.; Hamann, M.T. The Marine Bromotyrosine Derivatives. *Alkaloids Chem. Biol.* **2005**, *61*, 59–262.
13. Rama Rao, M.; Venkatesham, U.; Sridevi, K.V.; Venkateswarlu, Y. Chemical constituents and their biological activities of the sponge family Aplysinellidae: A review. *Ind. J. Chem.* **2000**, *39B*, 723–733.
14. Erwin, P.M.; Thacker, R.W. Phylogenetic analyses of marine sponges within the order Verongida: A comparison of morphological and molecular data. *Invertebr. Biol.* **2007**, *126*, 220–234. [CrossRef]
15. Hooper, J.N.; Van Soest, R.W. Systema Porifera. A guide to the classification of sponges. In *Systema Porifera*; Springer: Berlin/Heidelberg, Germany, 2020; pp. 1–7.
16. Thoms, C.; Schupp, P.J. Activated chemical defense in marine sponges—A case study on *Aplysinella Rhax*. *J. Chem. Ecol.* **2008**, *34*, 1242–1252. [CrossRef] [PubMed]
17. Thoms, C.; Wolff, M.; Padmakumar, K.; Ebel, R.; Proksch, P. Chemical defense of Mediterranean sponges *Aplysina cavernicola* and *Aplysina aerophoba*. *Z. Naturforsch.* **2004**, *59c*, 113–122. [CrossRef]
18. Ortlepp, S.; Sjogren, M.; Dahlstrom, M.; Weber, H.; Ebel, R.; Edrada, R.; Thoms, C.; Schupp, P.; Bohlin, L.; Proksch, P. Antifouling activity of bromotyrosine-derived sponge metabolites and synthetic analogues. *Mar. Biotechnol.* **2007**, *9*, 776–785. [CrossRef] [PubMed]
19. Teeyapant, R.; Woerdenbag, H.J.; Kreis, P.; Hacker, J.; Wray, V.; Witte, L.; Proksch, P. Antibiotic and cytotoxic activity of brominated compounds from the marine sponge *Verongia aerophoba*. *Z. Naturforsch.* **1993**, *48c*, 939–945. [CrossRef]
20. Wang, Q.; Tang, X.L.; Luo, X.C.; de Voog, N.J.; Li, P.L.; Li, G.Q. Aplysinopsin-type and Bromotyrosine-derived Alkaloids from the South China Sea Sponge *Fascaplysinopsis reticulata*. *Sci. Rep.* **2019**, *9*, 1–10. [CrossRef] [PubMed]
21. Nuñez, C.V.; de Almeida, E.V.R.; Granato, A.C.; Marques, S.O.; Santos, K.O.; Pereira, F.R.; Macedo, M.L.; Ferreira, A.G.; Hajdu, E.; Pinheiro, U.S.; et al. Chemical variability within the marine sponge *Aplysina fulva*. *Biochem. Syst. Ecol.* **2008**, *36*, 283–296. [CrossRef]
22. Ciminiello, P.; Fattorusso, E.; Forino, M.; Magno, S. Chemistry of Verongida sponges VIII Bromocompounds from the Mediterranean sponges *Aplysina aerophoba* and *Aplysina cavernicola*. *Tetrahedron* **1997**, *18*, 6565–6572. [CrossRef]
23. Ciminiello, P.; Fattorusso, E.; Magno, S.; Pansini, M. Chemistry of Verongiida sponges VI Comparison of the secondary metabolic composition of *Aplysina insularis* and *Aplysina fulva*. *Biochem. Syst. Ecol.* **1996**, *24*, 105–113. [CrossRef]
24. Quinoa, E.; Crews, P. Phenolic constituents of psammaplysilla. *Tetrahedron Lett.* **1987**, *28*, 3229–3232. [CrossRef]
25. Kumar, M.S.L.; Ali, K.; Chaturvedi, P.; Meena, S.; Datta, D.; Panda, G. Design, synthesis and biological evaluation of oxime lacking Psammaplin inspired chemical libraries as anti-cancer agents. *J. Mol. Struct.* **2021**, *1225*, 129173. [CrossRef]

26. Jing, Q.; Hu, X.; Ma, Y.; Mu, J.; Liu, W.; Xu, F.; Li, Z.; Bai, J.; Hua, H.; Li, D. Marine-Derived Natural Lead Compound Disulfide-Linked Dimer Psammaplin A: Biological Activity and Structural Modification. *Mar. Drugs* **2019**, *17*, 384. [CrossRef] [PubMed]
27. Bao, Y.; Xu, Q.; Wang, L.; Wei, Y.; Hu, B.; Wang, J.; Liu, D.; Zhao, L.; Jing, Y. Studying Histone Deacetylase Inhibition and Apoptosis Induction of Psammaplin A Monomers with Modified Thiol Group. *ACS Med. Chem. Lett.* **2021**, *12*, 39–47. [CrossRef] [PubMed]
28. Mayer, A.; Rodríguez, A.D.; Taglialatela-Scafati, O.; Fusetani, N. Marine pharmacology in 2009–2011: Marine compounds with antibacterial, antidiabetic, antifungal, anti-inflammatory, antiprotozoal, antituberculosis, and antiviral activities; affecting the immune and nervous systems, and other miscellaneous mechanisms of action. *Mar. Drugs* **2013**, *11*, 2510–2573.
29. Lebouvier, N.; Jullian, V.; Desvignes, I.; Maurel, S.; Parenty, A.; Dorin-Semblat, D.; Doerig, C.; Sauvain, M.; Laurent, D. Antiplasmodial activities of homogentisic acid derivative protein kinase inhibitors isolated from a Vanuatu marine sponge *Pseudoceratina* sp. *Mar. Drugs* **2009**, *7*, 640–653. [CrossRef] [PubMed]
30. Mayer, A.; Rodríguez, A.D.; Taglialatela-Scafati, O.; Fusetani, N. Marine pharmacology in 2012–2013: Marine compounds with antibacterial, antidiabetic, antifungal, anti-inflammatory, antiprotozoal, antituberculosis, and antiviral activities; affecting the immune and nervous systems, and other miscellaneous mechanisms of action. *Mar. Drugs* **2017**, *15*, 273.
31. Mayer, A.; Guerrero, A.J.; Rodríguez, A.D.; Taglialatela-Scafati, O.; Nakamura, F.; Fusetani, N. Marine pharmacology in 2014–2015: Marine compounds with antibacterial, antidiabetic, antifungal, anti-inflammatory, antiprotozoal, antituberculosis, antiviral, and anthelmintic activities; affecting the immune and nervous systems, and other miscellaneous mechanisms of action. *Mar. Drugs* **2020**, *18*, 5.
32. Xu, M.; Davis, R.A.; Feng, Y.; Sykes, M.L.; Shelper, T.; Avery, V.M.; Camp, D.; Quinn, R.J. Ianthelliformisamines A-C, antibacterial bromotyrosine-derived metabolites from the marine sponge *Suberea ianthelliformis*. *J. Nat. Prod.* **2012**, *75*, 1001–1005. [CrossRef]
33. Pieri, C.; Borselli, D.; Di Giorgio, C.; De Meo, M.; Bolla, J.-M.; Vidal, N.; Combes, S.; Brunel, J.M. New ianthelliformisamine derivatives as antibiotic enhancers against resistant Gram-negative bacteria. *J. Med. Chem.* **2014**, *57*, 4263–4272. [CrossRef]
34. Mani, L.; Jullian, V.; Mourkazel, B.; Valentin, A.; Dubois, J.; Cresteil, T.; Folcher, E.; Hooper, J.N.A.; Erpenbeck, D.; Aalbersberg, W.; et al. New antiplasmodial bromotyrosine derivatives from *Suberea ianthelliformis*. *Chem. Biodivers.* **2012**, *9*, 1436–1451. [CrossRef]
35. Buchanan, M.S.; Carroll, A.R.; Wessling, D.; Jobling, M.; Avery, V.M.; Davis, R.A.; Feng, Y.; Hooper, J.N.A.; Quinn, R.J. Clavatadines C-E Guanidine alkaloids from the Australian sponge *Suberea clavata*. *J. Nat. Prod.* **2009**, *72*, 973–975. [CrossRef] [PubMed]
36. Buchanan, M.S.; Carroll, A.R.; Wessling, D.; Jobling, M.; Avery, V.M.; Davis, R.A.; Feng, Y.; Xue, Y.; Oster, L.; Fex, T.; et al. Clavatadine A, A natural product with selective recognition and irreversible inhibition of factor XIa. *J. Med. Chem.* **2008**, *51*, 3583–3587. [CrossRef] [PubMed]
37. Feng, Y.; Bowden, B.F.; Kapoor, V. Ianthellamide A, a selective kynurenine-3-hydroxylase inhibitor from the Australian marine sponge *Ianthella quadrangulata*. *Bioorg. Med. Chem. Lett.* **2012**, *22*, 3398–3401. [CrossRef] [PubMed]
38. Tian, L.W.; Feng, Y.; Shimizu, Y.; Pfeifer, T.; Wellington, C.; Hooper, J.N.; Quinn, R.J. Aplysinellamides A-C, bromotyrosine-derived metabolites from an Australian *Aplysinella* sp. *marine sponge*. *J. Nat. Prod.* **2014**, *77*, 1210–1214. [CrossRef]
39. Mohanty, I.; Tapadar, S.; Moore, S.G.; Biggs, J.S.; Freeman, C.J.; Gaul, D.A.; Garg, N.; Agarwal, V. Presence of bromotyrosine alkaloids in marine sponges is independent of metabolic and microbiome architectures. *Msystems* **2021**, *6*, 1–17. [CrossRef]
40. Nicacio, K.J.; Ioca, L.P.; Froes, A.M.; Leomil, L.; Appolinario, L.R.; Thompson, C.C.; Thompson, F.L.; Ferreira, A.G.; Williams, D.E.; Andersen, R.J.; et al. Cultures of the Marine Bacterium *Pseudovibrio denitrificans* Ab134 Produce Bromotyrosine-Derived Alkaloids Previously Only Isolated from Marine Sponges. *J. Nat. Prod.* **2017**, *80*, 235–240. [CrossRef]
41. Thompson, J.E.; Barrow, K.D.; Faulkner, J.D. Localization of two brominated metabolites aerothionin and homoaerothionin in spherulous cells of the marine sponge *Aplysina fistularis*. *Acta. Zool.* **1983**, *64*, 199–210. [CrossRef]
42. Turon, X.; Becerro, M.A.; Uriz, M.J. Distribution of brominated compounds within the sponge *Aplysina aerophoba*: Coupling of X-ray microanalysis with cryofixation techniques. *Cell Tissue Res.* **2000**, *301*, 311–322. [CrossRef]
43. Ebel, R.; Brenzinger, M.; Kunze, A.; Gross, H.J.; Proksch, P. Wound activation of protoxins in marine sponge *Aplysina aerophoba*. *J. Chem. Ecol.* **1997**, *23*, 1451–1462. [CrossRef]
44. Pita, L.; Turon, X.; Lopez-Legentil, S.; Erwin, P.M. Host rules: Spatial stability of bacterial communities associated with marine sponges (*Ircinia* spp.) in the Western Mediterranean Sea. *FEMS Microbiol. Ecol.* **2013**, *86*, 268–276. [CrossRef] [PubMed]
45. Cardenas, C.A.; Bell, J.J.; Davy, S.K.; Hoggard, M.; Taylor, M.W. Influence of environmental variation on symbiotic bacterial communities of two temperate sponges. *FEMS Microbiol. Ecol.* **2014**, *88*, 516–527. [CrossRef] [PubMed]
46. Steinert, G.; Taylor, M.W.; Deines, P.; Simister, R.L.; de Voogd, N.J.; Hoggard, M.; Schupp, P.J. In four shallow and mesophotic tropical reef sponges from Guam the microbial community largely depends on host identity. *PeerJ* **2016**, *4*, e1936. [CrossRef]
47. Steinert, G.; Rohde, S.; Janussen, D.; Blaurock, C.; Schupp, P.J. Host-specific assembly of sponge-associated prokaryotes at high taxonomic ranks. *Sci. Rep.* **2017**, *7*, 1–9. [CrossRef] [PubMed]
48. Pita, L.; Rix, L.; Slaby, B.M.; Franke, A.; Hentschel, U. The sponge holobiont in a changing ocean: From microbes to ecosystems. *Microbiome* **2018**, *6*, 1–18. [CrossRef] [PubMed]
49. Nardo, G.D. De Spongiis. *Isis von Oken* **1834**, 714–716.
50. Bergquist, P.R. Dictyoceratida, Dendroceratida and Verongida from the New Caledonia Lagoon (Porifera: Demospongiae). *Mem. Qld. Mus.* **1995**, *38*, 1–51.

51. Salim, A.A.; Khalil, Z.G.; Capon, R.J. Structural and stereochemical investigations into bromotyrosine-derived metabolites from southern Australian marine sponges, *Pseudoceratina* spp. *Tetrahedron* **2012**, *68*, 9802–9807. [CrossRef]
52. Ragini, K.; Fromont, J.; Piggott, A.M.; Karuso, P. Enantiodivergence in the Biosynthesis of Bromotyrosine Alkaloids from Sponges? *J. Nat. Prod.* **2017**, *80*, 215–219. [CrossRef]
53. Carter, H.J. Descriptions of Sponges from the Neighbourhood of Port Phillip Heads, South Australia. *Ann. Mag. Nat. Hist.* **1885**, *15*, 107–117. [CrossRef]
54. Higgin, T. On a new sponge of the genus *Luffaria*, from Yucatan, in the Liverpool Free Museum. *Ann. Mag. Nat. Hist.* **1875**, *16*, 223–227. [CrossRef]
55. De Lamarck, J.B. Sur les polypiers empâtés. *Ann. Mus. Natl. d'Hist. Nat.* **1814**, *20*, 294–312.
56. Gray, J.E. Note on *Ianthella*, a new genus of keratose sponges. *Proc. Zool. Soc. Lond.* **1869**, *1869*, 49–51. [CrossRef]
57. Hyatt, A. Revision of the North American Poriferae; with Remarks upon Foreign Species. Part I. *Mem. Boston Soc. Nat. Hist.* **1875**, *2*, 399–408.
58. Topsent, E. Matériaux pour servir à l'étude de la faune des spongiaires de France. *Mémoires Société Zool. France* **1896**, *9*, 113–133.
59. Bergquist, P.R. A revision of the supraspecific classification of the orders Dictyoceratida, Dendroceratida and Verongida (class Demospongiae). *N. Zealand J. Zool.* **1980**, *7*, 443–503. [CrossRef]
60. De Laubenfels, M.W. *The Sponges of the West-Central Pacific*; Oregon State Monographs: Studies in Zoology; Oregon State College: Corvallis, OR, USA, 1954; pp. 35–41.
61. Verrill, A.E. The Bermuda Islands: Part V. An account of the Coral Reefs (Characteristic Life of the Bermuda Coral Reefs). Porifera: Sponges. *Trans. Conn. Acad. Arts Sci.* **1907**, *12*, 330–344.
62. Teeyapant, R.; Proksch, P. Biotransformation of brominated compounds in the marine sponge *Verongia aerophoba*—Evidence for an induced chemical defense? *Sci. Nat.* **1993**, *80*, 369–370. [CrossRef]
63. Teeyapant, R.; Kreis, P.; Wray, V.; Witte, L.; Proksch, P. Brominated secondary compounds from the marine sponge *Verongia aerophoba* and the sponge feeding gastropod *Tylodina perversa*. *Z. Naturforsch.* **1993**, *48*, 640–644. [CrossRef]
64. Kunze, K.; Niemann, H.; Ueberlein, S.; Schulze, R.; Ehrlich, H.; Brunner, E.; Proksch, P.; van Pee, K.H. Brominated skeletal components of the marine demosponges, *Aplysina cavernicola* and *Ianthella basta*: Analytical and biochemical investigations. *Mar. Drugs* **2013**, *11*, 1271–1287. [CrossRef]
65. Ocean Biodiversity Information System. 2021. Available online: https://obis.org/ (accessed on 21 March 2021).
66. Van Soest, R.W.M.; Boury-Esnault, N.; Hooper, J.N.A.; Rutzler, K.; de Voogd, N.J.; Alvarez, B.; Hajdu, E.; Pisera, A.B.; Manconi, R.; Schonberg, C.; et al. World Porifera Database. 2021. Available online: http://www.marinespecies.org/porifera (accessed on 6 June 2021).
67. Yagi, H.; Matsunaga, S.; Fusetani, N. Purpuramines A-I, New bromotyrosine-derived metabolites from the marine sponge *Psammaplysilla purpurea*. *Tetrahedron* **1993**, *49*, 3749–3754. [CrossRef]
68. Tsukamoto, S.; Kato, H.; Hirota, H.; Fusetani, N. Ceratinamides A and B: New antifouling dibromotyrosine derivatives from the marine sponge *Pseudoceratina purpurea*. *Tetrahedron* **1996**, *52*, 8181–8186. [CrossRef]
69. Tsukamoto, S.; Kato, H.; Hirota, H.; Fusetani, N. Ceratinamine: An unprecedented antifouling cyanoformamide from the marine sponge *Pseudoceratina purpurea*. *J. Org. Chem.* **1996**, *61*, 2936–2937. [CrossRef] [PubMed]
70. Jang, J.H.; van Soest, R.W.M.; Fusetani, N.; Matsunaga, S. Pseudoceratins A and B, antifungal bicyclic bromotyrosine-derived metabolites from the marine sponge *Pseudoceratina purpurea*. *J. Org. Chem.* **2007**, *72*, 1211–1217. [CrossRef]
71. Ma, K.; Yang, Y.; Deng, Z.; de Voogd, N.J.; Proksch, P.; Lin, W. Two new bromotyrosine derivatives from the marine sponge *Pseudoceratina* sp. *Chem. Biodivers.* **2008**, *5*, 1313–1320. [CrossRef]
72. Huang, X.-P.; Deng, Z.-W.; van Soest, R.W.M.; Lin, W.-H. Brominated derivatives from the Chinese sponge *Pseudoceratina* sp. *J. Asian Nat. Prod. Res.* **2008**, *10*, 239–242. [CrossRef]
73. Li, H.; Yu, H.; Wu, W.; Sun, P. Chemical constituents of sponge *Pseudoceratina* sp.; their chemotaxonomic significance. *Biochem. Syst. Ecol.* **2020**, *89*, 104002. [CrossRef]
74. Jimenez, C.; Crews, P. Novel marine sponge derived amino acids 13. additional psammaplin derivatives from *Psammplysilla purpurea*. *Tetrahedron* **1991**, *47*, 2097–2102. [CrossRef]
75. Kijjoa, A.; Bessa, J.; Wattanadilok, R.; Sawangwong, P.; Nascimento, N.S.J.; Pedro, M.; Silva, A.M.S.; Eaton, G.; van Soest, R.; Herz, W. Dibromotyrosine derivatives, a maleimide, aplysamine-2 and other constituents of the marine sponge *Pseudoceratina purpurea*. *Z. Naturforsch.* **2005**, *60*, 904–908. [CrossRef]
76. Morris, S.A.; Anderson, R.J. Brominated bis(indole) alkaloids from the marine sponge *Hexadella* sp. *Tetrahedron* **1990**, *46*, 715–720. [CrossRef]
77. Morris, S.A.; Anderson, R.J. Nitrogenous metabolites from the deep water sponge *Hexadella* sp. *Can. J. Chem.* **1989**, *67*, 677–681. [CrossRef]
78. Ichiba, T.; Scheuer, P.J. Three Bromotyrosine Derivatives, One Terminating in an Unprecedented Diketocyclopentenylidene Enamine. *J. Org. Chem.* **1993**, *58*, 4149–4150. [CrossRef]
79. Van Soest, R.W.; Boury-Esnault, N.; Vacelet, J.; Dohrmann, M.; Erpenbeck, D.; De Voogd, N.J.; Santodomingo, N.; Vanhoorne, B.; Kelly, M.; Hooper, J.N. Global diversity of sponges (Porifera). *PLoS ONE* **2012**, *7*, e35105. [CrossRef]
80. Carter, H.J. Report on Specimens dredged up from the Gulf of Manaar and presented to the Liverpool Free Museum by Capt.W.H. Cawne Warren. *Ann. Mag. Nat. Hist.* **1880**, *6*, 35–61. [CrossRef]

81. Kernan, M.R.; Cambie, R.C. Chemistry of sponges, VII. 11, 19-Dideoxyfistularin 3 and 11-hydroxyaerothionin, bromotyrosine derivatives from Pseudoceratina durissima. *J. Nat. Prod.* **1990**, *53*, 615–622. [CrossRef]
82. Benharref, A.; Pais, M. Bromotyrosine alkaloids from the sponge *Pseudoceratina verrucosa*. *J. Nat. Prod.* **1996**, *59*, 177–180. [CrossRef]
83. Tran, T.D.; Pham, N.B.; Fechner, G.; Hooper, J.N.; Quinn, R.J. Bromotyrosine alkaloids from the Australian marine sponge *Pseudoceratina verrucosa*. *J. Nat. Prod.* **2013**, *76*, 516–523. [CrossRef]
84. Kassuhlke, K.E.; Faulkner, J.D. Two new dibromotyrosine derivatives from the Caribbean sponge pseudoceratina crassa. *Tetrahedron* **1991**, *47*, 1809–1814. [CrossRef]
85. Albrizio, S.; Ciminiello, P.; Fattorusso, E.; Magno, S. Chemistry of Verongida sponges. I. constituents of the caribbean sponge *Pseudoceratina crassa*. *Tetrahedron* **1994**, *50*, 783–788. [CrossRef]
86. Ciminiello, P.; Fattorusso, E.; Magno, S. Chemistry of Verongida sponges, IV. comparison of the secondary metabolite composition of several specimens of *Pseudoceratina crassa*. *J. Nat. Prod.* **1995**, *58*, 689–696. [CrossRef]
87. Rahelivao, M.P.; Lubken, T.; Gruner, M.; Kataeva, O.; Ralambondrahety, R.; Andriamanantoanina, H.; Checinski, M.P.; Bauer, I.; Knolker, H.J. Isolation and structure elucidation of natural products of three soft corals and a sponge from the coast of Madagascar. *Org. Biomol. Chem.* **2017**, *15*, 2593–2608. [CrossRef]
88. Keller, C. Die Spongienfauna des rothen Meeres (I. Hälfte). *Z. Wiss. Zool.* **1889**, *48*, 311–405.
89. Badhr, J.M.; Shaala, L.A.; Abou-Shoer, M.I.; Tawfik, M.K.; Abdel-Azim, H.M. Bioactive brominated metabolites from the Red Sea sponge *Pseudoceratina arabica*. *J. Nat. Prod.* **2008**, *71*, 1472–1474. [CrossRef]
90. Shaala, L.A.; Youssef, D.T.; Sulaiman, M.; Behery, F.A.; Foudah, A.I.; Sayed, K.A. Subereamolline A as a potent breast cancer migration, invasion and proliferation inhibitor and bioactive dibrominated alkaloids from the Red Sea sponge *Pseudoceratina arabica*. *Mar. Drugs* **2012**, *10*, 2492–2508. [CrossRef]
91. Shaala, L.A.; Youssef, D.T.A.; Badr, J.M.; Sulaiman, M.; Khedr, A.; El Sayed, K.A. Bioactive alkaloids from the Red Sea marine Verongid sponge *Pseudoceratina arabica*. *Tetrahedron* **2015**, *71*, 7837–7841. [CrossRef]
92. Bergquist, P.R.; Kelly-Borges, M. Systematics and biogeography of the genus Ianthella (Demospongiae: Verongida: Ianthellidae) in the south-west Pacific. *Beagle Rec. Mus. Art Galleries North. Territ.* **1995**, *12*, 151–176.
93. Balansa, W.; Islam, R.; Gilbert, D.F.; Fontaine, F.; Xiao, X.; Zhang, H.; Piggott, A.M.; Lynch, J.W.; Capon, R.J. Australian marine sponge alkaloids as a new class of glycine-gated chloride channel receptor modulator. *Bioorg. Med. Chem.* **2013**, *21*, 4420–4425. [CrossRef] [PubMed]
94. Motti, C.A.; Freckelton, M.L.; Tapiolas, D.M.; Willis, R.H. FTICR-MS and LC-UV/MS-SPE-NMR Applications for the rapid dereplication of a crude extract from the sponge *Ianthella flabelliformis*. *J. Nat. Prod.* **2009**, *72*, 290–294. [CrossRef]
95. Carroll, A.R.; Kaiser, S.M.; Davis, R.A.; Moni, R.W.; Hooper, J.N.A.; Quinn, R.J. A Bastadin with Potent and Selective δ-Opioid Receptor Binding Affinity from the Australian Sponge *Ianthella flabelliformis*. *J. Nat. Prod.* **2010**, *73*, 1173–1176. [CrossRef]
96. Okamoto, Y.; Ojika, M.; Kato, S.; Sakagami, Y. Ianthesines A–D, Four Novel Dibromotyrosine-Derived Metabolites from a Marine Sponge, *Ianthella* sp. *Tetrahedron* **2000**, *56*, 5813–5818. [CrossRef]
97. Jaspars, M.; Rali, T.; Laney, M.; Schatzman, R.C.; Diaz, M.C.; Schmitz, F.J.; Pordesimo, E.O.; Crews, P. The search for inosine 5′-Phosphate dehydrogenase (IMPDH) inhibitors from marine sponges. Evaluation of the bastadin alkaloids. *Tetrahedron* **1994**, *50*, 7367–7374. [CrossRef]
98. Pallas, P.S. Elenchus zoophytorum sistens generum adumbrationes generaliores et specierum cognitarum succintas descriptiones, cum selectis auctorum synonymis. In *Fransiscum Varrentrapp Hagae*; Hagae-Comitum: Apud Petrum van Cleef: Hagae, The Netherlands, 1766.
99. Pordesimo, E.O.; Schmitz, F.J. New bastadins from the sponge *Ianthella Basta*. *J. Org. Chem.* **1990**, *55*, 4704–4709. [CrossRef]
100. Masuno, M.N.; Hoepker, A.C.; Pessah, I.N.; Molinski, T.F. 1-*O*-Sulfatobastadins-1 and -2 from *Ianthella basta* (Pallas). Antagonists of the RyR1-FKBP12 Ca^{2+} Channel. *Mar. Drugs* **2004**, *2*, 176–184. [CrossRef]
101. Miao, S.; Anderson, R.J. Cytotoxic metabolites from the sponge *Ianthella basta* collected in Papua New Guinea. *J. Nat. Prod.* **1990**, *53*, 1441–1446. [CrossRef] [PubMed]
102. Pettit, G.R.; Butler, M.S.; Bass, C.G.; Doubek, D.L.; Williams, M.D.; Schmidt, J.M.; Pettit, R.K.; Hooper, J.N.A.; Tackett, L.P.; Filiatrault, M.J. Antineoplastic agents, 326. The stereochemistry of bastadins 8, 10, and 12 from the Bismarck Archipelago marine sponge *Ianthella basta*. *J. Nat. Prod.* **1995**, *58*, 680–688. [CrossRef]
103. Pettit, G.R.; Butler, M.S.; Williams, M.D.; Filiatrault, M.J.; Pettit, R.K. Isolation and Structure of Hemibastadinols 1−3 from the Papua New Guinea Marine Sponge *Ianthella basta*. *J. Nat. Prod.* **1996**, *59*, 927–934. [CrossRef] [PubMed]
104. Eguchi, K.; Kato, H.; Fujiwara, Y.; Losung, F.; Mangindaan, R.E.; de Voogd, N.J.; Takeya, M.; Tsukamoto, S. Bastadins, brominated-tyrosine derivatives, suppress accumulation of cholesterol ester in macrophages. *Bioorg. Med. Chem. Lett.* **2015**, *25*, 5389–5392. [CrossRef] [PubMed]
105. Park, S.K.; Jurek, J.; Carney, J.R.; Scheuer, P.J. Two more bastadins, 16 and 17, from an Indonesian sponge *Ianthella basta*. *J. Nat. Prod.* **1994**, *57*, 407–410. [CrossRef]
106. Mathieu, V.; Wauthoz, N.; Lefranc, F.; Niemann, H.; Amighi, K.; Kiss, R.; Proksch, P. Cyclic versus hemi-bastadins. pleiotropic anti-cancer effects: From apoptosis to anti-angiogenic and anti-migratory effects. *Molecules* **2013**, *18*, 3543–3561. [CrossRef]
107. Niemann, H.; Lin, W.; Muller, W.E.; Kubbutat, M.; Lai, D.; Proksch, P. Trimeric hemibastadin congener from the marine sponge *Ianthella basta*. *J. Nat. Prod.* **2013**, *76*, 121–125. [CrossRef]

108. Park, S.K.; Park, H.; Scheuer, P.J. Isolation and structure determination of a new bastadin from an Indonesian sponge *Ianthella Basta*. *Bull. Korean Chem. Soc.* **1994**, *15*, 534–537.
109. Aoki, S.; Cho, S.H.; Hiramatsu, A.; Kotoku, N.; Kobayashi, M. Bastadins, cyclic tetramers of brominated-tyrosine derivatives, selectively inhibit the proliferation of endothelial cells. *J. Nat. Med.* **2006**, *60*, 231–235. [CrossRef]
110. Mack, M.M.; Molinski, T.F.; Buck, E.D.; Pessah, I.N. Novel modulators of skeletal muscle FKBP12/calcium channel complex from *Ianthella basta*. *J. Biol. Chem.* **1994**, *269*, 23236–23249. [CrossRef]
111. Kazlauskas, R.; Lidgard, R.O.; Murphy, P.T.; Wells, R.J.; Blount, J.F. Brominated tyrosine-derived metabolites from the sponge *Ianthella basta*. *Aust. J. Chem.* **1981**, *34*, 765–786. [CrossRef]
112. Butler, M.S.; Lim, T.K.; Capon, R.J.; Hammond, L.S. The Bastadins Revisited: New Chemistry From the Australian Marine Sponge *Ianthella basta*. *Aust. J. Chem.* **1991**, *44*, 287–296. [CrossRef]
113. Franklin, M.A.; Penn, S.G.; Lebrilla, C.B.; Lam, T.H.; Pessah, I.N.; Molinski, T.F. Bastadin 20 and Bastadin O-Sulfate Esters from *Ianthella basta*: Novel Modulators of the Ry1R FKBP12 Receptor Complex. *J. Nat. Prod.* **1996**, *59*, 1121–1127. [CrossRef]
114. Gartshore, C.J.; Salib, M.N.; Renshaw, A.A.; Molinski, T.F. Isolation of bastadin-6-O-sulfate and expedient purifications of bastadins-4, -5 and -6 from extracts of *Ianthella basta*. *Fitoterapia* **2018**, *126*, 16–21. [CrossRef] [PubMed]
115. Greve, H.; Meis, S.; Kassack, M.U.; Kehraus, S.; Krick, A.; Wright, A.D.; Konig, G.M. New Iantherans from the Marine Sponge *Ianthella quadrangulata* Novel Agonists of the P2Y11 Receptor. *J. Med. Chem.* **2007**, *50*, 5600–5607. [CrossRef]
116. Greve, H.; Kehraus, S.; Krick, A.; Kelter, G.; Maier, A.; Fiebig, H.-H.; Wright, A.D.; Konig, G.M. Cytotoxic Bastadin 24 from the Australian Sponge *Ianthella quadrangulata*. *J. Nat. Prod.* **2008**, *71*, 309–312. [CrossRef] [PubMed]
117. Coll, J.C.; Kearns, P.S.; Rideout, J.A.; Sankar, V. Bastadin 21, a Novel Isobastarane Metabolite from the Great Barrier Reef Marine Sponge *Ianthella quadrangulata*. *J. Nat. Prod.* **2002**, *65*, 753–756. [CrossRef] [PubMed]
118. Okamoto, Y.; Ojika, M.; Suzuki, S.; Murakami, M.; Sakagami, Y. Iantherans A and B, unique dimeric polybrominated benzofurans as Na, K-ATPase inhibitors from a marine sponge, *Ianthella* sp. *Bioorg. Med. Chem.* **2001**, *9*, 179–183. [CrossRef]
119. Okamoto, Y.; Ojika, M.; Sakagami, Y. Iantheran A, a dimeric polybrominated benzofuran as a Na,K-ATPase inhibitor from a marine sponge, *Ianthella* sp. *Tetrahedron Lett.* **1999**, *40*, 507–510. [CrossRef]
120. Zhang, H.; Conte, M.M.; Huang, X.C.; Khalil, Z.; Capon, R.J. A search for BACE inhibitors reveals new biosynthetically related pyrrolidones, furanones and pyrroles from a southern Australian marine sponge, *Ianthella* sp. *Org. Biomol. Chem.* **2012**, *10*, 2656–2663. [CrossRef]
121. Zhang, H.; Conte, M.M.; Khalil, Z.; Huang, X.-C.; Capon, R.J. New dictyodendrins as BACE inhibitors from a southern Australian marine sponge, *Ianthella* sp. *RSC Adv.* **2012**, *2*, 4209–4214. [CrossRef]
122. Carter, H.J. Notes introductory to the study and classification of the Spongida. Part II. Proposed classification of the Spongida. *Ann. Mag. Nat. Hist.* **1875**, *4*, 126–145. [CrossRef]
123. Nardo, G.D. Auszug aus einem neuen System der Spongiarien, wonach bereits die Aufstellung in der Universitäts-Sammlung zu Padua gemacht ist. *Isis, Order Encyclopadische Zeitung Coll (Oken: Jena)* **1833**, 519–523. Available online: http://ras.biodiversity.aq/aphia.php?p=sourcedetails=7979 (accessed on 1 October 2021).
124. Vacelet, J. Répartition générale des éponges et systématique des éponges cornées de la région de Marseille et de quelques stations méditerranéennes. *Recl. Trav. Stn. Mar. d'Endoume* **1959**, *16*, 39–101.
125. Putz, A.; Kloeppel, A.; Pfannkuchen, M.; Brummer, F.; Proksch, P. Depth-related alkaloid variation in Mediterranean *Aplysina* sponges. *Z. Naturforsch.* **2009**, *64c*, 279–287. [CrossRef]
126. Sacristan-Soriano, O.; Banaigs, B.; Becerro, M.A. Relevant spatial scales of chemical variation in *Aplysina aerophoba*. *Mar. Drugs* **2011**, *9*, 2499–2513. [CrossRef] [PubMed]
127. Sacristan-Soriano, O.; Banaigs, B.; Becerro, M.A. Temporal trends in the secondary metabolite production of the sponge *Aplysina aerophoba*. *Mar. Drugs* **2012**, *10*, 677–693. [CrossRef]
128. Reverter, M.; Perez, T.; Ereskovsky, A.V.; Banaigs, B. Secondary Metabolome Variability and Inducible Chemical Defenses in the Mediterranean Sponge *Aplysina cavernicola*. *J. Chem. Ecol.* **2016**, *42*, 60–70. [CrossRef]
129. Silva, M.M.; Bergamasco, J.; Lira, S.P.; Lopes, N.P.; Hajdu, E.; Peixinho, S.; Berlinck, R.G.S. Dereplication of bromotyrosine-derived metabolites by LC-PDA-MS and analysis of the chemical profile of 14 *Aplysina* sponge specimens from the Brazilian coastline. *Aust. J. Chem.* **2010**, *63*, 886–894. [CrossRef]
130. Ciminiello, P.; Costantino, V.; Fattorusso, E.; Magno, S.; Mangoni, A. Chemistry of Verongida sponges, II. Constituents of the Caribbean sponge *Aplysina Fistularis forma fulva*. *J. Nat. Prod.* **1994**, *57*, 705–712. [CrossRef]
131. Rogers, E.W.; Fernanda de Oliveira, M.; Berlinck, R.G.S.; Konig, G.M.; Molinski, T.F. Stereochemical Heterogeneity in Verongid Sponge Metabolites. Absolute Stereochemistry of (+)-Fistularin-3 and (+)-11-epi-Fistularin-3 by Microscale LCMS-Marfey's Analysis. *J. Nat. Prod.* **2005**, *68*, 891–896. [CrossRef] [PubMed]
132. Rogers, E.W.; Molinski, T.F. Highly polar spiroisoxazolines from the sponge *Aplysina fulva*. *J. Nat. Prod.* **2007**, *70*, 1191–1194. [CrossRef]
133. Gunasekera, M.; Gunasekera, S.P. Dihydroxyaerothionin and aerophobin 1. Two brominated tyrosine metabolites from the deep water marine sponge *Verongula rigida*. *J. Nat. Prod.* **1989**, *52*, 753–756. [CrossRef]
134. Mierzwa, R.; King, A.; Conover, M.A.; Tozzi, S.; Puar, M.S.; Patel, M.; Coval, S.J. Verongamine, a novel bromotyrosine-derived histamine H3-Antagonist from the marine sponge *Verongula gigantea*. *J. Nat. Prod.* **1994**, *57*, 175–177. [CrossRef] [PubMed]

135. Ciminiello, P.; Fattorusso, E.; Magno, S. Chemistry of Verongida sponges, III. Constituents of a Caribbean *Verongula* sp. *J. Nat. Prod.* **1994**, *57*, 1564–1569. [CrossRef]
136. Galeano, E.; Thomas, O.P.; Robledo, S.; Munoz, D.; Martinez, A. Antiparasitic bromotyrosine derivatives from the marine sponge *Verongula rigida*. *Mar. Drugs* **2011**, *9*, 1902–1913. [CrossRef]
137. Ciminiello, P.; Dell'Aversano, C.; Fattorusso, E.; Magno, S.; Pansini, M. Chemistry of Verongida Sponges. 10. Secondary Metabolite Composition of the Caribbean Sponge *Verongula gigantea*. *J. Nat. Prod.* **2000**, *63*, 263–266. [CrossRef] [PubMed]
138. Kochanowska, A.J.; Rao, K.V.; Childress, S.; El-Alfy, A.; Matsumoto, R.R.; Kelly, M.; Stewart, G.S.; Sufka, K.J.; Hamann, M.T. Secondary Metabolites from Three Florida Sponges with Antidepressant Activity. *J. Nat. Prod.* **2008**, *71*, 186–189. [CrossRef] [PubMed]
139. Jiso, A.; Kittiwisut, S.; Chantakul, R.; Yuenyongsawad, S.; Putchakarn, S.; Schaberle, T.F.; Temkitthaworn, P.; Ingkaninan, K.; Chaithirayanon, K.; Plubrukarn, A. Quintaquinone, a Merosesquiterpene from the Yellow Sponge *Verongula* cf *rigida* Esper. *J. Nat. Prod.* **2020**, *83*, 532–536. [CrossRef] [PubMed]
140. Kochanowska-Karamyan, A.J.; Araujo, H.C.; Zhang, X.; El-Alfy, A.; Carvalho, P.; Avery, M.A.; Holmbo, S.D.; Magolan, J.; Hamann, M.T. Isolation and Synthesis of Veranamine, an Antidepressant Lead from the Marine Sponge *Verongula rigida*. *J. Nat. Prod.* **2020**, *83*, 1092–1098. [CrossRef]
141. Hwang, I.H.; Oh, J.; Zhou, W.; Park, S.; Kim, J.H.; Chittiboyina, A.G.; Ferreira, D.; Song, G.Y.; Oh, S.; Na, M.; et al. Cytotoxic activity of rearranged drimane meroterpenoids against colon cancer cells via down-regulation of beta-catenin expression. *J. Nat. Prod.* **2015**, *78*, 453–461. [CrossRef]
142. Graham, S.K.; Lambert, L.K.; Pierens, G.K.; Hooper, J.N.A.; Garson, M.J. Psammaplin Metabolites New and Old: An NMR Study Involving Chiral Sulfur Chemistry. *Aust. J. Chem.* **2010**, *63*, 867–872. [CrossRef]
143. Pham, N.B.; Butler, M.S.; Quinn, R.J. Isolation of Psammaplin A 11′-Sulfate and Bisaprasin 11′-Sulfate from the Marine Sponge *Aplysinella rhax*. *J. Nat. Prod.* **2000**, *63*, 393–395. [CrossRef] [PubMed]
144. Tabudravu, J.N.; Eijsink, V.G.H.; Gooday, G.W.; Jaspars, M.; Komander, D.; Legg, M.; Synstad, B.; van Aalten, D.M.F. Psammaplin A, a chitinase inhibitor isolated from the Fijian marine sponge *Aplysinella rhax*. *Bioorg. Med. Chem.* **2002**, *10*, 1123–1128. [CrossRef]
145. Shin, J.; Lee, H.-S.; Seo, Y.; Rho, J.-R.; Cho, K.W.; Paul, V.J. New Bromotyrosine Metabolites from the Sponge *Aplysinella rhax*. *Tetrahedron* **2000**, *56*, 9071–9077. [CrossRef]
146. Mudianta, I.W. Bioprospecting of the Balinese marine sponges and nudibranchs. *J. Phys. Conf. Ser.* **2018**, *1040*, 1–7. [CrossRef]
147. Mudianta, I.W.; Skinner-Adams, T.; Andrews, K.T.; Davis, R.A.; Hadi, T.A.; Hayes, P.Y.; Garson, M.J. Psammaplysin derivatives from the Balinese marine sponge *Aplysinella strongylata*. *J. Nat. Prod.* **2012**, *75*, 2132–2143. [CrossRef]
148. Mandi, A.; Mudianta, I.W.; Kurtan, T.; Garson, M.J. Absolute Configuration and Conformational Study of Psammaplysins A and B from the Balinese Marine Sponge *Aplysinella strongylata*. *J. Nat. Prod.* **2015**, *78*, 2051–2056. [CrossRef]
149. Ankudey, F.J.; Kiprof, P.; Stromquist, E.R.; Chang, L.C. New bioactive bromotyrosine-derived alkaloid from a marine sponge *Aplysinella* sp. *Planta Med.* **2008**, *74*, 555–559. [CrossRef]
150. Liu, S.; Schmitz, F.J.; Kelly-Borges, M. Psammaplysin F, a New Bromotyrosine Derivative from a Sponge, *Aplysinella* sp. *J. Nat. Prod.* **1997**, *60*, 614–615. [CrossRef] [PubMed]
151. Fu, X.; Schmitz, F.J. 7-Hydroxyceratinamine, a New Cyanoformamide-Containing Metabolite from a Sponge, *Aplysinella* sp. *J. Nat. Prod.* **1999**, *62*, 1072–1073. [CrossRef]
152. Shaala, L.A.; Youssef, D.T.A. Cytotoxic Psammaplysin Analogues from the Verongid Red Sea Sponge *Aplysinella* Species. *Biomolecules* **2019**, *9*, 841. [CrossRef] [PubMed]
153. Von Lendenfeld, R. *Descriptive Catalogue of the Sponges in the Australian Museum, Sidney*; Taylor & Francis: London, UK, 1888.
154. El-Demerdash, A.; Moriou, C.; Toullec, J.; Besson, M.; Soulet, S.; Schmitt, N.; Petek, S.; Lecchini, D.; Debitus, C.; Al-Mourabit, A. Bioactive Bromotyrosine-Derived Alkaloids from the Polynesian Sponge *Suberea ianthelliformis*. *Mar. Drugs* **2018**, *16*, 146. [CrossRef] [PubMed]
155. Pulitzer-Finali, G. Some new or little-known sponges from the Great Barrier Reef of Australia. *Boll. Musei Ist. Biol. Dell'universitá Genova* **1982**, *48*, 87–141.
156. Spalding, M.D.; Fox, H.E.; Allen, G.R.; Davidson, N.; Ferdana, Z.A.; Finlayson, M.; Halpern, B.S.; Jorge, M.A.; Lombana, A.; Lourie, S.A.; et al. Marine ecoregions of the world: A bioregionalization of coastal and shelf areas. *Bioscience* **2007**, *57*, 573–583. [CrossRef]
157. Kerr, R.; Kelly-Borges, M. Biochemical and morphological heterogeneity in the Caribbean sponge Xestospongia muta (Petrosida: Petrosiidae). In *Sponges in Time and Space*; van Soest, R.W.M., van Kempen, T.M.G., Braekman, J.C., Eds.; Balkema: Rotterdam, The Netherlands, 1994; pp. 65–73.
158. Liu, N.; Lai, J.; Lyu, C.; Qiang, B.; Wang, H.; Jin, H.; Zhang, L.; Liu, Z. Chemical Space, Scaffolds, and Halogenated Compounds of CMNPD: A Comprehensive Chemoinformatic Analysis. *J. Chem. Inf. Model.* **2021**, *61*, 3323–3336. [CrossRef] [PubMed]
159. Langdon, S.R.; Brown, N.; Blagg, J. Scaffold diversity of exemplified medicinal chemistry space. *J. Chem. Inf. Model.* **2011**, *51*, 2174–2185. [CrossRef]
160. Wiedenmayer, F. *Shallow-Water Sponges of the Western Bahamas*; Experientia Supplementum; Springer: Berlin/Heidelberg, Germany, 1977.
161. Kruger, F.; Stiefl, N.; Landrum, G.A. rdScaffoldNetwork: The Scaffold Network Implementation in RDKit. *J. Chem. Inf. Model.* **2020**, *60*, 3331–3335. [CrossRef] [PubMed]

162. Jeh, G.; Widom, J. Simrank: A measure of structural-context similarity. In Proceedings of the 8th ACM SIGKDD International Conference on Knowledge Discovery and Data Mining, Edmonton, AB, Canada, 23–26 June 2002; pp. 538–543.
163. OSIRIS Property Explorer. 2021. Available online: https://www.organic-chemistry.org/prog/peo/ (accessed on 21 March 2021).
164. Gonzalez-Medina, M.; Medina-Franco, J.L. Platform for Unified Molecular Analysis: PUMA. *J. Chem. Inf. Model.* **2017**, *57*, 1735–1740. [CrossRef]
165. DIFACQUIM: Computer-Aided drug design at UNAM. 2021. Available online: https://www.difacquim.com/d-tools/ (accessed on 12 March 2021).
166. Maggiora, G.M.; Bajorath, J. Chemical space networks: A powerful new paradigm for the description of chemical space. *J. Comput. Aided Mol. Des.* **2014**, *28*, 795–802. [CrossRef] [PubMed]
167. Zhao, C.; Sun, M.; Bennani, Y.L.; Gopalakrishnan, S.M.; Witte, D.G.; Miller, T.R.; Krueger, K.M.; Browman, K.E.; Thiffault, C.; Wetter, J.; et al. The alkaloid Conessine and Analogues as potent Histamine H3 Reseptor Antagonists. *J. Med. Chem.* **2008**, *51*, 5423–5430. [CrossRef]
168. Nodwell, M.; Zimmerman, C.; Roberge, M.; Andersen, R.J. Synthetic analogues of the microtubule-stabilizing sponge alkaloid ceratamine A are more active than the natural product. *J. Med. Chem.* **2010**, *53*, 7843–7851. [CrossRef]
169. Smith, S.E.; Dello Buono, M.C.; Carper, D.J.; Coleman, R.S.; Day, B.W. Structure elucidation of phase I metabolites of the microtubule perturbagens: Ceratamines A and B. *J. Nat. Prod.* **2014**, *77*, 1572–1578. [CrossRef]
170. Pan, X.; Tao, L.; Ji, M.; Chen, X.; Liu, Z. Synthesis and cytotoxicity of novel imidazo[4,5-d]azepine compounds derived from marine natural product ceratamine A. *Bioorg. Med. Chem. Lett.* **2018**, *28*, 866–868. [CrossRef]
171. Pahwa, S.; Kaur, S.; Jain, R.; Roy, N. Structure based design of novel inhibitors for histidinol dehydrogenase from *Geotrichum candidum*. *Bioorg. Med. Chem. Lett.* **2010**, *20*, 3972–3976. [CrossRef]
172. Gao, J.; Caballero-George, C.; Wang, B.; Rao, K.V.; Shilabin, A.G.; Hamann, M.T. 5-OHKF and NorKA, Depsipeptides from a Hawaiian Collection of *Bryopsis pennata*: Binding Properties for NorKA to the Human Neuropeptide Y Y1 Receptor. *J. Nat. Prod.* **2009**, *72*, 2172–2176. [CrossRef]
173. Fdhila, F.; Vazquez, V.; Luis Sanchez, J.; Riguera, R. DD-Diketopiperazines: Antibiotics Active against *Vibrio anguillarum* Isolated from Marine Bacteria Associated with Cultures of *Pecten maximus*. *J. Nat. Prod.* **2003**, *66*, 1299–1301. [CrossRef] [PubMed]
174. Li, X.; Liu, N.; Zhang, H.; Knudson, S.E.; Slayden, R.A.; Tonge, P.J. Synthesis and SAR studies of 1,4-benzoxazine MenB inhibitors: Novel antibacterial agents against *Mycobacterium tuberculosis*. *Bioorg. Med. Chem. Lett.* **2010**, *20*, 6306–6309. [CrossRef] [PubMed]
175. Campagnola, G.; Gong, P.; Peersen, O.B. High-throughput screening identification of poliovirus RNA-dependent RNA polymerase inhibitors. *Antivir. Res.* **2011**, *91*, 241–251. [CrossRef] [PubMed]
176. de F. Cesario, H.P.S.; Silva, F.C.O.; Ferreira, M.K.A.; de Menezes, J.; Dos Santos, H.S.; Nogueira, C.E.S.; de L. Silva, K.S.B.; Hajdu, E.; Silveira, E.R.; Pessoa, O.D.L. Anxiolytic-like effect of brominated compounds from the marine sponge Aplysina fulva on adult zebrafish (Danio rerio): Involvement of the GABAergic system. *Neurochem. Int.* **2021**, *146*, 105021. [CrossRef] [PubMed]
177. Orfanoudaki, M.; Hartmann, A.; Alilou, M.; Mehic, N.; Kwiatkowski, M.; Johrer, K.; Nguyen Ngoc, H.; Hensel, A.; Greil, R.; Ganzera, M. Cytotoxic Compounds of Two Demosponges (*Aplysina aerophoba* and *Spongia* sp.) from the Aegean Sea. *Biomolecules* **2021**, *11*, 723. [CrossRef]
178. Oluwabusola, E.T.; Tabudravu, J.N.; Al Maqbali, K.S.; Annang, F.; Perez-Moreno, G.; Reyes, F.; Jaspars, M. Antiparasitic Activity of Bromotyrosine Alkaloids and New Analogues Isolated from the Fijian Marine Sponge *Aplysinella rhax*. *Chem. Biodivers.* **2020**, *17*, 1–9. [CrossRef]
179. Shaala, L.A.; Youssef, D.T.A. Pseudoceratonic Acid and Moloka'iamine Derivatives from the Red Sea Verongiid Sponge *Pseudoceratina arabica*. *Mar. Drugs* **2020**, *18*, 525. [CrossRef]
180. Chen, M.; Yan, Y.; Ge, H.; Jiao, W.-H.; Zhang, Z.; Lin, H.-W. Pseudoceroximes A-E and Pseudocerolides A-E—Bromotyrosine Derivatives from a *Pseudoceratina* sp. Marine Sponge Collected in the South China Sea. *Eur. J. Org. Chem.* **2020**, *2020*, 2583–2591. [CrossRef]
181. Tintillier, F.; Moriou, C.; Petek, S.; Fauchon, M.; Hellio, C.; Saulnier, D.; Ekins, M.; Hooper, J.N.A.; Al-Mourabit, A.; Debitus, C. Quorum Sensing Inhibitory and Antifouling Activities of New Bromotyrosine Metabolites from the Polynesian Sponge *Pseudoceratina* n. sp. *Mar. Drugs* **2020**, *18*, 272. [CrossRef]
182. Moriou, C.; Lacroix, D.; Petek, S.; El-Demerdash, A.; Trepos, R.; Leu, T.M.; Florean, C.; Diederich, M.; Hellio, C.; Debitus, C.; et al. Bioactive Bromotyrosine Derivatives from the Pacific Marine Sponge *Suberea clavata* (Pulitzer-Finali, 1982). *Mar. Drugs* **2021**, *19*, 143. [CrossRef]
183. Van Eck, N.J.; Waltman, L. CitNetExplorer: A new software tool for analyzing and visualizing citation networks. *J. Informetr.* **2014**, *8*, 802–823. [CrossRef]
184. Massol, F.; Macke, E.; Callens, M.; Decaestecker, E. A methodological framework to analyse determinants of host-microbiota networks, with an application to the relationships between *Daphnia magna*'s gut microbiota and bacterioplankton. *J. Anim. Ecol.* **2021**, *90*, 102–119. [CrossRef]
185. Fruchterman, T.M.J.; Reingold, E.M. Graph drawing by Force-directed Placement. *Softw. Pract. Exp.* **1991**, *21*, 1129–1164. [CrossRef]
186. Jacomy, M.; Venturini, T.; Heymann, S.; Bastian, M. ForceAtlas2, a continuous graph layout algorithm for handy network visualization designed for the Gephi software. *PLoS ONE* **2014**, *9*, e98679. [CrossRef] [PubMed]

187. Wilkens, S.J.; Janes, J.; Su, A.I. HierS: Hierarchical Scaffold Clustering using Topological Chemical Graphs. *J. Med. Chem.* **2005**, *48*, 3182–3193. [CrossRef] [PubMed]
188. Galitz, A.; Nakao, Y.; Schupp, P.J.; Wörheide, G.; Erpenbeck, D. A Soft Spot for Chemistry–Current Taxonomic and Evolutionary Implications of Sponge Secondary Metabolite Distribution. *Mar. Drugs* **2021**, *19*, 448. [CrossRef] [PubMed]
189. Gao, K.; Nguyen, D.D.; Sresht, V.; Mathiowetz, A.M.; Tu, M.; Wei, G.-W. Are 2D fingerprints still valuable for drug discovery? *Phys. Chem. Chem. Phys.* **2020**, *22*, 8373–8390. [CrossRef]
190. Hert, J.; Willett, P.; Wilton, D.J.; Acklin, P.; Azzaoui, K.; Jacoby, E.; Schuffenhauer, A. Comparison of topological descriptors for similarity-based virtual screening using multiple bioactive reference structures. *Org. Biomol. Chem.* **2004**, *2*, 3256–3266. [CrossRef]

marine drugs

MDPI

Article

Investigation of Marine-Derived Natural Products as Raf Kinase Inhibitory Protein (RKIP)-Binding Ligands

Shraddha Parate [1], Vikas Kumar [2], Jong Chan Hong [1,*] and Keun Woo Lee [2,*]

[1] Division of Applied Life Science, Plant Molecular Biology and Biotechnology Research Center (PMBBRC), Gyeongsang National University (GNU), 501 Jinju-daero, Jinju 52828, Korea; parateshraddha@gmail.com
[2] Division of Life Sciences, Department of Bio & Medical Big Data (BK4 Program), Research Institute of Natural Sciences (RINS), Gyeongsang National University (GNU), 501 Jinju-daero, Jinju 52828, Korea; vikaspathania777@gmail.com
* Correspondence: jchong@gnu.ac.kr (J.C.H.); kwlee@gnu.ac.kr (K.W.L.)

Abstract: Raf kinase inhibitory protein (RKIP) is an essential regulator of the Ras/Raf-1/MEK/ERK signaling cascade and functions by directly interacting with the Raf-1 kinase. The abnormal expression of RKIP is linked with numerous diseases including cancers, Alzheimer's and diabetic nephropathy. Interestingly, RKIP also plays an indispensable role as a tumor suppressor, thus making it an attractive therapeutic target. To date, only a few small molecules have been reported to modulate the activity of RKIP, and there is a need to explore additional scaffolds. In order to achieve this objective, a pharmacophore model was generated that explores the features of locostatin, the most potent RKIP modulator. Correspondingly, the developed model was subjected to screening, and the mapped compounds from Marine Natural Products (MNP) library were retrieved. The mapped MNPs after ensuing drug-likeness filtration were escalated for molecular docking, where locostatin was regarded as a reference. The MNPs exhibiting higher docking scores than locostatin were considered for molecular dynamics simulations, and their binding affinity towards RKIP was computed via MM/PBSA. A total of five molecules revealed significantly better binding free energy scores than compared to locostatin and, therefore, were reckoned as hits. The hits from the present in silico investigation could act as potent RKIP modulators and disrupt interactions of RKIP with its binding proteins. Furthermore, the identification of potent modulators from marine natural habitat can act as a future drug-discovery source.

Keywords: RKIP; marine natural products; pharmacophore modeling; virtual screening; molecular docking; molecular dynamics simulations; binding free energy

Citation: Parate, S.; Kumar, V.; Hong, J.C.; Lee, K.W. Investigation of Marine-Derived Natural Products as Raf Kinase Inhibitory Protein (RKIP)-Binding Ligands. *Mar. Drugs* **2021**, *19*, 581. https://doi.org/10.3390/md19100581

Academic Editors: Susana P. Gaudencio and Florbela Pereira

Received: 24 September 2021
Accepted: 14 October 2021
Published: 18 October 2021

1. Introduction

Raf kinase inhibitory protein (RKIP), also recognized as phosphatidylethanolamine-binding protein 1 (PEBP1), is an evolutionarily conserved, small (23 kDa) cytosolic protein, originally purified from bovine brain [1]. RKIP is broadly expressed in normal human tissues and identified to have an essential role in numerous physiological processes including neural development, spermatogenesis, cardiac output and membrane biosynthesis [2]. RKIP has been shown to be a vital modulator of various cell signaling cascades including the G protein-coupled receptor (GPCR), mitogen-activated protein kinase (MAPK) and the nuclear factor κB (NF-κB) pathways [1,2]. In particular, RKIP was acknowledged as an endogenous regulator of the kinases involved in the aforementioned pathways. RKIP binds specifically to the cytoplasmic serine/threonine Raf-1 kinase [3] and obstructs the Raf-1 dependent activation of MAPK/extracellular signal-regulated kinase (ERK) kinase (MEK), thereby disturbing the activation of ERK [4]. Additionally, RKIP indirectly hampers GPCR, which is an upstream activator of Raf-1. Therefore, when RKIP is released from Raf-1 after phosphorylation by protein kinase C (PKC) at the Ser153 residue, it associates with the kinase involved in the GPCR pathway, G protein-coupled receptor kinase 2 (GRK2) [5].

The phosphorylated RKIP/GRK2 association results in an enhanced activation of GPCR, thereby contributing to the overactivation of MAPK and downstream targets, as Raf-1 will no longer be inhibited by RKIP. Moreover, RKIP can act as a negative modulator of NF-κB signaling pathway by associating with upstream kinases NIK (NF-κB inducing kinase), TAK (transforming growth factor beta (TGFB)-activated kinase 1), IKKα (inhibitory-κ kinase α), IKKβ (inhibitory-κ kinase β) and inhibiting their kinase activity [4].

Owing to its essential role as an intracellular signaling pathway modulator, the dysregulated RKIP expression is implicated in several diseases, including cancer [6,7]. Literature reviews suggested the association of RKIP with prostate cancer [8], glioma [9], breast cancer [10], melanoma [11], colorectal cancer [12], lung cancer [13], thyroid cancer [14] and nasopharyngeal carcinoma [15]. Additionally, dysregulated PEBP1 expression was also observed to contribute to Alzheimer's disease (AD) [16] and diabetic nephropathy [1,2]. Interestingly, RKIP was also identified as being a metastasis suppressor [17]. Subsequently, RKIP has become a novel diagnostic marker for the associated pathologies. It is, therefore, imperative to search for RKIP agonists or inhibitors, which might aid in developing drugs to treat cell signaling-related abnormalities. The development of new probes for RKIP will help in the effort of perturbing RKIP's function and to define its seemingly conflicting roles.

Presently, only a few small molecules have been identified to modulate RKIP's role in pathological illnesses by binding to its conserved ligand-binding pocket. This pharmacological modulation has been accomplished through drugs encompassing Locostatin [18,19], pranlukast [20], clofazimine [21] and suramin [22] (Figure 1). The non-antibacterial oxazolidinone derivative, UIC-1005, was identified as a cell sheet migration inhibitor of RKIP [23] and later renamed as locostatin after its capability to inhibit cell locomotion in multiple systems [24]. In particular, locostatin abrogates the ability of RKIP to interact with Raf-1 kinase and also with GRK2, thereby functioning as a protein–protein interaction inhibitor [18,19]. Additionally, Sun et al. reported a novel RKIP-binding ligand, pranlukast, via structure-based virtual screening and demonstrated its binding on the conserved ligand-binding RKIP pocket through NMR and fluorescence experiments [20]. Guo et al. and team additionally identified Clofazimine and Suramin binding to RKIP through a combination of NMR and molecular docking [21,22].

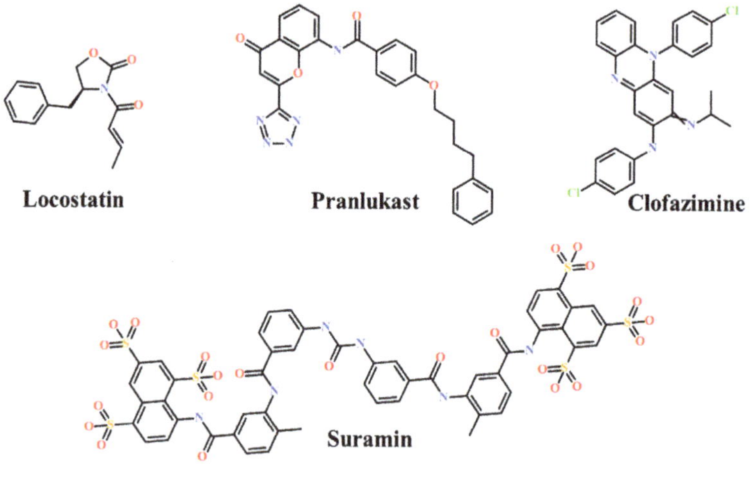

Figure 1. Chemical structures of small molecule RKIP modulators identified to date.

As secondary metabolites of microbes, plants, animals and marine organisms, natural products play predominant roles in self-defense, physiological homeostasis and propagation [25]. Moreover, they are prolific sources of active constituents in therapeutic drugs, featuring more structural diversity and complexity, fewer nitrogen or halogen atoms, more stereogenic centers and greater druggable pharmacophores than compared to synthetic molecules [26]. Marine organisms can be considered as the most abundant source of bioactive natural products as the diverse structures obtained from them reflect biodiversity of genes, species and ecosystems [27]. Drug discovery from marine natural products (MNP) has seen a resurgence in the past years with a growing number of molecules entering clinical trials [28,29]. A recent literature survey revealed strong anticancer biological activities concerning 170 MNPs and their semi-synthetic analogues [30]. MNPs have also exhibited neuroprotective effects on therapeutic targets of AD, Parkinson's disease (PD) and ischemic brain stroke [31].

The small number of RKIP-binding ligands in the literature and the structural diversity of compounds acquired from marine natural habitat prompted us to further explore potential therapeutics targeted for RKIP-related ailments. Accordingly, in the present in silico study, RKIP-binding ligands were identified via auto pharmacophore-based virtual screening of MNPs. Correspondingly, a pharmacophore model was generated by exploiting the features of a small molecule RKIP inhibitor, locostatin. Since locostatin has demonstrated exceptional results as an RKIP inhibitor, we intended to exploit the pharmacophore features manifested by its chemical scaffold. Subsequently, the attained model was escalated to screen the MNP library. The pharmacophore-mapped drug-like MNPs were further docked with the molecular structure of RKIP, and the compounds demonstrating better docking scores than locostatin were refined by computational simulations under physiological conditions. The MNPs exhibiting significantly better binding affinity scores than locostatin, as computed by Molecular Mechanics Poisson–Boltzmann Surface Area (MM/PBSA), were confirmed as hits and reported as potential therapeutics for RKIP-related diseases.

2. Results

The present investigation applied a sequence of computational methods for the identification of RKIP modulators via pharmacophore modeling from a single ligand structure of locostatin by using the below summarized workflow (Figure 2).

2.1. Generated Auto-Pharmacophore Model

A pharmacophore model was generated utilizing locostatin, the most potent RKIP inhibitor [18,19]. Prior to model generation, the *Feature Mapping* protocol in DS identified eight features encompassing four hydrogen bond acceptor (HBA), two hydrophobic (HyP) and two ring aromatic (RA) as the most occurring ones in locostatin. Subsequently, the generated model revealed a total of four features, with 2HBA, 1HyP and 1RA representing the most indispensable features of locostatin (Table 1). Upon scrupulous examination of the superimposed model on locostatin, it was observed that the 2-oxazolidinone core complements both the HBA features, the crotonyl moiety complements the HyP feature and the benzyl moiety complemented the RA feature [32] (Figure 3).

Table 1. Auto-pharmacophore model summary with its generated features.

Pharmacophore Model	Number of Features	Feature Set *
Pharmacophore hypothesis	4	2HBA, RA, HyP

* HBA: hydrogen bond acceptor; RA: ring aromatic; HyP: hydrophobic.

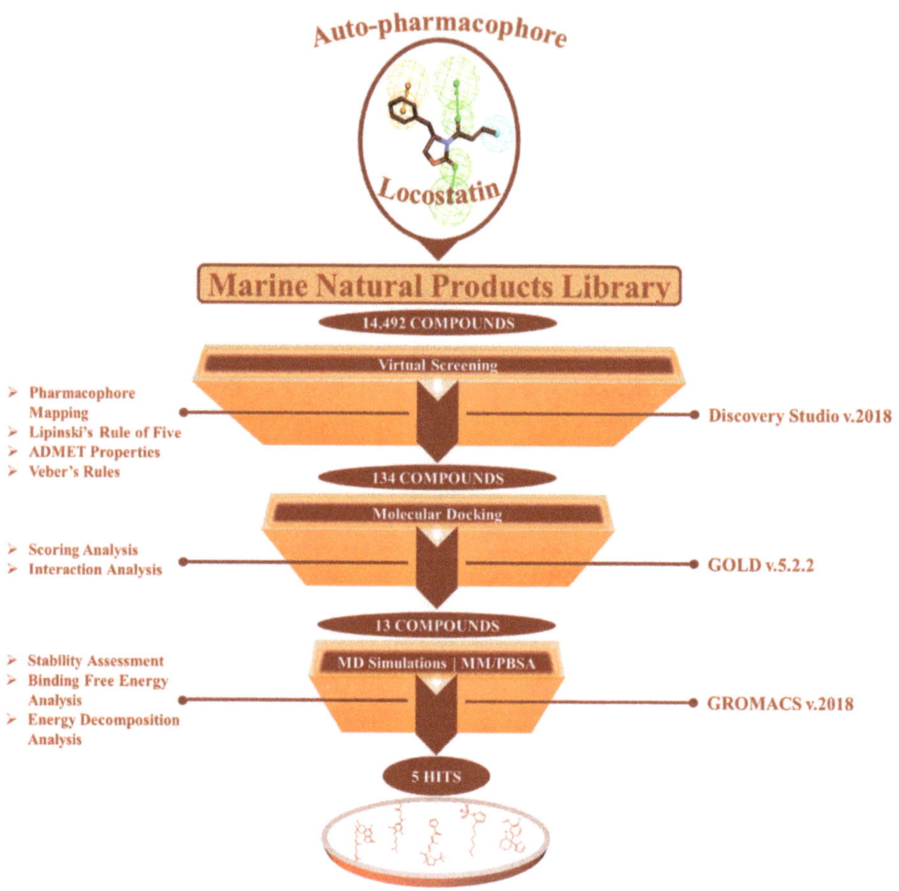

Figure 2. The in silico workflow depicting the sequence of computational techniques for identification of RKIP modulators.

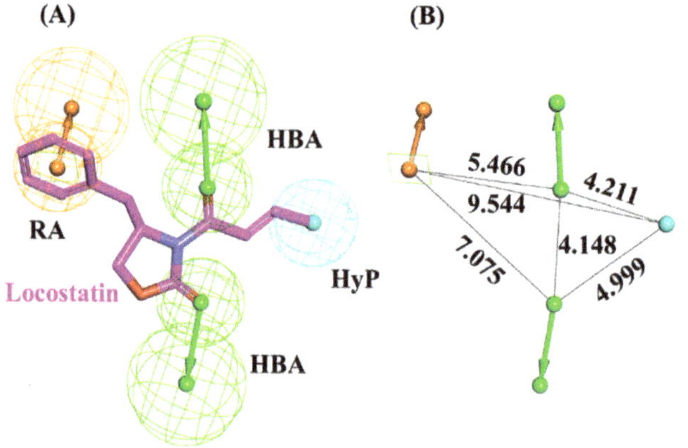

Figure 3. Auto-pharmacophore model exploiting locostatin. (**A**) Pharmacophore features demonstrated by locostatin- HBA (hydrogen bond acceptor), HyP (hydrophobic) and RA (ring aromatic). (**B**) Interfeature distance between the mapped features of locostatin.

2.2. Drug-Like Marine-Derived Compounds from Virtual Screening

From a total of 14,492 compounds available in the MNP library, the auto-pharmacophore model generated from the above analysis mapped an aggregate of 2557 MNPs representing the same features as acquired from locostatin. The large number of mapped compounds was further reduced by subsequent filtration on the basis of Lipinski's Rule of Five (Ro5) and Veber's rule. A total of 889 MNPs followed the collective Ro5 and Veber's rules demonstrating molecular weight <500 kDa, number of hydrogen bond donors ≤5, number of HBA ≤10, compound's lipophilicity (logP) ≤5 and number of rotatable bonds ≤10 [33,34]. Additionally, the evaluation of ADMET (absorption, distribution, metabolism, excretion and toxicity) properties further reduced the total number of compounds to 134 drug-like MNPs (Figure 2). These 134 MNPs displayed no blood–brain barrier (BBB) permeability, no CYP2D6 binding, no hepatotoxicity, good intestinal absorption and aqueous solubility. The procured 134 drug-like MNPs were escalated for molecular docking with the RKIP ligand-binding pocket.

2.3. Molecular Docking of Screening-Derived Compounds with RKIP

Molecular docking studies divulge into crucial information regarding the binding mode of ligands in the target protein pocket, thereby elucidating on the protein–ligand interaction. The validation of docking parameters resulted in reproducing similar docked poses as that observed for the co-crystallized PTR (Figure S1), establishing the efficiency of GOLD. The virtually screened 134 marine compounds were docked with RKIP along with locostatin as the reference (REF) compound. The REF compound demonstrated a Goldscore of 48.64 and a Chemscore of −26.48, while a total of thirteen drug-like MNPs exhibited higher Goldscores and lower Chemscores than compared to REF (Table 2). The thirteen compounds also displayed interactions with the key residues of RKIP ligand-binding pocket encompassing Asp70, Ala73, Pro74, Tyr81, Trp84, His86, Gly108, Gly110, Pro112, His118, Tyr120, Tyr181 and Leu184. Therefore, the stability of these compounds and the REF was confirmed in the RKIP ligand-binding pocket via processing them for molecular dynamics (MD) simulations.

Table 2. The docking scores of reference (REF) compound, locostatin and Marine Natural Product (MNP) library compounds with RKIP ligand-binding pocket (PDB ID: 2QYQ).

Compound No.	MNP ID (CAS No *)	Goldscore	Chemscore
1	62541-09-7	67.72	−33.37
2	799246-91-6	64.48	−31.02
3	383191-01-3	60.85	−28.18
4	313951-44-9	59.03	−35.95
5	61897-90-3	58.61	−27.03
6	302924-16-9	58.39	−29.14
7	182806-09-3	58.37	−27.80
8	587875-53-4	57.76	−28.71
9	142677-12-1	57.18	−35.13
10	144385-02-4	57.07	−30.29
11	853885-48-0	56.93	−27.96
12	853885-46-8	56.04	−34.01
13	58115-31-4	55.01	−37.15
14	133812-16-5 (REF)	48.64	−26.48

* CAS: Chemical Abstracts Service.

2.4. Molecular Dynamics Simulation Analyses

MD simulations were executed for the thirteen identified MNPs and REF, docked with RKIP, to elucidate their dynamic behavior at the physiological level. Along with performing MD simulations, the binding free energies (BFE) were also computed to assess the binding affinity of each ligand towards RKIP. This was instigated by the '*g_mmpbsa*' program, and the BFE scores of thirteen compounds were computed (Table S1). The REF compound, locostatin, exhibited a BFE score of −90.909 ± 9.155 kJ/mol, while five MNPs revealed better BFE scores. Therefore, the five MNPs were regarded as hits and were ranked according to their BFE scores (Table 3, Figure 4C).

Table 3. The entropic distribution of the total binding free energy (BFE) scores of reference (REF) compound, locostatin and identified hits from Marine Natural Products (MNP) library with RKIP (PDB ID: 2QYQ).

Hit No.	MNP ID (CAS No *)	Van Der Waals (kJ/mol)	Electrostatic (kJ/mol)	Polar Solvation (kJ/mol)	SASA Energy (kJ/mol)	BFE Scores ΔG_{bind} (kJ/mol)
HIT1	144385-02-4	−171.724 ± 13.242	−89.779 ± 8.171	143.371 ± 8.006	−17.151 ± 1.008	−135.283 ± 11.815
HIT2	799246-91-6	−159.666 ± 9.645	−66.487 ± 8.367	115.080 ± 11.961	−15.523 ± 0.756	−126.597 ± 8.883
HIT3	853885-46-8	−152.922 ± 10.576	−64.325 ± 7.461	117.843 ± 8.005	−15.684 ± 0.925	−115.088 ± 9.005
HIT4	383191-01-3	−144.389 ± 13.393	−68.213 ± 8.692	131.246 ± 6.782	−14.093 ± 0.641	−95.450±10.777
HIT5	587875-53-4	−118.918 ± 10.507	−78.010 ± 7.488	114.660 ± 4.794	−12.315 ± 0.793	−94.582 ± 8.703
HIT6	133812-16-5 (REF)	−149.624 ± 7.721	−62.839 ± 5.691	134.966 ± 6.467	−13.413 ± 0.628	−90.909 ± 9.155

* CAS: Chemical Abstracts Service.

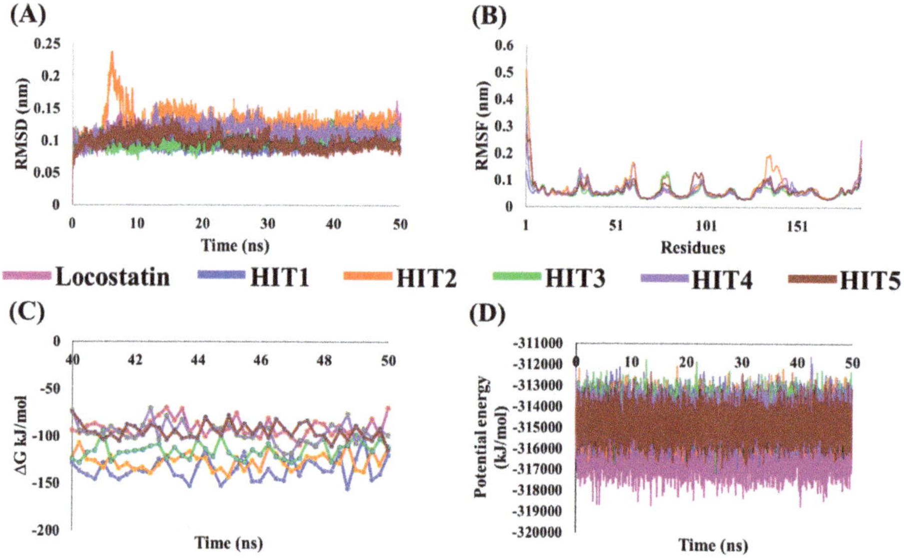

Figure 4. Molecular dynamics (MD) simulation analyses plots demonstrating the (**A**) backbone root mean square deviation (RMSD), (**B**) backbone root mean square fluctuation (RMSF), (**C**) binding free energy (ΔG_{bind}) values and (**D**) potential energy of the reference (REF) compound, locostatin and identified hits with RKIP.

The stability of hits and REF was determined on the basis of their backbone root mean square deviation (RMSD), root mean square fluctuation (RMSF) and potential energy plots. As perceived from the RMSD plots, it was observed that all the systems remained stable throughout the period of 50 ns, except for HIT2 which displayed slight instability towards the 6 ns (Figure 4A). The RMSF analysis also demonstrated the stability of all residues for the entire 50 ns of simulation run with an exception of HIT2, for which its residues (Asp134-Ser142) exhibited minor fluctuation (Figure 4B). Additionally, the energy of all the six systems remained stable as perceived from their potential energy plots (Figure 4D). In order to further gain insight into their mode of binding at the ligand-binding pocket of RKIP, the representative structures were extracted from the last 10 ns of stable MD trajectories and superimposed. The hits exhibited a similar binding mode as that observed for the locostatin (Figure 5).

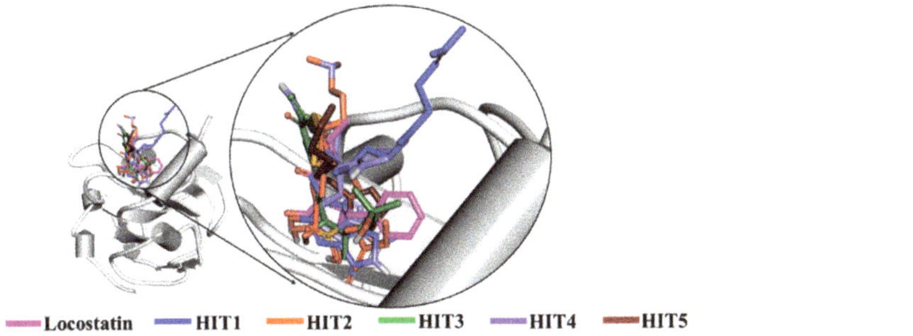

Figure 5. Binding mode of reference (REF) compound, locostatin and identified hits in the ligand-binding pocket of RKIP.

The characteristic binding interaction of the five hits and locostatin was examined on the basis of the average structure extracted from last 10 ns. The REF compound, locostatin, was observed to demonstrate one hydrogen bond with residue Tyr120 (bond length: 2.73 Å) (Figure 6A). In addition, REF also formed hydrophobic bonds with residues Trp84 (π–π stacked, bond length: 4.48 Å; π-alkyl, bond length: 4.97 Å), Val107 (π-alkyl, bond length: 5.05 Å) and Tyr181 (π–π T-shaped, bond length: 4.93 Å) (Figure S2A). The residues Asp70, Ala73, Pro74, Tyr81, His86, Gly108, Gly110, Pro111, Pro112, His118, Leu180 and Leu184 also supported locostatin, characterized by carbon–hydrogen bonds and van der Waals interactions (Figure S2A).

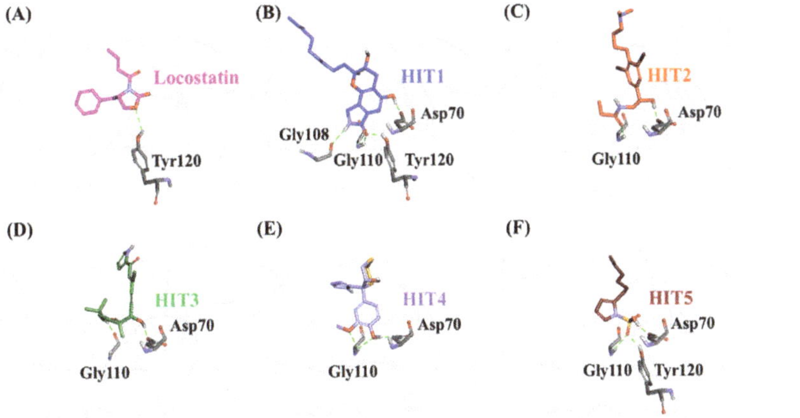

Figure 6. The three-dimensional (3D) intermolecular interactions of (**A**) reference (REF) compound, locostatin and the (**B**–**F**) identified hits with the key residues of RKIP. The hydrogen bonding interactions are displayed as dashed green lines.

The representative structure of HIT1 demonstrated hydrogen bonds with four RKIP residues: Asp70 (bond length: 1.70 Å), Gly108 (bond length: 2.28 Å), Gly110 (bond length: 1.86 Å) and Tyr120 (bond length: 1.80 Å) (Figure 6B). Additionally, HIT1 formed hydrophobic bonds with residues Trp84 (π–π stacked, bond length: 4.75 Å), Gly110 (amide π-stacked, bond length: 4.89 Å), Pro112 (alkyl, bond length: 4.51 Å), Tyr181 (π-alkyl, bond length: 4.10 Å) and Leu184 (alkyl, bond length: 5.13 Å) (Figure S2B). The residues Asp72, Ala73, Pro74, Tyr81, His86, Val107, Ser109, Pro111, His118, Gly143, Leu180 and Ser185 also assisted in the binding of HIT1 with RKIP via carbon–hydrogen bonds and van der Waals interactions (Figure S2B).

The average structure acquired for HIT2 exhibited hydrogen bonds with two RKIP residues: Asp70 (bond length: 1.68 Å) and Gly110 (bond length: 2.09 Å) (Figure 6C). Moreover, HIT2 exhibited hydrophobic interactions with Ala 73 (alkyl, bond length: 4.31 Å; π-alkyl, bond length: 5.17 Å), Pro74 (alkyl, bond length: 4.08 Å), Tyr81 (π-sigma, bond length: 3.74 Å), Trp84 (π-alkyl, bond length: 4.71 Å; π-alkyl, bond length: 5.28 Å; π-alkyl, bond length: 4.17 Å), Pro112 (π-alkyl, bond length: 5.09 Å) and Tyr181 (π-alkyl, bond length: 4.62 Å; π-alkyl, bond length: 5.40 Å) residues (Figure S2C). The carbon–hydrogen bonds, π-donor hydrogen bonds and van der Waals interactions with residues Pro74, Trp84, His86, Val107, Gly108, Ser109, Pro111, His118 and Tyr120 also played a vital role in supporting HIT2 in RKIP binding pocket (Figure S2C).

The representative HIT3 structure displayed hydrogen bonds with Asp70 (bond length: 1.69 Å) and Gly110 (bond length: 1.69 Å) (Figure 6D). The residues Pro74 (alkyl, bond length: 4.28 Å), Tyr81 (π-alkyl, bond length: 5.23 Å), Trp84 (π-alkyl, bond lengths: 3.53 Å and 4.46 Å), His86 (π-alkyl, bond lengths: 4.50 Å and 4.96 Å) and Tyr120 (π-alkyl, bond length: 5.38 Å) established hydrophobic bonds with RKIP (Figure S2D). Furthermore, residues Ala73, Val107, Ser109, Pro111, Pro112, His118, Val177, Leu180, Tyr181 and Leu184 also held a crucial role in assisting HIT3 via van der Waals interactions (Figure S2D).

The structure for HIT4, extracted as representative, exhibited hydrogen bonds with Asp70 (bond length: 1.68 Å) and Gly110 (bond lengths: 2.46 Å and 2.57 Å), similar to HIT2 and HIT3 (Figure 6E). Numerous types of hydrophobic bonds were formed by residues- Ala73 (π-alkyl, bond length: 4.98 Å), Tyr81 (π-alkyl, bond length: 4.95 Å), Trp84 (π-π stacked, bond length: 4.90 Å), Gly110 (amide-π stacked, bond length: 4.05 Å), Pro112 (alkyl, bond length: 5.49 Å) and Tyr181 (π–π T-shaped, bond length: 4.66 Å) (Figure S2E). The residue His86 established a carbon–hydrogen bond, while Val107, Gly108, Ser109, Pro111, His118, Tyr120, Leu180 and Leu184 interacted via van der Waals bonds (Figure S2E).

The representative structure of HIT5 attained from MD analysis showed hydrogen bonds with residues Asp70 (bond length: 1.62 Å), Gly110 (bond length: 2.42 Å) and Tyr120 (bond length: 1.96 Å) (Figure 6F). The residues Trp84 (π–π stacked, bond length: 4.77 Å) and His86 (π-sulfur, bond length: 5.22 Å) established hydrophobic bonds (Figure S2F). Additional residues including His86, Pro112 and His118 supported HIT5 via carbon–hydrogen bonds, while numerous residues such as Ala73, Pro74, Tyr81, Pro111, Tyr181 and Leu184 formed van der Waals interactions (Figure S2F).

The above overall analyses suggests that our hits displayed stability throughout 50 ns of MD run and also formed interactions with vital residues of the RKIP ligand-binding pocket. Most importantly, our hits demonstrated better binding affinity towards RKIP, as observed from their binding free energies. We, therefore, anticipate that our identified hits can provide potential scaffolds as RKIP agonists or inhibitors.

3. Discussion

RKIP/PEBP1 is involved in regulating several signaling pathways including Raf-1/MEK/ERK, NF-κB and GPCR by directly interacting with and inhibiting Raf-1, MEK and ERK protein kinases of the pathways, respectively [35]. RKIP was identified to contribute to dysregulated expression in numerous diseases as well as recognized as being a metastasis suppressor [17]. Only a few RKIP modulators have been identified to date encompassing locostatin, pranlukast, clofazimine and suramin (Figure 1), and there is still a need to search for additional ligands modulating the function of RKIP. Taking these views into account, we pursued our research towards exploring the features of the most potent cell sheet migration inhibitor of RKIP, locostatin [19]. As the X-ray crystallographic structure of RKIP/locostatin is difficult to obtain owing to locostatin's function to partially aggregate in vitro [18,19], the single structure of locostatin was adapted for our study. Therefore, an auto-pharmacophore model of locostatin was generated, which resulted in a four-featured model (Figure 3). Since marine extracts have displayed a remarkable potential as being a source of new drugs and is a relatively unexplored habitat, a MNP library of 14,492 compounds by Prof. Encinar (http://docking.umh.es/chemlib/mnplib accessed on 21 June 2021) was utilized for our study. Consequently, the library was screened using the pharmacophore model, retrieving a total of 2557 compounds that mapped the features of the pharmacophore. A drug-like database was generated from the above large number of compounds by employing Lipinski's Ro5, ADMET and Veber's rules, reducing the number to 134 compounds. The 134 drug-like compounds were taken forward for molecular docking with the crystal structure of RKIP in complex with o-phosphotyrosine (PTR) (PDB ID: 2QYQ) [36]. The RKIP/PTR is the first molecular structure providing a model of how a ligand would possibly bind in the ligand-binding pocket of RKIP [18]. Molecular docking of aforementioned 134 drug-like ligands into the binding pocket of RKIP resulted in the identification of thirteen compounds, which demonstrated better docking scores (Goldscore and Chemscore) than locostatin (Table 2). Moreover, the thirteen compounds also displayed similar interactions with RKIP, as observed for locostatin. Although molecular docking is computationally proficient, its prediction of the protein-ligand binding pose is not usually accurate. Therefore, these compounds were escalated to check their stability in the RKIP binding pocket via MD simulations. The simulations were also supplemented by calculating the binding affinity of each compound towards RKIP, and this was performed via MM/PBSA. The MM/PBSA method has been extensively used to gauge the poses from docking, determine their stability, predict the affinity towards the target protein and also to identify the hotspots responsible for the affinity [37]. From a total of thirteen drug-like compounds, five exhibited better binding affinities towards RKIP than that of locostatin (Table S1). With the locostatin BFE value of −90.909 kJ/mol, HIT1, HIT2, HIT3, HIT4 and HIT5 demonstrated the values of −135.283 kJ/mol, −126.597 kJ/mol, −115.088 kJ/mol, −95.450 kJ/mol and −94.582 kJ/mol, respectively (Table 3). The total number of free energy scores for each RKIP/HIT complex was characterized by individual scores of van der Waals, electrostatic, polar solvation and SASA energy. It was observed that the van der Waals and electrostatic forces played a major role in total binding free energy, thereby explaining that the van der Waals and hydrophobic interactions have a vital role in assisting the binding of hits with RKIP. From the RMSD, RMSF and potential energy analysis, it was perceived that our hits also remained stable in the binding pocket of RKIP (Figure 4). The representative structure was extracted from the last 10 ns of stable trajectory for all hits as well as locostatin, and the interaction pattern was scrutinized. Literature survey revealed that the conserved ligand-binding pocket of RKIP can be defined by 16 residues at the protein surface: Asp70, Ala73, Pro74, Tyr81, Trp84, His86, Val107, Gly108, Gly110, Pro111, Pro112, His118, Tyr120, Leu180, Tyr181 and Leu184 [38]. In the present study, our hits were observed to form bonds with the above-mentioned residues, characterized by hydrogen, hydrophobic and van der Waals interactions. Most notably, hydrogen bonds were perceived with residues Asp70, Gly108, Gly110 and Tyr120 of the RKIP binding pocket (Figure 6). Furthermore, interactions with residues Ala73, Pro74, Tyr81, His86, Val107, Gly108, Pro111, Pro112, His118, Leu180, Tyr181 and Leu184 were mostly driven by van der Waals, hydrophobic or carbon–hydrogen bonds (Figure S2). In order to identify the individual residues contributing considerably to the total binding free energy of each compound, the per-residue energy decomposition was estimated by MM/PBSA. The residues Trp84 and Tyr181 appeared to play an indispensable role in the affinity of all hits towards RKIP (Figure 7). These two residues were also identified as major contributing factors by Rudnitskaya et al. for RKIP/locostatin binding by MD simulation and quantum mechanics/molecular mechanics (QM/MM) [19]. The above overall analyses provide ample support for our hits as potential lead molecules to modulate RKIP. Individually, the identified hits portrayed the pharmacophoric features displayed by locostatin (Figures 3 and S3).

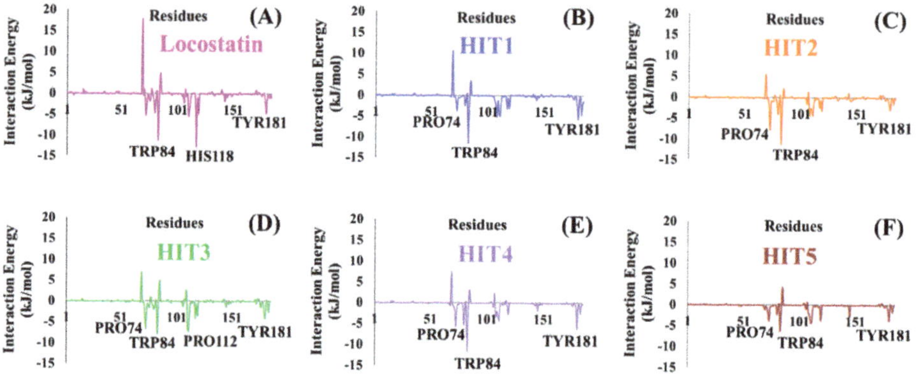

Figure 7. Energy decomposition of individual residues in RKIP contributing to the total binding free energy of (**A**) Locostatin, (**B**) HIT1, (**C**) HIT2, (**D**) HIT3, (**E**) HIT4 and (**F**) HIT5, computed by MM/PBSA.

As a final evaluation and on the basis of IUPAC names of thirteen drug-like compounds (Table S1), their source of origin was identified (Table 4). The hit compounds-HIT1, HIT2 and HIT5 were identified as alkaloids derived from a fungus *Stachybotrys* sp. [39], sponge *Psammaplysilla purpurea* [40] and annelid *Cirriformia tentaculata* [41], respectively. HIT3 was identified as a metabolite of a marine sediment and obtained from *Streptomyces* sp. [42], while HIT4 was isolated from the ascidian *Hypsistozoa fasmeriana* [42]. The chemical names and the source of additional molecules which demonstrated less binding free energy scores towards RKIP were also identified and reported in our study (Table 4). Overall, we believe that our hits can be utilized as potential alternatives to modulate the role of RKIP. Even though the experimental validation is required to validate our findings, auto-pharmacophore modeling from a single structure of a ligand can be helpful for designing potent molecules with similar efficacies. Additionally, our study represents a crucial platform for future drug optimization strategies from aquatic habitat.

Table 4. Molecular structures and chemical source of identified marine-derived drug-like compounds.

HIT/CAS No *	Chemical Name (Source)	Reference	Molecular Structure
HIT1 (144385-02-4)	Stachybotrin B (*Stachybotrys* sp.)	[39]	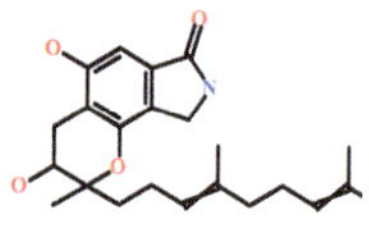
HIT2 (799246-91-6)	Purpurealidin G (*Psammaplysilla purpurea*)	[40]	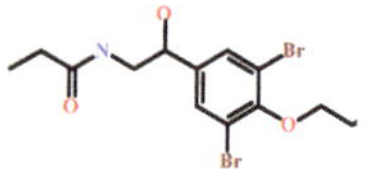
HIT3 (853885-46-8)	Glaciapyrrole A (*Streptomyces* sp.)	[42,43]	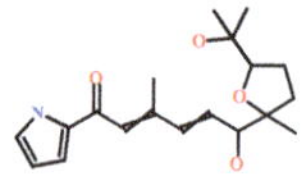
HIT4 (383191-01-3)	(*Hypsistozoa fasmeriana*)	[42]	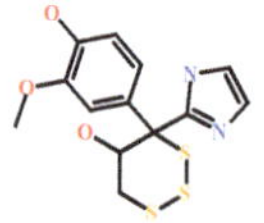

Table 4. *Cont.*

HIT/CAS No *	Chemical Name (Source)	Reference	Molecular Structure
HIT5 (587875-53-4)	2-Hexylpyrrole sulfamate (*Cirriformia tentaculata*)	[41,42]	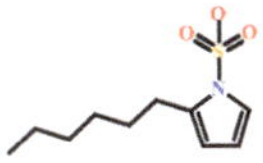
58115-31-4	Aurantiamide	[44]	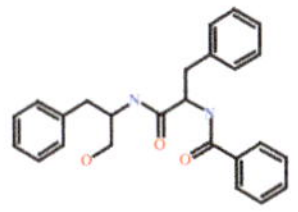
182806-09-3	Hemibastadinol 1 (*Ianthella basta*)	[45]	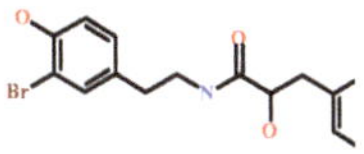
61897-90-3	Fumitremorgin H. (*Aspergillus fumigatus*)	[42]	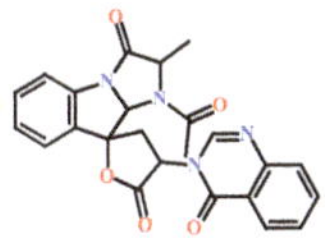
142677-12-1	(*Chondria* sp.)	[46]	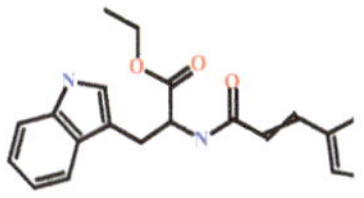
313951-44-9	Lorneamide A	[46,47]	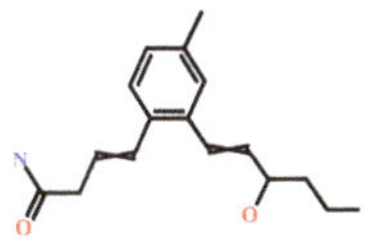
302924-16-9	Secobipinnatin J (*Pseudopterogorgia bipinnata*)	[42]	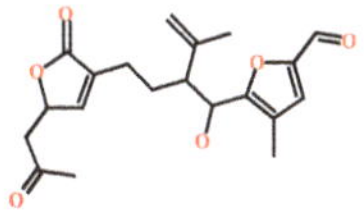
853885-48-0	Glaciapyrrole B (*Streptomyces* sp.)	[42,43]	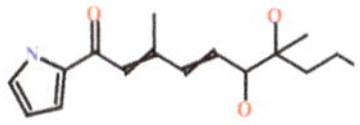
62541-09-7	Dehydrocoelenterazine (*Watasenia dehydropreluciferin*)	[42]	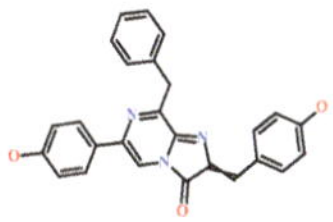

* CAS: Chemical Abstracts Service.

4. Materials and Methods

4.1. Auto-Pharmacophore Model Generation

Locostatin is a well-known inhibitor of cell migration and cell–substratum adhesion, covalently binding RKIP and disrupting its association with Raf-1 kinase as well as GRK2 [19]. The α,β-unsaturated carbonyl functionality of locostatin renders it potently reactive towards RKIP and sterically hinders the binding of other ligands in the pocket [18]. Therefore, the chemical features shared by its 2-oxazolidinone core were exploited by employing the *Auto Pharmacophore Generation* module in Discovery Studio (DS) v.2018 (Accelrys Inc. San Diego, CA, USA). This module predominantly considers the hydrogen bond acceptor (HBA), hydrogen bond donor (HBD), hydrophobic (HyP), negative ionizable (NEG_IONIZABLE), positive ionizable (POS_IONIZABLE) and ring aromatic (RA) features to generate a selective pharmacophore model from a single ligand. Moreover, the module elects the pharmacophore with the highest selectivity depending on the prediction by Genetic Function Approximation (GFA) model.

4.2. Virtual Screening of Marine-Derived Natural Products

The auto-pharmacophore model generated from the above step was utilized as a 3D-query to retrieve the compounds, complementing the features of the model, from a Marine Natural Products (MNP) library. The MNP library comprising a total of 14,492 natural compounds was screened using the generated model by employing the *Ligand Pharmacophore Mapping module* in DS [48]. The resulting MNPs complementing the pharmacophore features were filtered by Lipinski's Rule of Five (Ro5) [33,49] and Veber's rules [34], followed by further filtering their absorption, distribution, metabolism, excretion and toxicity (ADMET) properties. Accordingly, the *Filter by Lipinski and Veber Rules* and *ADMET Descriptors* modules implanted in DS were employed for retrieving the drug-like MNPs. Subsequently, the obtained drug-like MNPs were escalated for the next process of molecular docking with the ligand-binding pocket of RKIP.

4.3. Molecular Docking of Drug-Like Molecules with RKIP Ligand-Binding Pocket

Molecular docking techniques are established in silico methods that are applied widely in drug discovery for identifying novel compounds of therapeutic interest and predicting their interactions within the catalytic sites of macromolecular target proteins [50]. The drug-like MNPs acquired from the above virtual screening were further subjected to molecular docking with the crystal structure of RKIP (PDB ID: 2QYQ) [36] in Genetic Optimisation for Ligand Docking (GOLD) v5.2.2 docking software (CCDC software ltd., Cambridge, UK) [51]. The drug-like MNPs were assessed on the basis of two default scoring functions, implanted in GOLD-Goldscore and Chemscore [52–54]. Prior to docking, the retrieved 3D crystallographic RKIP structure was prepared by employing the *Clean Protein* module in DS and further removing the water molecules as well as the bound o-phosphotyrosine (PTR). Consequently, both the RKIP protein structure and drug-like MNPs were minimized by employing the *Minimization* and *Minimize Ligands* modules in DS [55]. A total of 50 conformers per ligand were allowed to generate for the drug-like MNPs and locostatin, which was considered as reference (REF). Each compound was examined on the basis of its obtained conformation in the largest cluster, high Goldscore, low Chemscore and molecular interactions with the vital residues of the RKIP binding pocket. Only the drug-like MNPs demonstrating better scores than locostatin and similar interactions were retained from this process and escalated for molecular dynamics (MD) simulation studies.

4.4. Molecular Dynamics Simulation of Identified Marine-Derived Natural Products

MD simulation studies are widely used to provide the dynamical structural information on biomacromolecules as well as knowledge about protein–ligand interactions at the physiological level [56]. The docked complexes resulting from the above docking process were subjected to MD simulations with GROningen MAchine for Chemical Simulations (GROMACS) v2018 (University of Groningen, Netherlands; Royal Institute of Technology; Uppsala University, Uppsala, Sweden) [57]. The topologies for RKIP and the compounds were generated with CHARMm27 force field [58] and SwissParam (Swiss Institute of Bioinformatics) [59] fast force field generation tool, respectively. The solvation of all systems was performed via a dodecahedron water box and TIP3P (transferable intermolecular potential with 3 points) water model. Further neutralization of systems was carried out by supplementing them with Cl^- ions. Bad contacts in the systems were dodged by performing initial energy minimization followed by a two-step equilibration. The first step encompassed the NVT (constant number of particles, volume and temperature) equilibration at 300 K with a V-rescale thermostat for 500 ps. The second step involved NPT (constant number of particles, pressure and temperature) equilibration at 1 bar pressure with a Parrinello–Rahman barostat for 1000 ps [60]. Two algorithms, namely the LINear Constraint Solver (LINCS) [61] and SETTLE [62], were employed in order to monitor bond constraints and the geometry of water molecules. The long-range electrostatic interactions were computed by an $N \cdot \log(N)$ method known as Particle mesh Ewald (PME) [63]. The systems after equilibration by both NVT and NPT were subjected to production simulation runs of 50 ns each. The results acquired after the production run were visualized in visual molecular dynamics (VMD, University of Illinois, Urbana, IL, USA) in order to interpret the stability of ligands in the RKIP pocket throughout the run [64]. Furthermore, the stability of all systems was also assessed by plotting their root mean square deviation (RMSD), root mean square fluctuation (RMSF) and potential energy plots for the entire 50 ns run [65].

4.5. Binding Free Energy Calculations of Identified Hits

The estimation of binding affinities of inhibitors with their macromolecular targets plays a quintessential role in drug discovery [66]. The binding free energy (BFE) estimation program, compatible with GROMACS, was utilized to predict the binding affinity of each ligand with RKIP. The molecular mechanics/Poisson–Boltzmann surface area (MM/PBSA) program is extensively utilized in drug discovery paradigms to compute the BFE of protein–ligand complexes and has been revealed to be a precise estimator in terms of correlation between experimental and theoretical values [67,68]. For computing this BFE, 25 snapshots of RKIP-ligand complexes were selected evenly from 40 to 50 ns of MD trajectories, and the resultant energy ΔG_{bind} was calculated on the basis of the following equation.

$$\Delta G_{bind} = G_{complex} - \left(G_{protein} + G_{ligand}\right) \quad (1)$$

The resulting RKIP-compound complexes with better BFE scores than RKIP-locostatin were considered as hits from the present in silico investigation.

5. Conclusions

An auto-pharmacophore model, exploiting the features of the most potent RKIP inhibitor, locostatin, revealed key pharmacophoric features imperative for binding RKIP. An orderly virtual screening process with the generated model as a 3D query, retrieved 2557 compounds from the Marine Natural Products (MNP) library and consequent filtration by Lipinski's, Veber's and ADMET was able to procure a total of 134 drug-like MNPs. The process of molecular docking of drug-like MNPs with the ligand-binding pocket of RKIP resulted in thirteen compounds with better docking scores than locostatin as well as noteworthy intermolecular interactions with vital residues of the pocket. From a total of thirteen compounds, only five demonstrated better binding free energy scores towards RKIP than that obtained for locostatin. Therefore, the five compounds were deemed as hit molecules from the current analysis. The per-residue energy contribution unveiled Trp84 as the most significant residue contributing to binding affinity towards RKIP. The biological origins of all thirteen compounds acquired from the present investigation was identified as either marine sponge, coral or fungus. Above all, we believe that our marine-derived hits provide scaffolds for future drug optimization studies against RKIP-related diseases. In conclusion, bioactive compounds from marine natural origin provide diverse scaffolds and represent a crucial platform for imminent drug discovery against various pathological complications.

Supplementary Materials: The following are available online at https://www.mdpi.com/article/10.3390/md19100581/s1, Figure S1: Validation of GOLD docking parameters using co-crystallized ligand, PTR (orange) and its docked pose (pink). Figure S2: The two-dimensional (2D) intermolecular interactions of reference (REF) compound, locostatin and the identified hits with the key residues of RKIP. Figure S3: The mapping of identified Marine Natural Products (MNP) hits onto the generated pharmacophore model. All hits display the hydrogen bond acceptor (HBA), hydrophobic (HyP) and ring aromatic (RA) pharmacophoric features. Table S1: The binding free energy (BFE) scores of reference (REF) locostatin and drug-like Marine Natural Products (MNP) with RKIP (PDB ID: 2QYQ) along with their IUPAC names.

Author Contributions: Conceptualization, S.P.; methodology, S.P.; software, S.P.; validation, S.P.; formal analysis, S.P. and V.K.; investigation, S.P.; resources, K.W.L.; data curation, S.P.; writing—original draft preparation, S.P.; writing—review and editing, S.P.; visualization, S.P.; supervision, K.W.L. and J.C.H.; project administration, K.W.L.; funding acquisition, J.C.H. All authors have read and agreed to the published version of the manuscript.

Funding: This research was supported by Basic Science Research Program through the National Research Foundation of Korea (NRF) funded by the Ministry of Education (2020R1A6A1A03044344).

Institutional Review Board Statement: Not applicable.

Informed Consent Statement: Not applicable.

Data Availability Statement: Data are contained within the article.

Conflicts of Interest: The authors declare no conflict of interest.

References

1. Al-Mulla, F.; Bitar, M.S.; Taqi, Z.; Yeung, K.C. RKIP: Much more than Raf Kinase inhibitory protein. *J. Cell. Physiol.* **2013**, *228*, 1688–1702. [CrossRef]
2. Keller, E.T.; Fu, Z.; Brennan, M. The role of Raf kinase inhibitor protein (RKIP) in health and disease. *Biochem. Pharmacol.* **2004**, *68*, 1049–1053.
3. Parate, S.; Rampogu, S.; Lee, G.; Hong, J.C.; Lee, K.W. Exploring the Binding Interaction of Raf Kinase Inhibitory Protein With the N-Terminal of C-Raf Through Molecular Docking and Molecular Dynamics Simulation. *Front. Mol. Biosci.* **2021**, *8*, 1. [CrossRef] [PubMed]
4. Gabriela-Freitas, M.; Pinheiro, J.; Raquel-Cunha, A.; Cardoso-Carneiro, D.; Martinho, O. Rkip as an inflammatory and immune system modulator: Implications in cancer. *Biomolecules* **2019**, *9*, 769. [CrossRef]
5. Lorenz, K.; Lohse, M.J.; Quitterer, U. Protein kinase C switches the Raf kinase inhibitor from Raf-1 to GRK-2. *Nature* **2003**, *426*, 574–579. [CrossRef]
6. Farooqi, A.A.; Li, Y.; Sarkar, F.H. The biological complexity of RKIP signaling in human cancers. *Exp. Mol. Med.* **2015**, *47*, e185. [CrossRef]
7. Yesilkanal, A.E.; Rosner, M.R. Targeting raf kinase inhibitory protein regulation and function. *Cancers* **2018**, *10*, 306. [CrossRef]
8. Fu, Z.; Kitagawa, Y.; Shen, R.; Shah, R.; Mehra, R.; Rhodes, D.; Keller, P.J.; Mizokami, A.; Dunn, R.; Chinnaiyan, A.M.; et al. Metastasis suppressor gene Raf kinase inhibitor protein (RKIP) is a novel prognostic marker in prostate cancer. *Prostate* **2006**, *66*, 248–256. [CrossRef] [PubMed]
9. Martinho, O.; Granja, S.; Jaraquemada, T.; Caeiro, C.; Miranda-Gonçalves, V.; Honavar, M.; Costa, P.; Damasceno, M.; Rosner, M.R.; Lopes, J.M.; et al. Downregulation of RKIP is associated with poor outcome and malignant progression in gliomas. *PLoS ONE* **2012**, *7*, e30769. [CrossRef] [PubMed]
10. Hagan, S.; Al-Mulla, F.; Mallon, E.; Oien, K.; Ferrier, R.; Gusterson, B.; Curto García, J.J.; Kolch, W. Reduction of Raf-1 kinase inhibitor protein expression correlates with breast cancer metastasis. *Clin. Cancer Res.* **2005**, *11*, 7392–7397. [CrossRef] [PubMed]
11. Schuierer, M.M.; Bataille, F.; Hagan, S.; Kolch, W.; Bosserhoff, A.K. Reduction in Raf kinase inhibitor protein expression is associated with increased Ras-extracellular signal-regulated kinase signaling in melanoma cell lines. *Cancer Res.* **2004**, *64*, 5186–5192. [CrossRef] [PubMed]
12. Wang, Y.; Wang, L.Y.; Feng, F.; Zhao, Y.; Huang, M.Y.; Shao, Q.; Chen, C.; Sheng, H.; Chen, D.L.; Zeng, Z.L.; et al. Effect of Raf kinase inhibitor protein expression on malignant biological behavior and progression of colorectal cancer. *Oncol. Rep.* **2015**, *34*, 2106–2114. [CrossRef] [PubMed]
13. Wang, A.; Duan, G.; Zhao, C.; Gao, Y.; Liu, X.; Wang, Z.; Li, W.; Wang, K.; Wang, W. Reduced RKIP expression levels are associated with frequent non-small cell lung cancer metastasis and STAT3 phosphorylation and activation. *Oncol. Lett.* **2017**, *13*, 3039–3045. [CrossRef]
14. Kim, H.S.; Kim, G.Y.; Lim, S.J.; Kim, Y.W. Raf-1 kinase inhibitory protein expression in thyroid carcinomas. *Endocr. Pathol.* **2010**, *21*, 253–257. [CrossRef] [PubMed]
15. Yuan, L.; Yi, H.M.; Yi, H.; Qu, J.Q.; Zhu, J.F.; Li, L.N.; Xiao, T.; Zheng, Z.; Lu, S.S.; Xiao, Z.Q. Reduced RKIP enhances nasopharyngeal carcinoma radioresistance by increasing ERK and AKT activity. *Oncotarget* **2016**, *7*, 11463–11477. [CrossRef] [PubMed]
16. George, A.J.; Holsinger, R.M.D.; McLean, C.A.; Tan, S.S.; Scott, H.S.; Cardamone, T.; Cappai, R.; Masters, C.L.; Li, Q.X. Decreased phosphatidylethanolamine binding protein expression correlates with Aβ accumulation in the Tg2576 mouse model of Alzheimer's disease. *Neurobiol. Aging* **2006**, *27*, 614–623. [CrossRef]
17. Granovsky, A.E.; Rosner, M.R. Raf kinase inhibitory protein: A signal transduction modulator and metastasis suppressor. *Cell Res.* **2008**, *18*, 452–457. [CrossRef]

18. Beshir, A.B.; Argueta, C.E.; Menikarachchi, L.C.; Gascón, J.A.; Fenteany, G. Locostatin disrupts association of Raf kinase inhibitor protein with binding proteins by modifying a conserved histidine residue in the ligand-binding pocket. *For. Immunopathol. Dis. Therap.* **2011**, *2*, 47–58. [CrossRef] [PubMed]
19. Rudnitskaya, A.N.; Eddy, N.A.; Fenteany, G.; Gascón, J.A. Recognition and reactivity in the binding between Raf kinase inhibitor protein and its small-molecule inhibitor locostatin. *J. Phys. Chem. B* **2012**, *116*, 10176–10181. [CrossRef] [PubMed]
20. Sun, T.; Wu, Z.; Luo, M.; Lin, D.; Guo, C. Pranlukast, a novel binding ligand of human Raf1 kinase inhibitory protein. *Biotechnol. Lett.* **2016**, *38*, 1375–1380. [CrossRef]
21. Guo, C.; Chang, T.; Sun, T.; Wu, Z.; Dai, Y.; Yao, H.; Lin, D. Anti-leprosy drug Clofazimine binds to human Raf1 kinase inhibitory protein and enhances ERK phosphorylation. *Acta Biochim. Biophys. Sin.* **2018**, *50*, 1062–1067. [CrossRef] [PubMed]
22. Guo, C.; Wu, Z.; Lin, W.; Xu, H.; Chang, T.; Dai, Y.; Lin, D. Suramin Targets the Conserved Ligand-Binding Pocket of Human Raf1 Kinase Inhibitory Protein. *Molecules* **2021**, *26*, 1151. [CrossRef]
23. Mc Henry, K.T.; Ankala, S.V.; Ghosh, A.K.; Fenteany, G. A Non-Antibacterial Oxazolidinone Derivative that Inhibits Epithelial Cell Sheet Migration. *ChemBioChem* **2002**, *3*, 1105–1111. [CrossRef]
24. Zhu, S.; Mc Henry, K.T.; Lane, W.S.; Fenteany, G. A chemical inhibitor reveals the role of Raf kinase inhibitor protein in cell migration. *Chem. Biol.* **2005**, *12*, 981–991. [CrossRef]
25. Atanasov, A.G.; Zotchev, S.B.; Dirsch, V.M.; Orhan, I.E.; Banach, M.; Rollinger, J.M.; Barreca, D.; Weckwerth, W.; Bauer, R.; Bayer, E.A.; et al. Natural products in drug discovery: Advances and opportunities. *Nat. Rev. Drug Discov.* **2021**, *20*, 200–216. [CrossRef]
26. Bauer, R.A.; Wurst, J.M.; Tan, D.S. Expanding the range of "druggable" targets with natural product-based libraries: An academic perspective. *Curr. Opin. Chem. Biol.* **2010**, *14*, 308–314. [CrossRef]
27. Jiménez, C. Marine Natural Products in Medicinal Chemistry. *ACS Med. Chem. Lett.* **2018**, *9*, 959–961. [CrossRef]
28. Molinski, T.F.; Dalisay, D.S.; Lievens, S.L.; Saludes, J.P. Drug development from marine natural products. *Nat. Rev. Drug Discov.* **2009**, *8*, 69–85. [CrossRef] [PubMed]
29. Shinde, P.; Banerjee, P.; Mandhare, A. Marine natural products as source of new drugs: A patent review (2015–2018). *Expert Opin. Ther. Pat.* **2019**, *29*, 283–309. [CrossRef] [PubMed]
30. Matulja, D.; Wittine, K.; Malatesti, N.; Laclef, S.; Turks, M.; Markovic, M.K.; Ambrožić, G.; Marković, D. Marine Natural Products with High Anticancer Activities. *Curr. Med. Chem.* **2020**, *27*, 1243–1307. [CrossRef] [PubMed]
31. Choi, D.Y.; Choi, H. Natural products from marine organisms with neuroprotective activity in the experimental models of Alzheimer's disease, Parkinson's disease and ischemic brain stroke: Their molecular targets and action mechanisms. *Arch. Pharm. Res.* **2015**, *38*, 139–170. [CrossRef]
32. Shemon, A.N.; Eves, E.M.; Clark, M.C.; Heil, G.; Granovsky, A.; Zeng, L.; Imamoto, A.; Koide, S.; Rosner, M.R. Raf kinase inhibitory protein protects cells against locostatin-mediated inhibition of migration. *PLoS ONE* **2009**, *4*, e6028. [CrossRef] [PubMed]
33. Lipinski, C.A. Lead- and drug-like compounds: The rule-of-five revolution. *Drug Discov. Today Technol.* **2004**, *1*, 337–341. [CrossRef]
34. Veber, D.F.; Johnson, S.R.; Cheng, H.Y.; Smith, B.R.; Ward, K.W.; Kopple, K.D. Molecular properties that influence the oral bioavailability of drug candidates. *J. Med. Chem.* **2002**, *45*, 2615–2623. [CrossRef]
35. Zaravinos, A.; Bonavida, B.; Chatzaki, E.; Baritaki, S. RKIP: A key regulator in tumor metastasis initiation and resistance to apoptosis: Therapeutic targeting and impact. *Cancers* **2018**, *10*, 287. [CrossRef]
36. Simister, P.C.; Burton, N.M.; Brady, R.L. Phosphotyrosine recognition by the raf kinase inhibitor protein. *For. Immunopathol. Dis. Therap.* **2011**, *2*, 59–70. [CrossRef]
37. Wang, E.; Sun, H.; Wang, J.; Wang, Z.; Liu, H.; Zhang, J.Z.H.; Hou, T. End-Point Binding Free Energy Calculation with MM/PBSA and MM/GBSA: Strategies and Applications in Drug Design. *Chem. Rev.* **2019**, *119*, 9478–9508. [CrossRef] [PubMed]
38. Tavel, L.; Jaquillard, L.; Karsisiotis, A.I.; Saab, F.; Jouvensal, L.; Brans, A.; Delmas, A.F.; Schoentgen, F.; Cadene, M.; Damblon, C. Ligand binding study of human PEBP1/RKIP: Interaction with nucleotides and raf-1 peptides evidenced by NMR and mass spectrometry. *PLoS ONE* **2012**, *7*, e36187. [CrossRef] [PubMed]
39. Xu, X.; de Guzman, F.S.; Gloer, J.B.; Shearer, C.A. Stachybotrins A and B: Novel Bioactive Metabolites from a Brackish Water Isolate of the Fungus Stachybotrys sp. *J. Org. Chem.* **1992**, *57*, 6700–6703. [CrossRef]
40. Tilvi, S.; Rodrigues, C.; Naik, C.G.; Parameswaran, P.S.; Wahidhulla, S. New bromotyrosine alkaloids from the marine sponge Psammaplysilla purpurea. *Tetrahedron* **2004**, *60*, 10207–10215. [CrossRef]
41. Barsby, T.; Kicklighter, C.E.; Hay, M.E.; Sullards, M.C.; Kubanek, J. Defensive 2-alkylpyrrole sulfamates from the marine annelid Cirriformia tentaculata. *J. Nat. Prod.* **2003**, *66*, 1110–1112. [CrossRef]
42. Blunt, J.W.; Munro, M.H.G. *Dictionary of Marine Natural Products with CD-ROM*, 1st ed.; Chapman and Hall/CRC: Boca Raton, FL, USA, 2007; Available online: https://www.routledge.com/Dictionary-of-Marine-Natural-Products-with-CD-ROM/Blunt-Munro/p/book/9780849382161 (accessed on 26 May 2021).
43. Macherla, V.R.; Liu, J.; Bellows, C.; Teisan, S.; Nicholson, B.; Lam, K.S.; Potts, B.C.M. Glaciapyrroles A, B, and C, pyrrolosesquiterpenes from a Streptomyces sp. isolated from an Alaskan marine sediment. *J. Nat. Prod.* **2005**, *68*, 780–783. [CrossRef] [PubMed]

44. CAS 58115-31-4 Aurantiamide—BOC Sciences. Available online: https://www.bocsci.com/aurantiamide-cas-58115-31-4-item-189189.html (accessed on 26 May 2021).
45. Pettit, G.R.; Butler, M.S.; Williams, M.D.; Filiatrault, M.J.; Pettit, R.K. Isolation and structure of hemibastadinols 1-3 from the Papua New Guinea marine sponge Ianthella basta. *J. Nat. Prod.* **1996**, *59*, 927–934. [CrossRef]
46. Dictionary of Alkaloids with CD-ROM—Google Books. Available online: https://books.google.co.kr/books?id=mynNBQAAQBAJ&pg=PA1033&lpg=PA1033&dq=142677-12-1&source=bl&ots=JLw2aSbhuf&sig=ACfU3U1C5GJjiqtHw9UXnh_gnToAhdYrZQ&hl=en&sa=X&ved=2ahUKEwj6wZ-a_ubwAhUdx4sBHcR2DpgQ6AEwAXoECAIQAw#v=onepage&q=142677-12-1&f=false (accessed on 26 May 2021).
47. Capon, R.J.; Skene, C.; Lacey, E.; Gill, J.H.; Wicker, J.; Heiland, K.; Friedel, T. Lorneamides A and B: Two New Aromatic Amides from a Southern Australian Marine Actinomycete. *J. Nat. Prod.* **2000**, *63*, 1682–1683. [CrossRef] [PubMed]
48. Parate, S.; Kumar, V.; Lee, G.; Rampogu, S.; Hong, J.C.; Lee, K.W. Marine-Derived Natural Products as ATP-Competitive mTOR Kinase Inhibitors for Cancer Therapeutics. *Pharmaceuticals* **2021**, *14*, 282. [CrossRef] [PubMed]
49. Lipinski, C.A.; Lombardo, F.; Dominy, B.W.; Feeney, P.J. Experimental and computational approaches to estimate solubility and permeability in drug discovery and development settings. *Adv. Drug Deliv. Rev.* **2001**, *46*, 3–26. [CrossRef]
50. Pinzi, L.; Rastelli, G. Molecular docking: Shifting paradigms in drug discovery. *Int. J. Mol. Sci.* **2019**, *20*, 4331. [CrossRef]
51. Jones, G.; Willett, P.; Glen, R.C.; Leach, A.R.; Taylor, R. Development and validation of a genetic algorithm for flexible docking. *J. Mol. Biol.* **1997**, *267*, 727–748. [CrossRef] [PubMed]
52. Verdonk, M.L.; Cole, J.C.; Hartshorn, M.J.; Murray, C.W.; Taylor, R.D. Improved protein-ligand docking using GOLD. *Proteins Struct. Funct. Genet.* **2003**, *52*, 609–623. [CrossRef] [PubMed]
53. Parate, S.; Kumar, V.; Hong, J.C.; Lee, K.W. Computational Investigation Identified Potential Chemical Scaffolds for Heparanase as Anticancer Therapeutics. *Int. J. Mol. Sci.* **2021**, *22*, 5311. [CrossRef] [PubMed]
54. Kumar, V.; Parate, S.; Yoon, S.; Lee, G.; Lee, K.W. Computational Simulations Identified Marine-Derived Natural Bioactive Compounds as Replication Inhibitors of SARS-CoV-2. *Front. Microbiol.* **2021**, *12*, 583. [CrossRef]
55. Parate, S.; Kumar, V.; Hong, J.C.; Lee, K.W. Identification of Flavonoids as Putative ROS-1 Kinase Inhibitors Using Pharmacophore Modeling for NSCLC Therapeutics. *Molecules* **2021**, *26*, 2114. [CrossRef]
56. Liu, X.; Shi, D.; Zhou, S.; Liu, H.; Liu, H.; Yao, X. Molecular dynamics simulations and novel drug discovery. *Expert Opin. Drug Discov.* **2018**, *13*, 23–37. [CrossRef] [PubMed]
57. Abraham, M.J.; Murtola, T.; Schulz, R.; Páll, S.; Smith, J.C.; Hess, B.; Lindah, E. Gromacs: High performance molecular simulations through multi-level parallelism from laptops to supercomputers. *SoftwareX* **2015**, *1–2*, 19–25. [CrossRef]
58. Zhu, X.; Lopes, P.E.M.; Mackerell, A.D. Recent developments and applications of the CHARMM force fields. *Wiley Interdiscip. Rev. Comput. Mol. Sci.* **2012**, *2*, 167–185. [CrossRef] [PubMed]
59. Zoete, V.; Cuendet, M.A.; Grosdidier, A.; Michielin, O. SwissParam: A fast force field generation tool for small organic molecules. *J. Comput. Chem.* **2011**, *32*, 2359–2368. [CrossRef] [PubMed]
60. Parrinello, M.; Rahman, A. Polymorphic transitions in single crystals: A new molecular dynamics method. *J. Appl. Phys.* **1981**, *52*, 7182–7190. [CrossRef]
61. Hess, B.; Bekker, H.; Berendsen, H.J.C.; Fraaije, J.G.E.M. LINCS: A linear constraint solver for molecular simulations. *J. Comput. Chem.* **1997**, *18*, 1463–1472. [CrossRef]
62. Miyamoto, S.; Kollman, P.A. Settle: An analytical version of the SHAKE and RATTLE algorithm for rigid water models. *J. Comput. Chem.* **1992**, *13*, 952–962. [CrossRef]
63. Darden, T.; York, D.; Pedersen, L. Particle mesh Ewald: An N·log(N) method for Ewald sums in large systems. *J. Chem. Phys.* **1993**, *98*, 10089–10092. [CrossRef]
64. Humphrey, W.; Dalke, A.; Schulten, K. VMD: Visual molecular dynamics. *J. Mol. Graph.* **1996**, *14*, 33–38. [CrossRef]
65. Kumar, V.; Kumar, R.; Parate, S.; Yoon, S.; Lee, G.; Kim, D.; Lee, K.W. Identification of ACK1 Inhibitors as Anticancer Agents by using Computer-Aided Drug Designing. *J. Mol. Struct.* **2021**, 130200. [CrossRef]
66. Yang, C.Y.; Sun, H.; Chen, J.; Nikolovska-Coleska, Z.; Wang, S. Importance of ligand reorganization free energy in protein-ligand binding-affinity prediction. *J. Am. Chem. Soc.* **2009**, *131*, 13709–13721. [CrossRef] [PubMed]
67. Kumari, R.; Kumar, R.; Lynn, A. G-mmpbsa -A GROMACS tool for high-throughput MM-PBSA calculations. *J. Chem. Inf. Model.* **2014**, *54*, 1951–1962. [CrossRef] [PubMed]
68. Huang, K.; Luo, S.; Cong, Y.; Zhong, S.; Zhang, J.Z.H.; Duan, L. An accurate free energy estimator: Based on MM/PBSA combined with interaction entropy for protein-ligand binding affinity. *Nanoscale* **2020**, *12*, 10737–10750. [CrossRef] [PubMed]

marine drugs

MDPI

Article

Saliniquinone Derivatives, Saliniquinones G−I and Heraclemycin E, from the Marine Animal-Derived *Nocardiopsis aegyptia* HDN19-252

Luning Zhou [1], Xuedong Chen [1], Chunxiao Sun [1], Yimin Chang [1], Xiaofei Huang [1], Tianjiao Zhu [1], Guojian Zhang [1,2], Qian Che [1,*] and Dehai Li [1,2,*]

1 School of Medicine and Pharmacy, Ocean University of China, Qingdao 266003, China; 18895692529@163.com (L.Z.); chenxuedong1206@163.com (X.C.); sunchunxiao93@163.com (C.S.); yiminchang@163.com (Y.C.); hxf17853102898@163.com (X.H.); zhutj@ouc.edu.cn (T.Z.); zhangguojian@ouc.edu.cn (G.Z.)

2 Laboratory for Marine Drugs and Bioproducts of Qingdao National Laboratory for Marine Science and Technology, Qingdao 266237, China

* Correspondence: cheqian064@ouc.edu.cn (Q.C.); dehaili@ouc.edu.cn (D.L.); Tel.: +86-532-82031619 (D.L.)

Abstract: Four new anthraquinone derivatives, namely saliniquinones G−I (**1–3**) and heraclemycin E (**4**), were obtained from the Antarctic marine-derived actinomycete *Nocardiopsis aegyptia* HDN19-252, guided by the Global Natural Products Social (GNPS) molecular networking platform. Their structures, including absolute configurations, were elucidated by extensive NMR, MS, and ECD analyses. Compounds **1** and **2** showed promising inhibitory activity against six tested bacterial strains, including methicillin-resistant coagulase-negative *staphylococci* (MRCNS), with MIC values ranging from 3.1 to 12.5 μM.

Keywords: anthraquinone derivatives; GNPS; *Nocardiopsis aegyptia*; MRCNS

Citation: Zhou, L.; Chen, X.; Sun, C.; Chang, Y.; Huang, X.; Zhu, T.; Zhang, G.; Che, Q.; Li, D. Saliniquinone Derivatives, Saliniquinones G−I and Heraclemycin E, from the Marine Animal-Derived *Nocardiopsis aegyptia* HDN19-252. *Mar. Drugs* **2021**, *19*, 575. https://doi.org/10.3390/md19100575

Academic Editors: Susana P. Gaudencio and Florbela Pereira

Received: 25 September 2021
Accepted: 10 October 2021
Published: 14 October 2021

1. Introduction

Saliniquinones are renowned antibiotics featuring a typical anthraquinone-γ-pyrone skeleton [1] and a side chain with different substituents, such as methyl and allyl groups. Since being first described in 1956, [2] more than 50 saliniquinone derivatives have been isolated from various genera, mainly *Streptomyces*. As optically active metabolites, most of them featured *R* configuration at C-15, with only six derivatives assigned as having *S* configuration naturally. Saliniquinones show various biological activities, including cytotoxic [3], antimicrobial [4], and DNA synthesis inhibitory effects [5], etc.

During our efforts in obtaining new bioactive metabolites from actinomycetes, *Nocardiopsis aegyptia* HDN19-252 was selected for the intriguing UV absorption of EtOAc extract. A comprehensive examination of EtOAc extract using the Global Natural Product Social Molecular Networking (GNPS) platform [6,7], LC-MS-UV, and MarinLit database indicated that the strain *N. aegyptia* HDN19-252 has potential saliniquinone derivatives in the metabolite profile. Moreover, a number of nodes that could not be retrieved in the GNPS platform [6,7] or other databases indicated the existence of new saliniquinone analogues. Followed up by HPLC-UV and LC-MS profiles, three saliniquinone derivatives and one new heraclemycin analogue (Figure 1) were isolated from the crude extract of *N. aegyptia* HDN19-252. Among them, **1–3** represent the first discovery of saliniquinones produced by *Nocardia* sp., and all of them possess the rare *S* configuration at C-15. Compounds **1–4** were evaluated for antibacterial activity against six bacterial strains, including methicillin-resistant coagulase-negative *staphylococci* (MRCNS), *B. subtilis*, *Proteus* sp., *B. cereus*, *Escherichia coli*, and *Mycobacterium phlei*. As a result, compounds **1** and **2** showed broad inhibitory effects. Herein, we report the details of the isolation, structure elucidation, and bioactivities of these compounds.

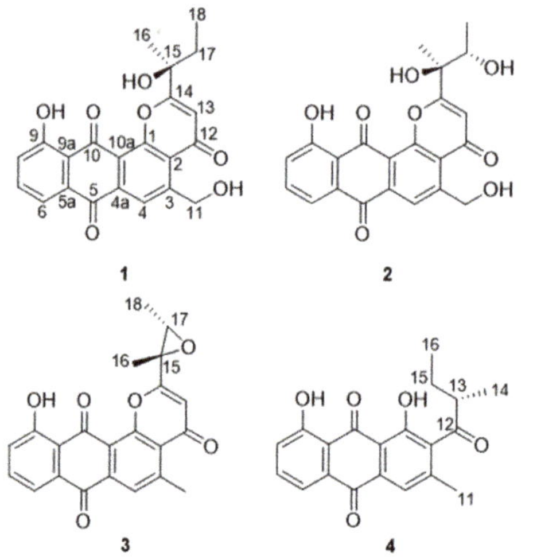

Figure 1. Structures of **1–4**.

2. Results

The actinomycete strain *N. aegyptia* HDN19-252 was isolated from an unidentified animal (Figure S1) collected form the Antarctic sea. The strain was cultured under static conditions, and the EtOAc extract (10.2 g) was fractionated by vacuum-liquid chromatography (VLC) using an ODS column to obtain seven subfractions, which were further analyzed via the GNPS web platform. A concentrated cluster with nodes attributed to subfractions 1–7 was spotted within the whole molecular network (Figure 2a). Combining LC-MS-UV analysis and the MarinLit database retrieval (http://pubs.rsc.org/marinlit, 15 June 2021) using the *m/z* values of 389.067 and 425.124 suggested the reasonable candidate molecules heraclemycin B [8] and bleomycin B [9]. Further analysis of the related molecular cluster indicated a series of putative new saliniquinone-related analogues through MarinLit database and SciFinder searches. Guided by LC-MS-UV, three undescribed saliniquinones, named saliniquinones G-I (**1–3**), and a new heraclemycin E (**4**) were obtained by repeated separation by column chromatography using silica gel, LH-20, and HPLC with an ODS column.

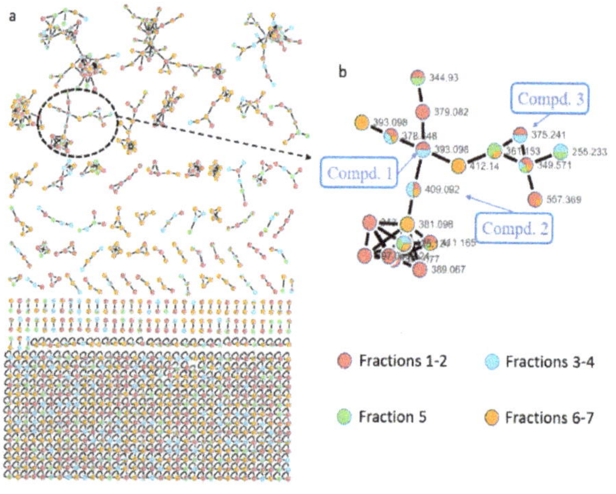

Figure 2. (**a**) Molecular network of all subfractions from *Nocardiopsis aegyptia* HDN19-252; (**b**) cluster corresponding to compounds of the saliniquinone family observed in the molecular network.

Saliniquinone G (**1**) was obtained as yellow powder with a molecular formula of $C_{22}H_{18}O_7$ deduced by HRESIMS, indicating fourteen degrees of unsaturation. The 1D NMR data of **1** (Tables 1 and 2) are similar to those of saliniquinone F. [1] The difference was the replacement of methyl at C-5 in saliniquinone F [1] by a hydroxymethyl (C-11, δ_C 62.8, H_2-11 δ_H 5.18) group, which was supported by the COSY correlation from OH-11 (δ_H 5.74) to H-11 (δ_H 5.18) and the HMBC correlation from H-11 to C-3 (δ_C 153.9), as well as the replacement of an allyl group on C-15 by an ethyl group (Tables 1 and 2, Figure 3). The absolute configuration of C-15 was determined as 15*S* based on the CD data, which showed two negative Cotton effects at 267 nm and 372 nm (Figure S4), similar to those of saliniquinone F [1].

Table 1. ^{1}H NMR (600 MHz) spectroscopic data of **1–4** in DMSO-d_6 (δ in ppm, *J* in Hz).

No.	1	2	3	4
4	8.55, s	8.55, s	8.01, s	7.60, s
6	7.73, d (7.5)	7.74, d (7.0)	7.73, d (6.3)	7.70, d (7.5)
7	7.81, t (8.0)	7.81, t (7.2)	7.81, t (8)	7.79, t (7.4)
8	7.43, d (8.8)	7.44, d (7.0)	7.44, d (8.4)	7.38, d (8.4)
11	5.18, d (6.3)	5.19, d (4.0)	2.93, s	2.28, s
13	6.49, s	6.54, s	6.22, s	3.00, m
14	-	-	-	1.07, d (7.2)
15	-	-	-	1.73, m, 1.34, m
16	1.61, s	1.51, s	1.85, s	0.88, t (7.5)
17	1.84, m 2.07, m	4.20, m	3.48, q (5.0)	-
18	0.83, t (7.5)	1.20, d (6.0)	1.22, d (5.2)	-
11-OH	5.74, t	5.73, t	-	-
15-OH	5.59, s	5.42, s	-	-
17-OH	-	4.67, d	-	-

Table 2. ^{13}C NMR (150 MHz) spectroscopic data of **1–4** in DMSO-d_6 (δ in ppm).

No.	1	2	3	4
1	174.7, C	174.9 C	176.0, C	158.7, C
2	124.5, C	124.6, C	126.3, C	145.5, C
3	153.9, C	153.9, C	156.4, C	136.0, C
4	119.3, CH	119.4, CH	125.6, CH	121.8, CH
4a	120.5, C	120.5, C	120.5, C	114.9, C
5	182.5, C	182.3, C	182.1, C	181.7, C
5a	132.9, C	132.9, C	132.8, C	133.9, C
6	119.3, CH	119.3, CH	119.3, CH	120.0, CH
7	137.3, CH	137.3, CH	137.5, CH	138.1, CH
8	125.3, CH	125.3, CH	125.4, CH	125.1, CH
9	161.9, C	163.3, C	161.8, C	161.9, C
9a	117.5, C	117.4, C	117.4, C	116.6, C
10	187.8, C	187.7, C	187.8, C	192.3, C
10a	136.8, C	136.7, C	137.3, C	153.2, C
11	62.8, CH_2	62.9, CH_2	24.1, CH_3	20.3, CH_3
12	179.0, C	179.1, C	178.5, C	208.9, C
13	109.4, CH	110.2, CH	111.2, CH	48.2, CH
14	174.7, C	174.9, C	165.7, C	15.0, CH_3
15	73.3, C	76.5, C	59.9, C	24.9, CH_2
16	27.4, CH_3	23.7, CH_3	20.8, CH_3	12.0, CH_3
17	33.6, CH_2	70.9, CH	62.2, CH	-
18	8.5, CH_3	17.4, CH_3	13.7, CH_3	-

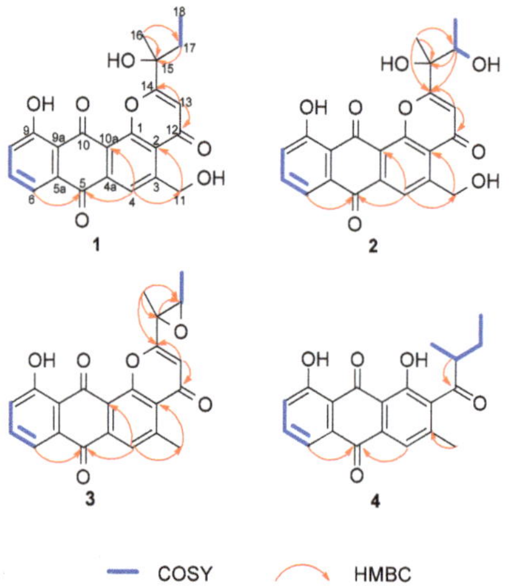

Figure 3. The key HMBC and COSY correlations in **1–4**.

Saliniquinone H (**2**), obtained as red-yellow powder, has a molecular formula of $C_{22}H_{18}O_8$, according to the (−)-HRESIMS *m*/*z* 409.0931 [M−H]$^-$ (calcd. for $C_{22}H_{17}O_8$, 409.0929). Examination of the NMR data (Tables 1 and 2) showed considerable resemblance to those of **1**. The differences between **2** and **1** were the presence of an additional hydroxyl group at C-17 (δ_C 70.9) and the absence of one methylene on the side chain at C-15 (δ_C 76.5), which was supported by the downfield shift of C-17 (Table 2) and the COSY correlation from 17-OH (δ_H 4.67)/H-17(δ_H 4.20)/H_3-18 (δ_H 1.20) (Table 1, Figure 3), as well as HMBC correlations from H-18 to C-15 (δ_C 76.5) and C-17, H-17 to C-14 (δ_C 174.9), C-15, and C-16 (δ_C 23.7), and H_3-16 (δ_H 1.51) to C-14, C-15, and C-17. However, it was a challenge to determine the absolute configurations of C-15 and C-17 due to a free rotation of the C15–C17 single bond. Detailed analysis the ECD curve of **1** and saliniquinone C [1] allowed us to draw the conclusion that the negative Cotton effect around 263 nm and 372 nm indicated an *S* configuration. Accordingly, the hydroxy stereocenter at C-15 was an *S* configuration due to its negative Cotton effect around 263 nm and 372 nm. Hence, there are two relative configurations, named (15*S**, 17*S**)-**2a** and (15*S**, 17*R**)-**2b**, theoretically. The ^{13}C NMR chemical shifts for the two possible isomers were calculated at the B3LYP/6-31+G(d)//B3LYP/6-311+G(d,p) levels and further checked by DP4+ probability [10,11]. The (15*S*, 17*S*)-**2a** isomer showed a striking predominance (100% probability) over the (15*S*, 17*R*)-**2b** isomer (Figure S6), which allowed us to assign the relative configuration of **2** as 15*S**, 17*S**. To determine the absolute configuration of C-15 and C-17 in **2**, the ECD calculations of the optimized conformation of (15*S*, 17*S*)-**2** obtained at the B3LYP/6-31+G(d) level were performed. The overall pattern of the experimental ECD spectrum was in reasonable agreement with the calculated one of (15*S*, 17*S*)-**2** (Figure 4), indicating the absolute configuration of C-15 and C-17 in **2** as 15*S*, 17*S*.

Saliniquinone I (**3**) was obtained as yellow powder with a molecular formula of $C_{22}H_{16}O_6$ by HRESIMS. The 1D (Tables 1 and 2) and 2D NMR (Figure 3) data indicated that **3** shares the same skeleton as **2**. Instead of the hydroxymethyl group in **2**, **3** has a methyl group (C-11, δ_C 24.1) at C-3, which was supported by HMBC correlation from H_3-11 (δ_H 2.93) to C-3 (δ_C 156.4) (Figure 3), and possesses an epoxide ring between C-15 (Figure 3) and C-17, which is in agreement with the molecular formula as well as higher chemical shift values of C-17 (δ_C 62.2 in **3** vs. 70.9 in **2**) and C-15 (δ_C 59.9 in **3** vs. 76.5 in **2**). The relative configurations of C-15 and C-17 in **3** was evidenced by the NOESY correlations from H-17 (δ_H 3.48) to H_3-16 (δ_H 1.85), which indicated 15*S** and 17*S** relative configurations of **3**. To determine the absolute configurations of C-15 and C-17, the optimized conformations of (15*S*, 17*S*)-**3** were obtained at the B3LYP/6-31+G(d) level and used for ECD calculations.

The agreement of the experimental and calculated ECD curves (Figure 5) indicated the 15*S* and 17*S* absolute configurations of **3**.

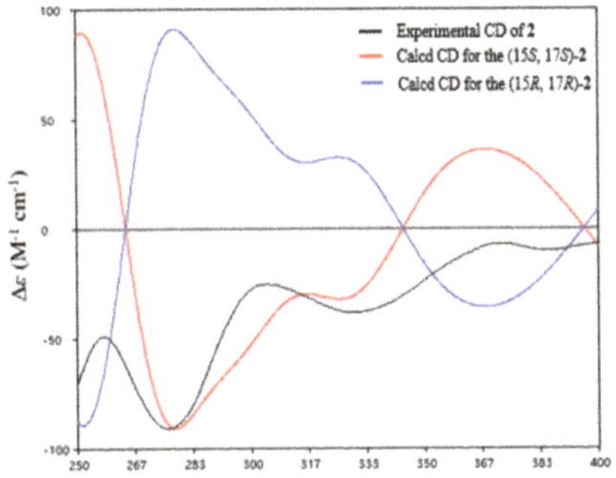

Figure 4. Experimental ECD spectra of compounds **2** and the calculated spectra for (15*S*, 17*S*)-**2**.

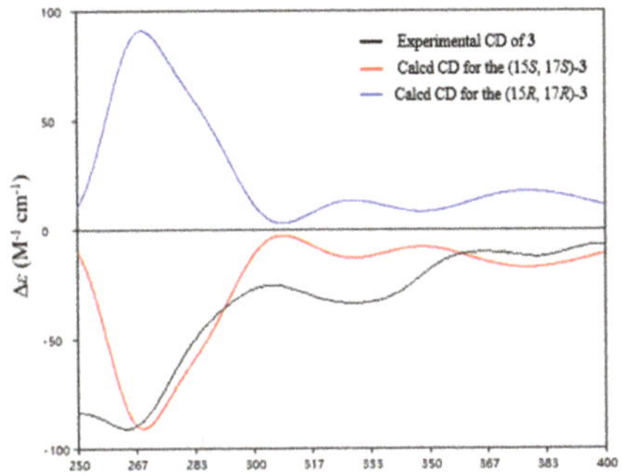

Figure 5. Experimental ECD spectra of compounds **3** and the calculated spectra for (15*S*, 17*S*)-**3**.

Heraclemycin E (**4**) was obtained as a brownish oil with a molecular formula of $C_{20}H_{18}O_5$, as evidenced by HRESIMS. Comparison of the ^1H and ^{13}C NMR data of **4** with those of the reported heraclemycin C [4] revealed that they shared a similar anthraquinone skeleton. The difference between heraclemycin C and **4** is the substituent on C-2, being 2-methylhexanoyl in the former and 2-methylbutanoyl in the latter. This was confirmed by the COSY correlations from H-14 (δ_H 1.07)/H-13 (δ_H 3.00)/H-15 (δ_H 1.73, 1.34)/H-16 (δ_H 0.88) and HMBC correlations from H-13, H-14, and H-15 to C-12 (δ_C 208.9). The absolute configuration of C-13 was determined to be *S* in **4** by comparison of the calculated and experimental ECD spectra of 13*S*-**4** (Figure 6).

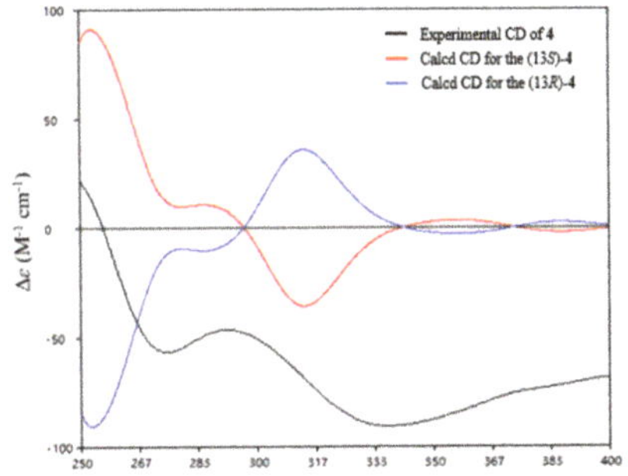

Figure 6. Experimental ECD spectrum of compound **4** and the calculated spectra for (13*S*)-**4**.

The new compounds (**1–4**) were evaluated for antibacterial activity against six bacterial strains, including methicillin-resistant coagulase-negative *staphylococci* (MRCNS), *B. subtilis*, *Proteus* sp., *B. cereus*, *Escherichia coli*, and *Mycobacterium phlei* [12]. Compounds **1** and **2** showed inhibitory effects against six strains, with MIC values ranging from 3.1 to 12.5 μM (Table 3). The structure activity relationship indicated the extra hydroxyl group at C-17 seems to play an important role for the inhibition activity (**1** vs. **2**). It was noted that the MIC values of **1** and **2** against MRCNS were 8-fold stronger than that of the positive control, ciprofloxacin (CPFX) [13].

Table 3. Inhibition effects of **1–4** against six pathogenic bacteria.

Compd.	MIC (μM)					
	MRCNS	***B. subtilis***	***P. species***	***B. cereus***	***E. coli***	***M. Phlei***
1	6.2	6.2	12.5	6.2	6.2	6.2
2	6.2	6.2	6.2	6.2	6.2	3.1
3	>50	>50	>50	>50	>50	>50
4	>50	>50	>50	>50	>50	>50
CPFX	50	0.01	0.2	3.1	3.1	1.5

3. Materials and Methods

3.1. General Experimental Procedures

The UV spectra were recorded on a Hitachi 5430 spectrophotometer (Hitachi Ltd., Tokyo, Japan). The ECD spectra and optical rotations were measured on a JASCO J-715 spectropolarimeter and a JASCOP-1020 digital (JASCO Corporation, Tokyo, Japan) polarimeter, respectively. IR spectra were obtained on a Bruker Tensor-27 (Bruker Corporation, Billerica, MA, USA). spectrophotometer in KBr discs. HRESIMS data were measured on a Thermo Scientific LTQ Orbitrap XL mass spectrometer (Thermo Fisher Scientific, Waltham, MA, USA). NMR spectra were collected on JEOLJN M-ECP 600 (JEOL Ltd., Tokyo, Japan and Agilent 500 MHz DD2 spectrometers (Agilent Technologies, Palo Alto, CA, USA), and tetramethylsilane was used as an internal standard. Sephadex LH-20 (Amersham Biosciences, NJ, USA) and silica gel (Qingdao Marine Chemical Factory, Qingdao, China) were used as stationary phases in column chromatography. An ODS column (YMC-Pack ODS-A, 10 × 250 mm, 5 μm, 3 mL/min, YMC Co., Ltd., Kyoto, Japan) was used for HPLC.

3.2. Actinomycete Material and Fermentation

Nocardiopsis aegyptia HDN19-252 (GenBank No. MN822699) was isolated from an animal sample collected from Antarctica (61°42′28″ S, 57°38′22″ W). The strain was aerobic and Gram-positive and produced beige to light-yellow aerial mycelium, brown substrate mycelium, and straight to flexuous hyphae but no specific spore chains [14]. It was deposited at the Key Laboratory of Marine Drugs, the Ministry of Education of China, School of Medicine and Pharmacy, Ocean University of China, Qingdao, People's Republic of China.

Nocardiopsis aegyptia HDN19-252 was cultured in 1 L Erlenmeyer flasks containing 200 g of culture medium composed of 80 g of rice and 120 g of seawater, pH = 7.0 (in seawater collected from Huiquan Bay, Yellow Sea) at 28 °C for 25 days on stable fermentation. A total of 130 bottles of the culture medium were extracted with EtOAc (3 × 20 L) to generate a crude extract (10.2 g).

3.3. LC-MS/MS and Molecular Networking Analysis

LC-MS/MS analysis was performed using a UHPLC system (Ultimate 3000, Thermo Scientific) combined with a hybrid Quadrupole-Orbitrap mass spectrometer (QExactive, Thermo Scientific). As a mobile phase, 0.1% formic acid in H_2O (A) and HPLC-grade MeCN (B) were used in negative-ionization conditions. The elution gradient conditions of LC-MS/MS were as follows, based on times (t): t = 0–1 min, hold at 10% B; t = 1–23 min, increased to 100% B linearly; t = 23–26 min, hold at 100% B; t = 26–30 min, returned to initial conditions and hold at 10% B to re-equilibrate the column. The elution velocity and injection volume were 0.25 mL/min and 3 µL, respectively. All MS/MS data were converted to mzXML format files by MSConvert software (Ver. 3.0.20169, MSConvert, ProteoWizard). Molecular networking was established by GNPS data analysis workflow and algorithms. The spectral network files were visualized through Cytoscape (Ver. 3.8.0, Cytoscape, NRNB.)

3.4. Isolation and Purification of Compounds

The crude extract was applied over a VLC column and eluted with mixtures of CH_2Cl_2-MeOH to give nine fractions (Fr.1–Fr.9). Fr.3–Fr.7 was combined as Fr.A, which was separated by HPLC using an ODS column to obtain ten subfractions (Fr.A.1–Fr.A.10). Fr.A.6 was purified by semi-preparative HPLC to obtain **2** (3 mg, t_R = 15 min). Fr.A.7 was purified by semi-preparative HPLC to afford **4** (2.5 mg, t_R = 13 min). Fr.A.8 was separated on the LH-20 column to obtain three subfractions (Fr.A.8.1–Fr.A.8.5). Fr.A.8.3 was purified by semi-preparative HPLC using a stepped gradient elution to obtain **1** (1.5 mg, t_R = 25 min). Fr.A.8.2 was purified by semi-preparative HPLC to afford **3** (2.1 mg, t_R = 27 min).

Saliniquinone G (1): yellow powder, $[\alpha]_D^{25}$ −12 (MeOH); UV (MeOH) λ_{max} 240 (1.6), 417 (0.3) nm; IR (KBr) ν_{max} 3414, 2926, 1679, 1211, 1139 cm^{-1}; ECD (*c* 1.5mM, DMSO λ_{max} (Δ ε) 264 (−1.01), 372 (−0.22) nm; ^1H and ^{13}C NMR data, Tables 1 and 2; HRESIMS *m/z* 393.0978 $[M-H]^-$ (calcd for $C_{22}H_{17}O_7$, 393.0980).

Saliniquinone H (2): red-yellow powder, $[\alpha]_D^{25}$ −83 (MeOH); UV (MeOH) λ_{max} (log ε) 240 (1.8), 419 (0.3) nm; IR (KBr) ν_{max} 3409, 2927, 1687, 1210, 1138 cm^{-1}; ECD (*c* 1.5mM, DMSO λ_{max} (Δ ε) 264 (−8.63), 335 (−3.32) nm, 385 (−1.02) nm; ^1H and ^{13}C NMR data, Tables 1 and 2; HRESIMS *m/z* 409.0931 $[M-H]^-$ (calcd for $C_{22}H_{17}O_8$, 409.0929).

Saliniquinone I (3): yellow powder, $[\alpha]_D^{25}$ −83 (MeOH); UV (MeOH) λ_{max} 241 (1.5), 417 (0.3) nm; IR (KBr) ν_{max} 3437, 2925, 1679, 1215, 1140 cm^{-1}; ECD (*c* 1.5mM, DMSO λ_{max} (Δ ε) 264 (−4.00), 335 (−1.37) nm, 385 (−0.53) nm; ^1H and ^{13}C NMR data, Tables 1 and 2; HRESIMS *m/z* 375.0881 $[M-H]^-$ (calcd for $C_{22}H_{15}O_6$, 375.0874).

Heraclemycin E (4): brownish oil, $[\alpha]_D^{25}$ −12 (MeOH); UV (MeOH) λ_{max} 225 (0.5), 380 (0.3) nm; IR (KBr) ν_{max} 3435, 2929, 1696, 1210, 1156 cm^{-1}; ECD (*c* 1.5mM, DMSO λ_{max} (Δ ε) 264 (−0.91), 335 (−0.86) nm; ^1H and ^{13}C NMR data, Tables 1 and 2; HRESIMS *m/z* 337.1075 $[M-H]^-$ (calcd for $C_{20}H_{17}O_5$, 337.1081).

3.5. Computation Section

Conformational searches were run, employing Spartan'14, [15] based on the MMFF (Merck Molecular Force Field). All conformers were further optimized with DFT calculations at the B3LYP/6-31+G(d) level by using the Gaussian 09 program [16]. TDDFT calculations were performed on the five lowest-energy conformations for **2**, the lowest-energy conformation for **3**, and the six lowest-energy conformations for **4** (>5% population). ECD spectra were obtained on the program SpecDis 1.71 software [17] by using a Gaussian band shape with a 0.25 eV width for **2**, a 0.3 eV width for **3**, and a 0.25 eV width for **4** from dipole-length rotational strengths. The calculated spectra were shifted by −25 nm for **2**, 32 nm for **3**, and 0 nm for **4** to facilitate comparison to the experimental data.

3.6. Assay of Antimicrobial Activity

Antibacterial activity of **1–4** was evaluated against MRCNS, *B. subtilis*, *Proteus* sp., *B. cereus*, *Escherichia coli*, *Mycobacterium phlei* by a conventional broth dilution assay. Six strains were cultured in 100 mL Erlenmeyer flasks at 28 °C for 24 h. Then, the culture medium was diluted to a concentration of 10^6 cfu/mL and added into 96-well plates. Ciprofloxacin was used as a positive control. The detailed methodologies for biological testing have been described in previous reports [14].

4. Conclusions

In summary, four new anthraquinone derivatives were isolated from *Nocardiopsis aegyptia* HDN19-252 under the guidance of GNPS. Compared with saliniquinone I (**3**), saliniquinone G (**1**) and saliniquinone H (**2**) exhibited significant antibacterial activity against six tested bacterial strains, suggesting that a free hydroxyl group is an important part of antibacterial activity. Compounds **1–3** represent a rare class of saliniquinones with *S* configuration at C-15, indicating a stereospecific ketoreductase in strain *N. aegyptia* HDN19-252. Additionally, this is also the first report of saliniquinones from *Nocardia* sp. Notably, **1** and **2** specifically inhibited the growth of a drug-resistant MRCNS strain with an MIC of 6.2 μM, which was even stronger than the positive control, CPFX (50 μM). Our results highlight the potential for screening and developing therapeutic molecules from actinomycete-derived saliniquinones.

Supplementary Materials: The following are available online at https://www.mdpi.com/article/10.3390/md19100575/s1, Figure S1: the picture of Antarctica animal, Figure S2: *Nocardiopsis aegyptia* HDN19-252; Figure S3: HPLC analysis of the crude extract of HDN19-252; Figure S4: the experimental curves of **1** and saliniquinones F; Figure S5: correlation plots of experimental ^{13}C NMR chemical shifts versus the corresponding calculated data for **2a** and **2b**; Figure S6: sDP4+, uDP4+ and DP4+ probabilities (%) for compound **2a** and **2b**; Figure S7-S38: 1D and 2D NMR spectra, HRESIMS spectra, IR spectra of compounds **1–4**; Table S1: deviations between the calculated and experimental ^{13}C NMR chemical shifts for stereoisomers **2a** and **2b**.

Author Contributions: The contributions of the respective authors are as follows: L.Z. drafted the work and performed isolation and structural elucidation of the extract. C.S., Y.C. and X.H. performed isolation and scale-up fermentation of the strain. Biological evaluations were performed by X.C., G.Z., Q.C., T.Z. and D.L. checked the procedures of this work. D.L. and Q.C. designed the project and contributed to the critical reading of the manuscript. All authors have read and agreed to the published version of the manuscript.

Funding: The National Natural Science Foundation of China (41876216, 41976105), the National Natural Science Foundation of China Major Project for Discovery of New Leading Compounds (81991522), National Key R&D Program of China (2018YFC1406705), The Youth Innovation Plan of Shandong province (2019KJM004), Taishan Scholar Youth Expert Program in Shandong Province (tsqn201812021), the Fundamental Research Funds for the Central Universities (201941001).

Institutional Review Board Statement: Not applicable.

Informed Consent Statement: Not applicable.

Data Availability Statement: The data presented in this study are available in this article and supplementary material.

Conflicts of Interest: The authors declare no conflict of interest.

References

1. Murphy, B.T.; Narender, T.; Kauffman, C.A. Saliniquinones A–F, new members of the highly cytotoxic anthraquinone-γ-pyrones from the marine actinomycete *Salinispora arenicola*. *Cheminform* **2010**, *41*, 929–934. [CrossRef]
2. Maeda, K.; Takeuchi, T.; Nitta, K.; Yagishita, K.; Utahara, R.; Osato, T.; Ueda, M.; Kondo, S.; Okami, Y.; Umezawa, H. A new antitumor substance, pluramycin; studies on antitumor substances produced by Actinomycetes. *J. Antibiot.* **1956**, *9*, 75–81.
3. Hsu, D.S.; Huang, J.Y. Total synthesis and determination of the absolute configuration of parimycin. *Org. Lett.* **2019**, *21*, 7665–7668. [CrossRef] [PubMed]
4. Liu, M.; Abdel-Mageed, W.M.; Ren, B.; He, W.; Huang, P.; Li, X.; Bolla, K.; Guo, H.; Chen, C.; Song, F.; et al. Endophytic *Streptomyces* sp. Y3111 from traditional Chinese medicine produced antitubercular pluramycins. *Appl. Microbiol. Biotechnol.* **2014**, *98*, 1077–1085. [CrossRef] [PubMed]
5. Schumacher, R.W.; Davidson, B.S.; Montenegro, D.A. Gamma-indomycinone, a new pluramycin metabolite from a deep-sea derived actinomycete. *J. Nat. Prod.* **1995**, *26*, 613–617. [CrossRef] [PubMed]
6. Kang, K.B.; Park, E.J.; Silva, R.R.; Kim, H.W.; Dorrestein, P.C.; Sung, S.H. Targeted isolation of neuroprotective dicoumaroyl neolignans and lignans from *Sageretia theezans* using in silico molecular network annotation propagation-based dereplication. *J. Nat. Prod.* **2018**, *81*, 1819–1828. [CrossRef] [PubMed]

7. Wang, M.; Carver, J.J.; Phelan, V.V.; Sanchez, L.M.; Garg, N.; Peng, Y.; Nguyen, D.D.; Watrous, J.; Kapono, C.A.; Luzzatto-Knaan, T.; et al. Sharing and community curation of mass spectrometry data with global natural products social molecular networking. *Nat. Biotechnol.* **2016**, *34*, 828–837. [CrossRef] [PubMed]
8. Jones, K.D.; Rixson, J.E.; Skelton, B.W.; Gericke, K.M.; Stewart, S.G. The total synthesis of heraclemycin B through β-ketosulfoxide and aldehyde annulation. *Asian J. Org. Chem.* **2015**, *4*, 936–942. [CrossRef]
9. Ojiri, K.; Saito, K.; Nakajima, S.; Suda, H. Substance BE-26554 from *Streptomyces* A26554 as Neoplasm Inhibitors. JP 06228121, 16 August 1994.
10. Zanardi, M.M.; Sarotti, A.M. Sensitivity analysis of DP4+ with the probability distribution terms: Development of a universal and customizable method. *J. Org. Chem.* **2021**, *86*, 8544–8548. [CrossRef] [PubMed]
11. Grimblat, N.; Zanardi, M.M.; Sarotti, A.M. Beyond DP4: An improved probability for the stereochemical assignment of isomeric compounds using quantum chemical calculations of NMR shifts. *J. Org. Chem.* **2015**, *80*, 12–34. [CrossRef] [PubMed]
12. Yu, G.; Wu, G.; Sun, Z.; Zhang, X.; Che, Q.; Gu, Q.; Zhu, T.; Li, D.; Zhang, G. Cytotoxic tetrahydroxanthone dimers from the mangrove-associated fungus *Aspergillus versicolor* HDN1009. *Mar. Drugs* **2018**, *16*, 335. [CrossRef] [PubMed]
13. Andrews, J.M. Determination of minimum inhibitory concentrations. *J. Antimicrob. Chemoth.* **2001**, *48*, 5–16. [CrossRef] [PubMed]
14. Sabry, S.A.; Ghanem, N.B.; Abu-Ella, G.A. *Nocardiopsis aegyptia* sp. nov. isolated from marine sediment. *Int. J. Syst. Evol. Microbiol.* **2004**, *54*, 453–456. [CrossRef] [PubMed]
15. *Spartan'14*; Wavefunction Inc.: Irvine, CA, USA, 2013.
16. Frisch, M.J.; Trucks, G.W.; Schlegel, H.B.; Scuseria, G.E.; Robb, M.A.; Cheeseman, J.R.; Scalmani, G.; Barone, V.; Mennucci, B.; Petersson, G.A.; et al. *Gaussian 09, Revision A.1*; Gaussian, Inc.: Wallingford, CT, USA, 2009.
17. Bruhn, T.; Hemberger, Y.; Schaumlöffel, A.; Bringmann, G. *SpecDis, Version 1.53*; University of Wuerzburg: Wuerzburg, Germany, 2011.

marine drugs

Article

Efficacy of Chondroprotective Food Supplements Based on Collagen Hydrolysate and Compounds Isolated from Marine Organisms †

Thomas Eckert [1,2,3,4,‡], Mahena Jährling-Butkus [2,5,‡], Helen Louton [6], Monika Burg-Roderfeld [2,3], Ruiyan Zhang [1,7], Ning Zhang [1,7,*], Karsten Hesse [8], Athanasios K. Petridis [9], Tibor Kožár [10], Jürgen Steinmeyer [11], Roland Schauer [12], Peter Engelhard [1], Anna Kozarova [13], John W. Hudson [13] and Hans-Christian Siebert [1,*]

1 RI-B-NT—Research Institute of Bioinformatics and Nanotechnology, Schauenburgerstr. 116, 24118 Kiel, Germany; thomasi-e@gmx.de (T.E.); zry147896@163.com (R.Z.); p.engelhard@kielnet.net (P.E.)
2 Institut für Veterinärphysiolgie und Biochemie, Fachbereich Veterinärmedizin, Justus-Liebig-Universität Gießen, Frankfurter Str. 100, 35392 Gießen, Germany; mahenabutkus0@gmail.com (M.J.-B.); monika.burg-roderfeld@hs-fresenius.de (M.B.-R.)
3 Department of Chemistry and Biology, University of Applied Sciences Fresenius, Limburger Str. 2, 65510 Idstein, Germany
4 RISCC—Research Institute for Scientific Computing and Consulting, Ludwig-Schunk-Str. 15, 35452 Heuchelheim, Germany
5 Tierarztpraxis Dr. Silke Fritscher, Bergstraße 104, 73441 Bopfingen, Germany
6 Animal Health and Animal Welfare, Faculty of Agricultural and Environmental Sciences, University of Rostock, Justus-von-Liebig-Weg 6b, 18059 Rostock, Germany; helen.louton@uni-rostock.de
7 Institute of BioPharmaceutical Research, Liaocheng University, Liaocheng 252059, China
8 Tierarztpraxis Dr. Karsten Hesse, Rathausstraße 16, 35460 Staufenberg, Germany; k.hesse@tiermedizin-drhesse.de
9 Medical School, Heinrich-Heine-Universität Düsseldorf, Universitätsstr. 1, 40225 Düsseldorf, Germany; opticdisc@aol.com
10 Center for Interdisciplinary Biosciences, Technology and Innovation Park, P. J. Šafárik University, Jesenná 5, 04001 Košice, Slovakia; tibor.kozar@upjs.sk
11 Laboratory for Experimental Orthopaedics, Department of Orthopaedics, Justus Liebig University Giessen, Paul-Meimberg-Str. 3, 35392 Giessen, Germany; Juergen.Steinmeyer@ortho.med.uni-giessen.de
12 Biochemisches Institut, Christian-Albrechts Universität Kiel, Olshausenstrasse 40, 24098 Kiel, Germany; e_schauer@t-online.de
13 Department of Biomedical Sciences, University of Windsor, Windsor, ON N9B 3P4, Canada; kozarova@uwindsor.ca (A.K.); jhudson@uwindsor.ca (J.W.H.)
* Correspondence: zhangning1111@126.com (N.Z.); hcsiebert@aol.com (H.-C.S.)
† We dedicate this article to the memory of our colleague Roland Schauer who passed away on 24 October 2019.
‡ Contributed equally.

Citation: Eckert, T.; Jährling-Butkus, M.; Louton, H.; Burg-Roderfeld, M.; Zhang, R.; Zhang, N.; Hesse, K.; Petridis, A.K.; Kožár, T.; Steinmeyer, J.; et al. Efficacy of Chondroprotective Food Supplements Based on Collagen Hydrolysate and Compounds Isolated from Marine Organisms. *Mar. Drugs* **2021**, *19*, 542. https://doi.org/10.3390/md19100542

Academic Editors: Susana P. Gaudencio, Florbela Pereira, Bill J. Baker and Orazio Taglialatela-Scafati

Received: 6 July 2021
Accepted: 23 September 2021
Published: 26 September 2021

Abstract: Osteoarthritis belongs to the most common joint diseases in humans and animals and shows increased incidence in older patients. The bioactivities of collagen hydrolysates, sulfated glucosamine and a special fatty acid enriched dog-food were tested in a dog patient study of 52 dogs as potential therapeutic treatment options in early osteoarthritis. Biophysical, biochemical, cell biological and molecular modeling methods support that these well-defined substances may act as effective nutraceuticals. Importantly, the applied collagen hydrolysates as well as sulfated glucosamine residues from marine organisms were strongly supported by both an animal model and molecular modeling of intermolecular interactions. Molecular modeling of predicted interaction dynamics was evaluated for the receptor proteins MMP-3 and ADAMTS-5. These proteins play a prominent role in the maintenance of cartilage health as well as innate and adapted immunity. Nutraceutical data were generated in a veterinary clinical study focusing on mobility and agility. Specifically, key clinical parameter (MMP-3 and TIMP-1) were obtained from blood probes of German shepherd dogs with early osteoarthritis symptoms fed with collagen hydrolysates. Collagen hydrolysate, a chondroprotective food supplement was examined by high resolution NMR experiments. Molecular modeling simulations were used to further characterize the interaction potency of collagen fragments and glucosamines with protein receptor structures. Potential beneficial effects of collagen hydrolysates, sulfated glycans (i.e., sulfated glucosamine from crabs and mussels) and lipids, especially, eicosapentaenoic acid (extracted from fish oil) on biochemical and physiological processes are discussed here in the context of human and veterinary medicine.

Keywords: osteoarthritis; collagen hydrolysate; sulfated *N*-acetyl glucosamine; sialic acids; eicosapentaenoic acid (EPA); MMP-3; ADAMTS-5

1. Introduction

Osteoarthritis is the most common joint disease in humans and animals and shows increased incidence in older patients. Generally, NSAIDs (Non-Steroidal Anti-Inflammatory Drugs) are used in the treatment of osteoarthritis [1,2]. However, their use is problematic in that side effects cannot be excluded and liver and/or kidney damage can be present, particularly in geriatric patients [2]. Therefore, conventional painkillers are of concern and alternatives with less or no side effects are being sought. Chondroprotective compounds are considered to be well tolerated and can be administered unhesitatingly over longer periods of time. In this context, glucosamine sulfate as well as a special diet with fish oil belongs to a standard therapy in veterinary medicine. However, collagen hydrolysate has not been used in the same way of so-called chondroprotective drugs such as glucosamine-based nutraceuticals [3]. Nevertheless, collagen hydrolysates were analyzed on a submolecular level in various conditions [4–10]. Clinical studies in which potential effects of collagen hydrolysate and sulfated glucosamine are directly compared with each other and discussed in relation to molecular mechanisms are still missing. Beneficial effects of collagen- and proteoglycan-fragments may be related to specific interactions with receptors like integrins, especially in the case of collagen fragments [4] and aggrecan [11–13]. Beside these specific interactions, unspecific contacts between collagen-strands [14–18], proteoglycans and fatty acids within the extracellular matrix of the cartilage could also play a crucial role when explaining the therapeutic effects on a sub-molecular size level. Therefore, we assessed the effect of the applied substances on the cartilage health of animals under study by a combination of biophysical, biochemical, cell-biological methods and molecular modeling tools. Such an arsenal of methods has previously been used to assess the beneficial therapeutic effects of other bio-medical-relevant macromolecules. These macromolecules are hyaluronic acid, proteoglycans and phospholipid species [19], sulfated poly- and oligosaccharides [20–23], polysialic acid and sialic acid containg oligosaccharides [24–28] as well as lysozymes and anti-microbial peptides in complex with oligosaccharides [29–31]. We analyzed structure–function relationships and focused on molecular modeling calculations that would allow us to better understand the details of intermolecular interactions between sialic acids and relevant proteins. The collagen hydrolysate under study [32–37] was examined with high resolution NMR experiments, especially, DOSY NMR [4,7]. Additionally, molecular modeling approaches such as molecular docking and molecular dynamics simulations were carried out in order to obtain more information about the interaction potency of collagen fragments and sulfated GlcNAc with receptor structures. As a result of this study we are now able to formulate efficient encapsulation strategies [38–40] for an oral application of peptides and proteins [41–44]. The concept of this study was to provide a comparative examination of the potential benefits of nutraceuticals as chondroprotective agents. Thereby, we tested two specific collagen hydrolysates of bovine and fish origin, sulfated glucosamine from marine organisms as well as fish oil in lipid and vitamin enriched dog food. Collagen-hydrolysate is not a standard therapy in veterinary medicine for the treatment of osteoarthritis symptoms. We therefore carried out this study in both dogs and horses which both suffer from similar osteoarthritis symptoms to compare its efficacy to standard therapy (sulfated GlcNAc). Molecular modeling studies of the applied nutraceuticals are essential since they provide valuable hints on how these substances could influence biochemical processes not only in dogs and horses but as an extension of this study also in humans.

The aim of this work was to examine and compare the influence of collagen hydrolysate and sulfated glucosamine in dogs with osteoarthritis with regard to their ability to alleviate pain and to reduce the associated clinical orthopedic symptoms. In addition, a smaller control group (trailing group) was employed in order to avoid a placebo group. This group was administered a special food developed for joint protection since, due to ethical considerations, it was necessary that all dogs under study were treated for the symptoms of early osteoarthritis. The study was combined with cell assays and molecular modeling calculations with the information obtained, providing a foundation on how the results of this clinical study may be applied or be useful in the treatment of other species (e.g., horses) with the same or different collagen hydrolysates (e.g., from fish skin or from jellyfish collagen).

2. Results

2.1. Drug Administration and Statistical Analysis od Dog Treatment

All dogs (Table 1) were examined at the beginning of our study for the characteristic symptoms of osteoarthritis. The body condition score (BCS) of the dogs is defined according to Mele [45]. Level 1 (cachectic) to level 9 (obese). Level 5 is considered ideal.

Table 1. Characteristics of studied dogs grouped according to their treatment. The table shows the individual dog number, the race, the age, the gender, the weight, the disease (coxosteoarthritis—CA, gonosteoarthritis—GA), the degree of lameness (DL) and the body condition score (BCS). The abbreviations regarding the gender of the dogs are: f: female, fc: female castrated, m: male, mc: male castrated. * problem with mocing but neither CA nor GA was diagnosed.

Group 1: Collagen Hydrolysate							
Dog Nr.	**Race**	**Age**	**Gender**	**Weight**	**Disease**	**DL**	**BCS**
2	Golden Retriever	10	m	43.7	CA	2	8
4	Cairn Terrier	8	m	11	CA	stiff movement	5
6	Boxer mix	13	fc	30.5	CA	1	5
14	Boerboel	3	f	45	GA	2	4
15	Magyar Vizsla	6	fc	24	CA	2	6
19	Leonberger	4	f	51	CA	0	7
20	Mixed breed	8	mc	16	GA	1	8
21	Bernese Mountain Dog	9	fc	38.6	CA	2	6
25	German Wirehaired Pointer	5	m	46	CA	0	7
26	Shepherd mix	13	fc	34.9	GA	2	6
27	Labrador	3	m	40	CA	0	5
33	Shepherd mix	11	mc	38	CA	3	7
34	German Shepherd	2	f	26	CA	0	4
35	Gordon Setter	10	m	29.4	CA	1	5
37	Poodle	13	fc	9.4	CA	3	7
40	Appenzeller	8	fc	37.8	CA	1	7
45	Samoyed	4	fc	24.8	*	1	4
49	German Shepherd mix	2	fc	23.4	CA	1	5
51	Mixed breed	14	mc	29.7	CA	1	5

Table 1. *Cont.*

Group 1: Collagen Hydrolysate							
Dog Nr.	**Race**	**Age**	**Gender**	**Weight**	**Disease**	**DL**	**BCS**
52	Border collie mix	2	fc	23.1	GA	0	3
	Summary:	**Ø 7.35**	**m: 5 mc: 3 f:3 fc: 9**	**Ø 31.1**	**CA: 15 GA: 4**	**Ø 1.23**	**Ø 5.7**
Group 2: Glucosamine							
Dog Nr.	**Race**	**Age**	**Gender**	**Weight**	**Disease**	**DL**	**BCS**
1	Schnauzer mix	5	mc	26.5	CA	2 to 3	6
3	Newfoundland Dog	7	fc	50	GA	2	6
5	Mixed breed	12	f	28	CA	3	7
7	Mixed breed	12	mc	28	CA/GA	3	5
8	Bernese Mountain Dog	6	m	41	CA	2	6
10	Mixed breed	8	m	40	CA	1	6
12	Mixed breed	7	mc	17	CA/GA	1	7
13	Cairn Terrier	8	mc	11	CA	stiff movement	5
16	Beagle	4	mc	16.8	CA	1	6
18	Swiss Mountain Dog	4	m	55	CA	stiff movement	5
22	Labrador	10	mc	32	CA	2	6
23	Newfoundland Dog	10	m	59	CA	2	3
28	Boxer	3	f	30	CA	2	5
29	Kangal	2.5	fc	50	CA	0	6
36	Yorkshire Terrier	6	fc	6.4	CA	2	5
39	German Shepherd	9	m	45.6	CA	1	7
41	Shepherd mix	6	m	32.2	CA	1	5
42	Belgian Shepherd Dog	10	f	36	CA	2	4
44	Ridgeback	1	fc	27.5	CA	2	3
48	Mixed breed	4	mc	29.4	CA	1	3
50	Labrador	8	fc	24.8	CA	0	3
	Summary:	**Ø 6,8**	**m: 6 mc: 7 f: 3 fc: 5**	**Ø 32.7**	**CA: 18 GA: 1 GA/CA: 2**	**Ø 1.45**	**Ø 5.2**
GROUP 3: Commercial Joint Diet							
Dog Nr.	**Race**	**Age**	**Gender**	**Weight**	**Disease**	**DL**	**BCS**
9	Shepherd mix	8	fc	42	GA	1	5
11	Shepherd mix	7	f	35	GA	2	5
17	German Shepherd	10	fc	34	CA	2	6
24	Mixed breed	9	m	23	CA	1	4
30	German Shepherd–Sennendog-Mix	5	mc	37	CA	1	7

Table 1. *Cont.*

Dog Nr.	Race	Age	Gender	Weight	Disease	DL	BCS
			GROUP 3: Commercial Joint Diet				
31	Mixed breed	5	fc	33	CA	0	6
32	German Shepherd–Husky-Mix	13	fc	40.5	CA	2	7
38	Pomeranian	8	mc	8	CA	2	8
43	Mixed breed	4	mc	38	GA	2	5
46	Golden Retriever	5	mc	29	CA	1	5
47	Mixed breed	10	fc	26	CA	1	6
	Summary:	**Ø 7.6**	**m: 1 mc: 4 f: 1 fc: 5**	**Ø 31.4**	**CA: 8 GA: 3**	**Ø 1.32**	**Ø 5.8**

Fifty-two dogs were treated during the 16 weeks of the therapy period. The treatment resulted in improvements in agility of animals found in all three groups. To assess pain, one of the symptoms of OA, and any therapeutic progress, palpation was performed independently for the left and right femoral joint throughout the study. Notably, a reduction in tenderness/pain was observed as early as four weeks into treatment (Figure 1). After 16 weeks (the end of the therapy), all groups (including the control group which contains only the half number of patients) exhibited a reduction in the sensitivity of their femoral joints to manipulation.

A key indicator of therapeutic value in any trial is the effect of the substances under study on the quality of life (QOL). We therefore assessed QOL using previously published guidelines [46–49]. The QOL score of dogs is shown on Figure 2. All substances under study (collagen hydrolysate, sulfated glucosamine as well as the special dog food enriched with fatty acids and vitamins) resulted in positive effects on the QOL score. Collagen hydrolysate led to the most promising results in terms of displaying moderate to minor symptoms or no joint problems at the focus of study.

Our observations suggest that the collagen hydrolysate applied in this dog-study contains bio-active fragments that have a beneficial effect on OA symptoms, similar to that observed for sulfated glucosamine. Cellular studies show that the collagen fragments in the hydrolysate are responsible for the effects within the extracellular matrix of the joint tissue. These effects can be supportive, non-supportive or even detrimental [8–10]. In order to establish the correlation between structure and function of bio-active components of the collagen hydrolysate applied in our study (Fortigel from Gelita) we further characterized the relationship by well-established protocols [4,7–10].

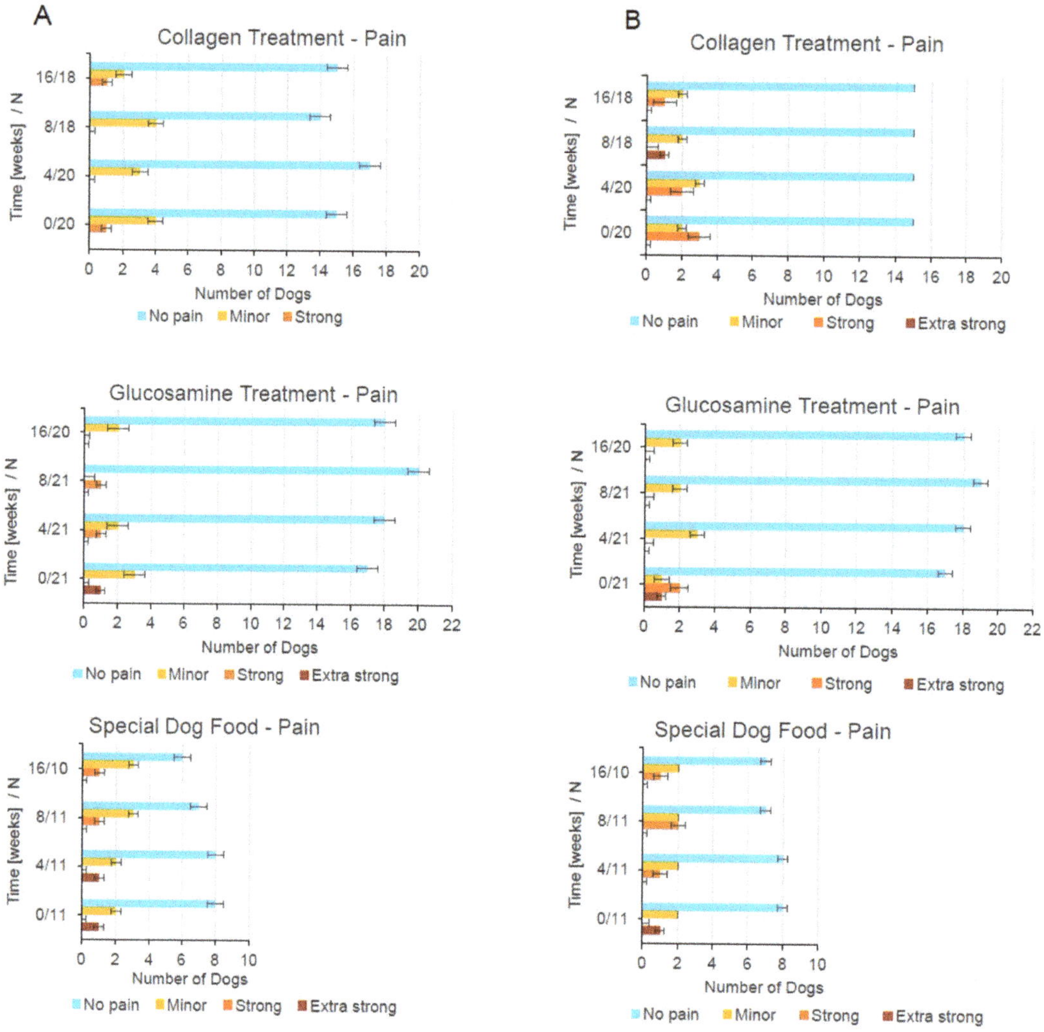

Figure 1. Canine dog patients with beginning OA symptoms were examined at the different time frames, i.e., beginning (0) and after 4, 8 and 16 weeks of treatment concerning pain in their (**A**) left or (**B**) right femoral joint. Pain symptoms during palpation were examined for all dogs in the three groups according to a clinical standard protocol. Four scores are given: no pain reaction (blue), minor (orange), strong (red) and extra strong pain reaction (dark red). N on the y-axis corresponds to the total number of dogs within a group.

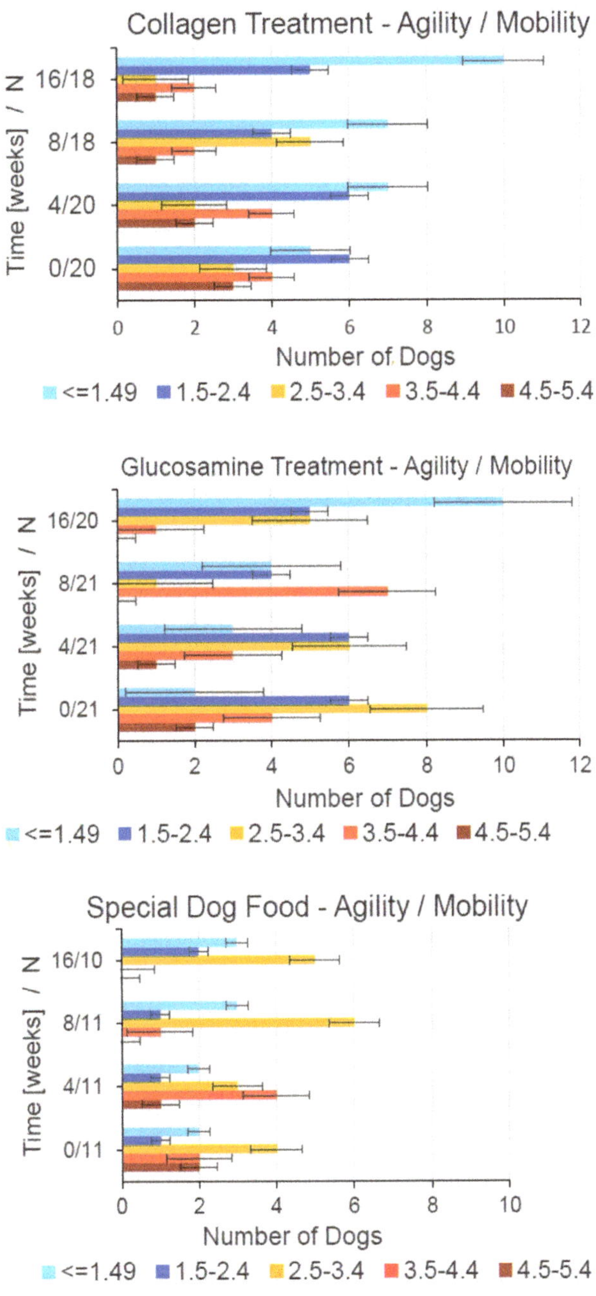

Figure 2. Agility and mobility of dogs with beginning OA symptoms. Marks/color coding: light blue—no problems, blue—minor problems, orange—moderate problems, red—large problems, dark red—extremely large problems. The marks were given by the animal-holders at different time-points (see Figure 1 for details) for the groups of dogs as indicated. These marks correlate with the QOL.

The grades, i.e., the degrees of lameness (DL) were determined by a veterinary expert. The orthopedic examination concerning joint pain symptoms (Figure 1) was carried out first. By presenting the dogs on a plane, non-slip floor covering at walk and trot, the degree of lameness was assessed. Both the orthopedic examination and the lameness assessment were documented on the standardized examination sheets by the veterinarian. The entire movement cycle (walk and trot) including walking upstairs was examined. Since dogs usually display a mixed lameness, it was not recorded whether this was a support-leg-lameness or a sloping-leg-lameness. The decisive factor is the degree of lameness, which is differentiated into five different degrees (zero means not detectable). The grade of lameness (DL) in dogs (Figure 3) with chronic musculoskeletal disorders is given on a scale from zero to four. Of the total of 52 dogs, 9 dogs showed no lameness during the entire study period (4 animals in the collagen group, 3 animals in the glucosamine group and 2 animals in the joint diet group). All other dogs were permanently or intermittently lame or had a stiff gait. DL 4 could not be determined in any of the test subjects. At week 0 (initial examination) a stiff gait could be observed in 3 dogs, DL 1 was present in 16 dogs and DL 2 was present in 22 patients. DL 3 was prevalent in two dogs. At week 16 (final examination), DL 3 was present in one dog, DL 2 in 15 animals, DL 1 in 11 animals and a stiff gait pattern in 2 dogs. A total of 19 dogs show no lameness (DL = 0).

Four dogs had to be removed from the study and were therefore not included in the final examination. No statistically significant differences were found in the distribution of the DL between the groups (p-value for week 0: 0.35; week 4: 0.85; week 8: 0.36; week 16: 0.59). There were roughly the same number of dogs free of lameness in all groups, with mild or moderate lameness. The lameness of the dogs decreased significantly during the investigation period (p-value 0.015), i.e., at the end of the investigation period significantly more animals were free of lameness than at the beginning of the investigation. The collagen and glucosamine groups had a comparable composition in regard to the degree of lameness. There were no statistically significant differences. Within the three groups, the distribution of the DL was shown as presented in Figure 3. In the group following the joint diet, only minor changes in the DL were found during the study period. During the final examination three animals were free of lameness, while at the beginning there were two in group 3. Within the other two groups, significantly more animals were free of lameness at week 16. In the younger dogs (2 to 5 years old), a relatively large number of them were still running free of lameness, despite the x-ray evidence of arthritis. With increased age of the animals, the number of dogs showing lameness increased. In particular, the proportion of dogs with DL 2 was frequently represented with advancing age. When comparing group 1 (collagen) with group 2 (glucosamine) at the end of the study period 9 in group 1 and 7 in group 2 are completely free from lameness.

The distribution of grades in regard to an assessment of complaints after invalidation/burden is shown differentially by color at 4-week intervals during the sixteen-week study period (Figure S1). The complaints of all dogs under study after prolonged exposure were rated with an average mark of 2.92 at the beginning of the study period. In the collagen, glucosamine and joint diet groups the average mark was initially 2.64, 3.38 and 2.16, respectively. At the end of the study period, the average mark of all dogs was rated 2.42. In the individual collagen, glucosamine and joint diet groups, the average marks were 1.93, 2.8 and 2.46, respectively. As the diagram shows, the dogs in the glucosamine group tend to have more severe symptoms after prolonged exercise.

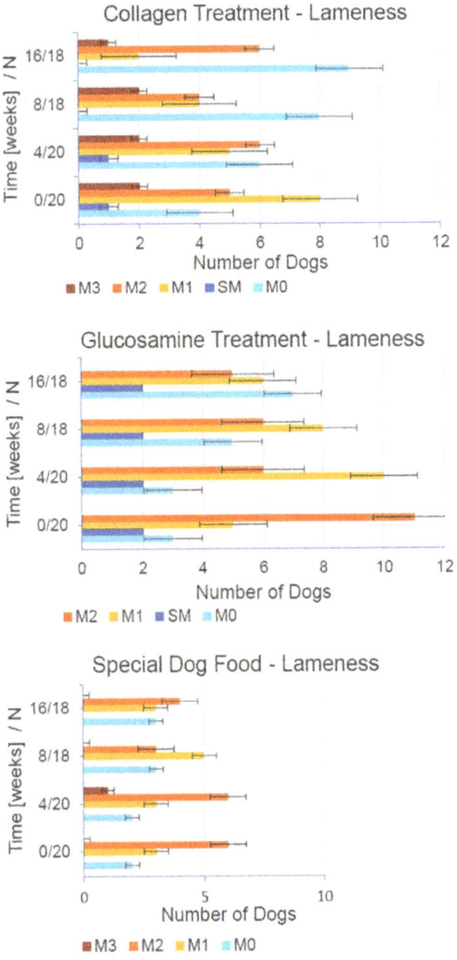

Figure 3. Lameness of dogs with beginning OA symptoms. The grades were given by a veterinarian not further involved in the study but viewing and evaluating the video footage at both the beginning and end of the therapy. Grades/color coding: light blue—no problems (M0), blue—minor problems (marked SM—stiff movement), yellow—moderate problems (M1), orange—large problems (M2), dark red—extremely large problems (M3).

The distribution of jumping ability is shown differentially by color at 4-week intervals during the sixteen-week study period (Figure S2). The average mark for jumping was rated with a mark of 3.24 at the beginning of the study period. In the individual collagen, glucosamine and joint diet groups the average marks were 3.0, 3.63 and 2.86, respectively. At the end of the study period the average mark was 2.6, with the collagen, glucosamine and joint groups displaying marks 2.34, 2.79 and 2.68, respectively. Figure S2 shows that the dogs in the glucosamine group tended to have more discomfort when jumping with a smaller number of animals jumping completely symptom-free.

The distribution of back pain sensitivity as revealed by the patient holders is shown differentially by color at 4-week intervals during the sixteen-week study period (Figure S3). The touch sensitivity of the back was rated with an average mark of 1.85 at the beginning of the study period. In the collagen, glucosamine and joint diet groups the averages were

1.89, 1.85 and 1.78, respectively. At the end of the study period, the average was 1.59 and characterized by a certain degree of homogeneity. At the same time the collagen, glucosamine and joint diet groups attained marks of 1.69, 1.48 and 1.63, respectively.

The distribution of joint pain sensitivity is shown differentially by color at 4-week intervals during the sixteen-week study period (Figure S4). The distribution of grades is shown differentially by color at 4-week intervals during the sixteen-week study period. The touch sensitivity of the affected joint was rated with an average mark of 2.19 at the beginning of the study period. In the collagen, glucosamine and joint diet groups the average was 2.63, 1.78 and 2.22, respectively. At the end of the study period the average was 1.97. In the collagen, glucosamine and joint diet the sensitivity score was 2.4, 1.63 and 1.94, respectively. By a descriptive point of view, a decrease in the sensitivity to touch was found in the collagen and glucosamine groups during the study. Overall, the difference in joint pain sensitivity between the groups was not striking at any time of the investigation (*p*-value 0.23 week 0 and 0.21 week 16). However, a possible trend is apparent with touch sensitivity decreasing for all three groups over the course of the study (grade 1.5–2.49).

The HCPI (Helsinki Chronic Pain Index [50]) of dog patients at the beginning and after 16 weeks of treatment is summarized in Table 2. We compared our data with the results of an article about the ameliorative effects of omega-3 concentrate in managing coxofemoral osteoarthritic pain in dogs [51]. Scores in the HCPI range from zero to four points, with four points corresponding to highest degree of pain. The points were averaged for each group with the expectation that with successful therapy the average score would decrease.

Table 2. HCPI (Helsinki Chronic Pain Index) of dog patients at the beginning and after 16 weeks of Collagen hydrolysate, or Glucosamine or Special dog-food treatment.

Behavior	Collagen Hydrolysate		Glucosamine		Special Dog-Food	
	Start	16 Weeks	Start	16 Weeks	Start	16 Weeks
Mind and mood	0.5	0.26	0.55	0.35	0.78	0.67
Vocalization	0.36	0.43	1	0.88	0	0
Joy of playing	1.31	1	1.72	1.35	1.25	1
Joy of running	1.5	0.76	1.83	0.94	1.78	1
Will to trot	1.56	1	1.89	1.47	1.33	0.89
Will to gallop	2.06	1.5	2.33	1.82	2.22	2
Jumping	2.25	1.71	2.72	2	2.22	2.11
Laying down	1.44	1.29	1.56	1.29	1.78	1.67
Standing up	2.13	1.79	2.61	2	2.33	2.22
Difficulty moving after a long break	2.38	2.14	2.61	1.94	2.22	2
Difficulty moving after exercise	2.07	1.58	2.94	2.5	2	2

The impact of drugs and nutritional supplements on the mobility of randomly selected dogs of the study (Table 3) was evaluated and documented by video at both the beginning and end of the therapy. Our current observations are in full agreement with a horse-study recently published [35].

Table 3. Characteristics of randomly selected dogs shown in video presentation.

Dog Name (#Number)	Treatment	Breed	Age (Years)	Weight (kg)
Buddy (#1)	glucosamine	Schnauzer-mix	5	26.5
Cora (#3)	glucosamine	Newfoundland Dog	7	50
Sarabi (#14)	collagen hydrolysate	Boerboel	3	45
Tobi (#20)	collagen hydrolysate	Mixed-breed	8	16
Emma	special dog-food with lipids and vitamins	German shepherd-mix	7	35

Representative videos (mp4 format) for two patients from the sulfated glucosamine group, two from the collagen hydrolysate group and one dog from the control group are available for download from the Supplementary Material.

Dog-patient handlers were able to easily perceive that dogs in the early stages of OA already exhibited difficulty with stair climbing. The videos clearly display this observation and demonstrate that sixteen weeks of therapy had a positive effect on the ability of these dogs to climb stairs along with no new outwardly discernable negative aspects or progression of disease.

2.2. X-ray and Statistics

X-ray data were recorded from each dog at the beginning of the study. There was no significant statistical deviation in the x-ray data when comparing the left with the right hip joint (Figure S6). This is also the case when comparing the left and the right knee joint (p-value left knee joint: 0.12; right knee joint: 0.13; left hip joint: 0.11; right hip joint: 0.15). We also recorded x-ray data from selected dogs at the end of the study. The number of dogs was limited due to the necessity of obtaining the permission of the patient holders. Furthermore, sedation of the dogs was necessary for X-ray imaging and our goal was always to reduce unecessary risk in the dogs under study. While the symptoms of pain and the QOL improved for a subset of the dogs under study, the X-ray data revealed that the damage to the bone in the affected joints was not improved with any of the treatments.

In relation to the X-ray analysis measurements of the left thigh circumference at the time of the initial examination resulted in an arithmetic mean of 39.7 cm (all patients combined). The smallest value was 24 cm, the largest 56 cm. The standard deviation was 8.1. A mean value of 38.5 cm was calculated for the collagen group, 39.6 cm for the glucosamine group and 42.5 cm for the joint diet group. At the final examination, the values were recorded in 46 patients. The mean value was 41.1 cm; the wingspan ranged from 21 cm to 57 cm. The mean value for the collagen group was 40.4 cm, for the glucosamine group it was also 40.4 cm and for the joint diet group it was 44.0 cm. The right thigh circumference at the time of the initial examination averaged 39.6 cm. In the collagen group it was 38.4 cm, in the glucosamine group it was 39.6 cm and in the joint diet group it was 42.2 cm. The smallest value was 24 cm, the largest 57 cm. During the final examination, the arithmetic mean of 40.98 cm was determined for all tested patients, 40.5 cm for the collagen group, 40.1 cm for the glucosamine group and 43.9 cm for the joint diet group. The wingspan ranged from 21 cm to 57 cm. The mean difference between the right and left thigh muscles at the initial examination, all groups combined, was 1.1 cm. The wingspan ranged from no difference up to 6 cm. In the collagen group the mean value was 1.3 cm, in the glucosamine group 0.9 cm, and in the joint diet group 1.1 cm. At the final examination, the arithmetic mean in the aggregation of all groups was 0.45 cm, in the collagen group 0.47 cm, in the glucosamine group 0.42 cm and in the joint diet group 0.5 cm. For the size of the left thigh muscles, the p-value for time was 0.0037 and the p-value for the groups was 0.67, i.e., there were only small differences between the groups that are not statistically significant. With regard to time, however, significant differences could be found, which means indicating a statistically significant increase in muscle size during the study period. The size of the right thigh muscles was similar. There were no statistically significant differences between the groups (p-value 0.68). Here, too, there was a significant increase in muscle size over time (p-value 0.01). The difference between the right and left thigh muscles (delta value) also shows no decisive differences in relation to the two main groups (p-value 0.33). Over time, however, there was a statistically significant reduction in the difference between right and left muscle circumference (p-value 0.0001).

X-ray data and measurements of the muscle circumferences provide physically measurable data, however, observation concerning pain symptoms and the mobility are also of high importance in the evaluation of the efficacy of nutraceuticals. The data were collected by the patient-holders (Figure 2 and Figures S1–S5) but also by experienced veterinarians (Figures 1 and 3) at the four examination times (initial examination, first examination—4 weeks, second examination—8 weeks, final examination—16 weeks).

2.3. Cell Biology Tests and Blood Parameters

The differentiation of canine as well as of equine chondrocytes was studied in the absence and in the presence of collagen hydrolysates and proteoglycan fragments. The distinct time-dependent differentiation pattern (e.g., with respect to the known sialic acid galactose linkage at the end of the saccharide chains of the corresponding glycoproteins is well established [24], and can be used to test the respective impact of various substances in cell culture very precisely [10]. A representative image displaying the expected pattern for equine chondrocytes grown on collagen is presented in Figure 4A.

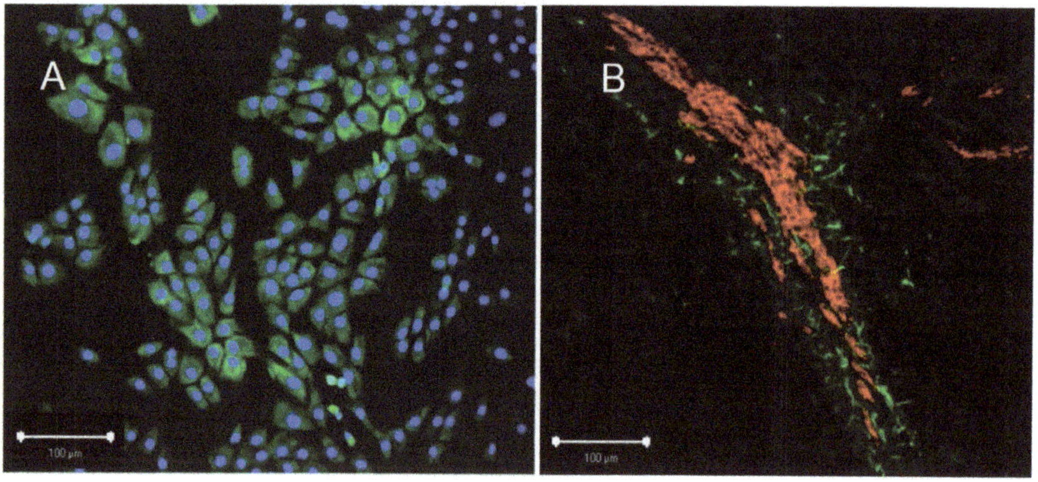

Figure 4. (**A**) Equine chondrocytes were grown on collagen media. The cell nuclei are highlighted by DAPI staining with the growing collagen strands around the nuclei stained in light green. (**B**) The polysialic acid molecules on progenitor cells from the subventricular zone of the mouse brain are colored in red. The glia cells are colored in dark green.

The induction of multi-directional differentiation processes of equine and canine chondrocytes strongly depends on the kind of collagen hydrolysate [10], as shown in Figure 4A with the collagen hydrolysate under study. Furthermore, the nerve cell progenitor assay can act as a test system to control the sialic acid dependent impact of collagen fragments on cell migration and differentiation [24,26,52,53]. Figure 4B shows an example of a progenitor cell assay from cells of the subventricular zone of the mouse brain. This indicates that sialic acid staining is a feasible method to control the collagen dependent differentiation of glia.

Blood samples were analyzed for a homogenous group of dog patients (23 German Shepherd dogs) in which collagen hydrolysate was tested as a food supplement. Previous studies were focused on a correlation between MMP-3 plasma levels and MMP-3 synovia levels for dogs suffering from osteoarthritis [46,47]. Since MMP-3 is a highly proteolytic enzyme, enhanced breakdown of cartilage tissue in the German shepherd dog OA group could occur via degradation of collagen types II, IX, X [54] and aggrecan [55]. Additionally, TIMPs are known inhibitors of MMP within tissues. We therefore examined MMP-3 (Figure 5A) and TIMP-1 levels (Figure 5B) in a back-to-back study of 23 German Shepherd dogs (guard and protection dogs of the police) which were fed over a time of 8 weeks with the same collagen hydrolysate provided to the 20 dogs in the collagen hydrolysate group described above. The analysis of MMP-3 and TIMP-1 levels (presented in Figure 5) was performed in accordance with Parkkonen et al. [56]. Notably, MMP-3 levels were significantly reduced ($p = 0.01$) after 8 weeks of treatment. We did not find a significant alteration in TIMP-1 levels during this same period.

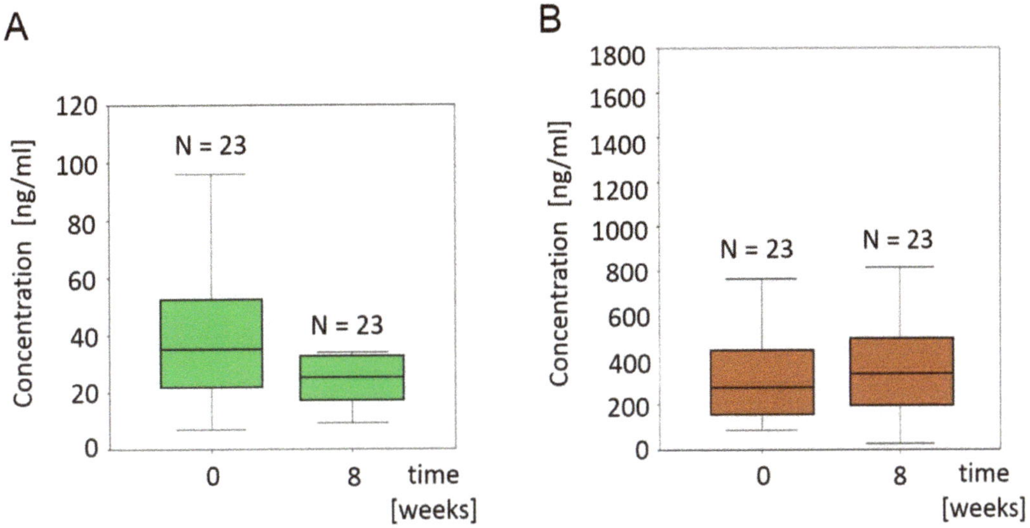

Figure 5. (**A**) MMP-3 and (**B**) TIMP-1 levels in 23 German shepherd dogs with early OA in which their diet was supplemented with collagen fragments. The concentration values (different scaling for MMP-3 and TIMP-1) at the y-axis correspond to ng/mL. Shown are the levels at the beginning and after 8 weeks of treatment. Data in box plots are presented as medians, 25th and 75th percentiles (boxes), and 10th and 90th percentiles (whiskers).

The data presented here also support the data gained earlier at Tierärztliche Hochschule Hannover [49]. Our results suggest that sulfated and non-sulfated glucosamines and small collagen fragments may have a direct influence on the activity of matrix metalloproteinases. Given this result, allosteric inhibition and stimulation as well as competitive inhibition were considered as an additional mechanism to be investigated when using collagen hydrolysates or proteoglycan fragments, i.e., sulfated and non-sulfated glucosamines as nutraceuticals.

2.4. NMR Analysis of Fortigel Collagen Hydrolysate

Our studies indicated that pain reducing effects are detectable by an evaluation of the mobility and agility of the animals under study. Furthermore, biochemical parameters are also altered as found in our analysis of the blood-probes with respect to osteoarthritis markers (e.g., TIMP-1, MMP-3). These observations are probably related to the occurrence of certain bio-active collagen fragments within the hydrolysates. It was therefore of interest to determine whether the positive effect on cartilage health for dog patients with beginning osteoarthritis symptoms can be correlated with the applied collagen fragment mixture. We therefore conducted TOCSY, NOESY and DOSY NMR experiments as described previously. Since the collagen hydrolysates differed in their composition, we further characterized them to provide a more detailed molecular analysis. In the present study, we used TOCSY and NOESY experiments to identify specific amino acid residues (e.g., Arg residues) of these bio-active compounds (Figure 6). This type of analysis allowed us to characterize the collagen hydrolysate unambiguously. The NMR results indicate that the size-range of the collagen fragments in the collagen hydrolysate food supplement is between 2.9 and 8.1 kDa, with no triple helical collagen structures present. Since the collagen hydrolysates differed in their composition, we further characterized them to provide a more detailed molecular analysis. In the present study, we used DOSY to identify specific amino acid residues (e.g., Arg residues) of these bio-active compounds (Figure 7). This type of analysis allowed us to characterize the collagen hydrolysate unambiguously.

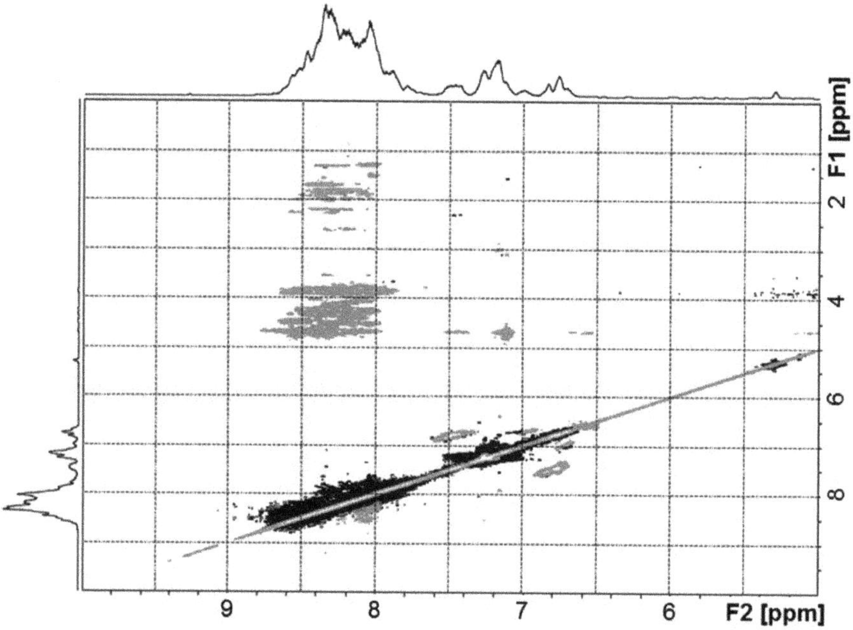

Figure 6. NOESY NMR spectrum of the collagen hydrolysate Fortigel® from Gelita applied in our dog study. F1 and F2 are the frequency axes which display both the chemical shifts of the aromatic- and NH-region of the collagen protons (in ppm).

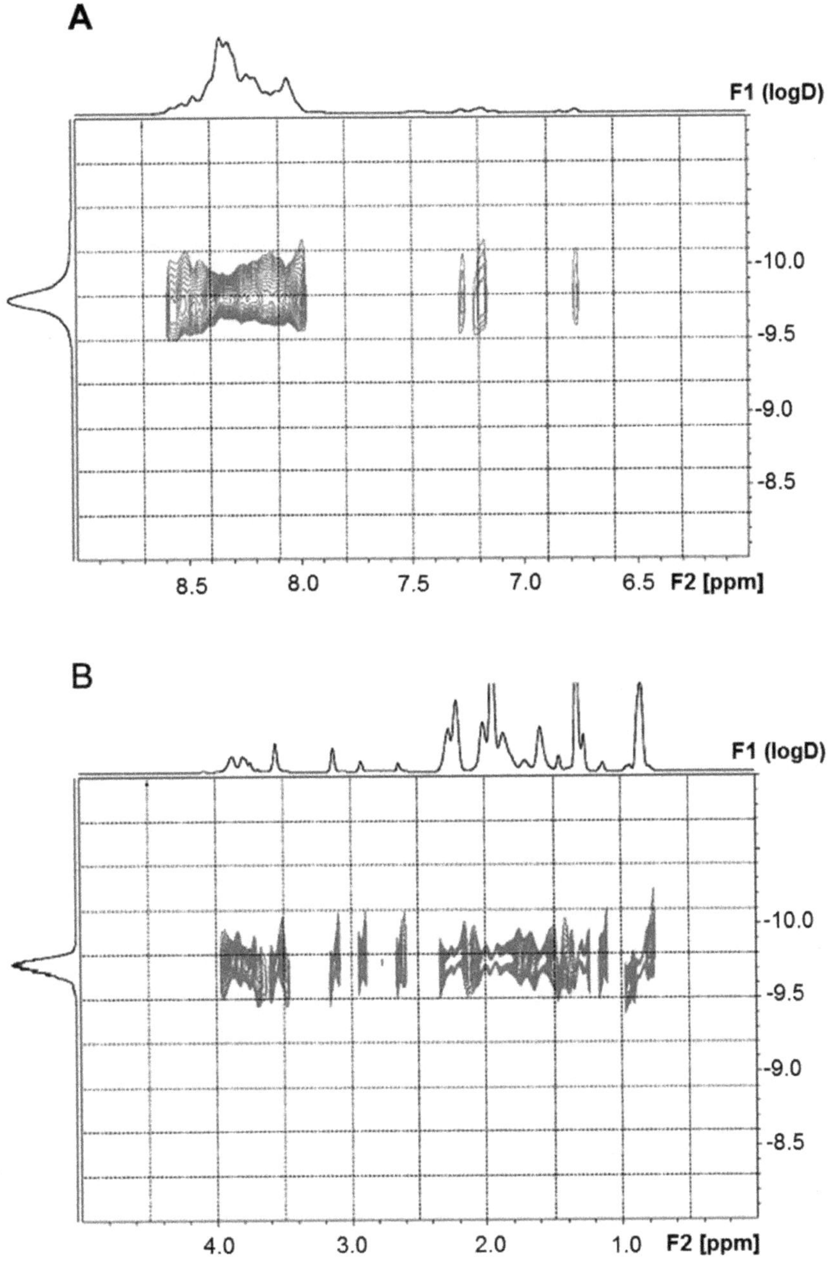

Figure 7. (**A**,**B**) Parts of a two-dimensional DOSY spectrum of the used collagen hydrolysate, Fortigel®. The aromatic- and NH-region (**A**) as well as the aliphatic region (**B**) were used to determine the diffusion constant. F2 displays the chemical shift of the collagen protons (in ppm). F1 is the frequency axis which provides information about the diffusion constant of the collagen fragments.

2.5. Molecular Modeling

We utilized the available PDB structural data for MMP-3 (2JT6.pdb) and ADAMTS-5 (2RJQ.pdb) as the starting geometries for molecular modeling tasks. Although their experimental geometries also exhibit ligands in their binding sites, we were also interested in how sialic acid and GlcNAc in standard and sulfated forms can bind to MMP-3 and ADAMTS-5. Thus, we were equally interested in the prediction of all possible binding sites (BS) for these two proteins. Three binding sites were predicted using the SiteMap program for MMP-3, whereas the prediction of BS for ADAMTS-5 was three times higher. The number of predicted binding sites is in agreement with the size/weight of these proteins (18.54 kDa for MMP-3 and 42.84 kDa for ADAMTS-5).

In the next step, we calculated how *N*-Acetyl glucosamine (GlcNAc) and *N*-Acetyl neuraminic acid (Neu5Ac) (both in standard and sulfated forms) can bind into all predicted binding sites. We used the Glide program to determine binding poses and the energetics of binding for the four carbohydrates.

The Glide analysis for all binding sites and all carbohydrates resulted in more than one thousand protein–ligand complexes. Table 4 presents the lowest energy binding poses for MMP-3 and ADAMTS-5.

Table 4. Summary of the lowest docking scores for carbohydrate–protein complexes for all predicted binding sites. The lower value in the comparison standard versus the sulfated form of the carbohydrates is shown in italics; the lowest binding scores in comparison to the four carbohydrates in the particular binding site are highlighted in bold. Carbohydrates bound to the MMP-3 binding site and three preferred binding sites for ADAMTS-5 (marked *) are visualized in Figure 8.

			Docking Score (kcal/mol)			
Protein	**PDB Code**	**Binding Site**	**GlcNAc**	**GlcNAc-sulf**	**Neu5Ac**	**Neu5Ac-sulf**
		BS1	−8.16	−8.23	−11.48 *	−8.76
MMP-3	2JT6	BS2	−9.20	−9.12	−8.68	−9.43 *
		BS3	−5.24	−6.27	−6.88	−7.42 *
		BS1	−6.28	−6.96	−7.61	−8.09*
		BS2	−7.05	−7.94	−9.00	−9.22 *
		BS3	−5.94	−5.45	−5.87	−5.78
		BS4	−7.25	−9.16	−8.61	−9.35 *
ADAMTS-5	2RJQ	BS5	−6.99	−5.73	−8.61	−7.73
		BS6			−4.47	−4.89
		BS7	−7.07	−7.31	−8.35	−8.88
		BS8	−6.07	−5.85	−8.86	−8.19
		BS9	−6.68	−6.81	−8.82	−7.93

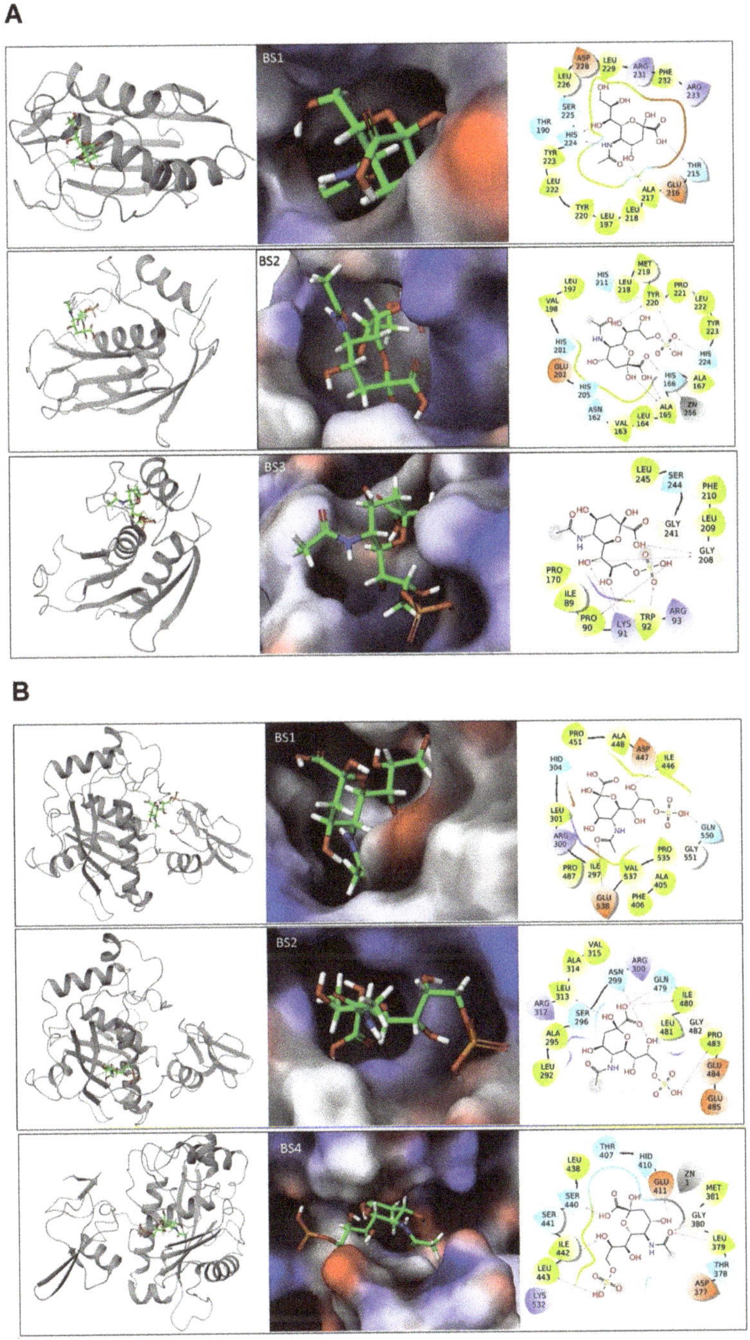

Figure 8. Glucosamines in binding sites of (**A**) MMP-3 (2JT6.pdb) and (**B**) ADAMTS-5 (2RJQ.pdb). The protein–ligand complexes are shown as a ribbon representation in the left set of figures; the protein surfaces (colored according the electrostatic potential) zoomed into binding sites are in the middle set of figures whereas the details of the protein–ligand interaction profiles are visualized in the right set of figures.

The ribbon presentation for MMP-3 together with the ligand–protein interaction analysis is illustrated in Figure 8A. Equivalent figures for ADAMTS-5 are presented in Figure 8B.

It is interesting to note Neu5Ac is predicted to bind preferably (apart from BS3 of ADAMTS-5) over GlcNAc. The sulfated forms of glucosamines in most cases bind better than the unsulfated molecules. The exception is Neu5Ac in BS1 of MMP-3. This is a special case (illustrated in Figure 8A-BS1) because this binding site appears below the protein loop and the carbohydrate molecule also interacts with the amino acids of the loop.

The next modeling step dealt with explicit modeling of the proteins with collagen fragments. We used the HEX program here to generate (based on shape and electrostatics complementarity) around 100 protein–collagen complexes for both proteins. The lowest-energy forms from the HEX modeling were used as the starting structures for molecular dynamics (MD) simulations.

MD simulations were performed in a water environment in order to evaluate the stability of the protein–collagen complexes. Figure 9 presents part of the results from a 50 ns simulation. The structure at the start of simulation plus 10 time-dependent structures extracted from the saved simulation trajectory at 5 ns intervals were superposed and are shown on Figure 9 in order to present the time-evolved conformational changes. The "simulation quality analysis" of Maestro/Desmond (Figures 8C and 9A) indicated that the standard deviation of all analyzed parameters like total energy, potential energy or volume is below 0.01% of the average value variables that were a result of the MD simulations.

PLIP analysis and the consequent Access processing of the MD trajectory geometries allowed a comparison of overall hydrogen bonding versus hydrophobic interactions for both MMP-3/collagen and ADAMTS-5 collagen. Similar data were obtained with both systems with hydrogen bonding predominating with an incidence of 68% for ADAMTS-5 and 66% for MMP-3 complexes. In comparison, hydrophobic interaction stabilization accounted for 34% in the case of MMP-3 and 32% in the case of ADAMTS-5.

The carbohydrate entity present on the protein surface in the case of ADAMTS-5 interacts with the collagen structure as shown in Figures 8D and 9B. Accordingly, the sulfate groups present at the glycan chains of proteoglycans can mediate interactions with collagen—triple helix structures of collagen present in cartilage.

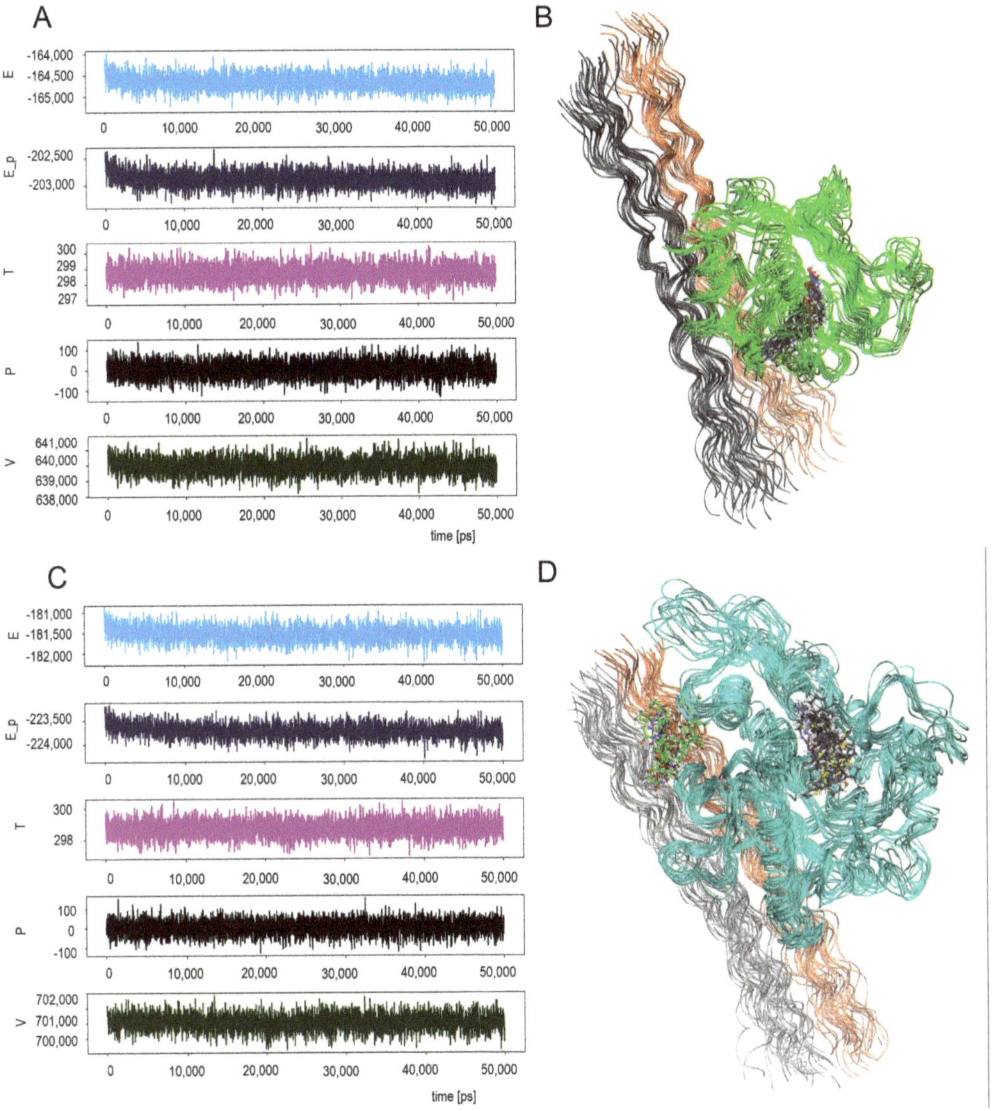

Figure 9. Molecular dynamics simulation results of solvated MMP-3/collagen (starting structure based on 2JT6.pdb + 1EI8.pdb) and ADAMTS-5/collagen (starting structure based on 2RJQ.pdb + 1EI8.pdb) supramolecular complexes. (**A**) and (**C**)—Simulation quality analysis of 50 ns DESMOND simulation as visualized in Maestro. Color coding: blue—total energy of the simulated system; dark blue—potential energy; violet—temperature; black—pressure; dark green—volume. (**B**,**D**)—Superposition of protein–collagen structures resulted from the MD simulations. Only selected structures (shown as ribbons) of the supramolecular complexes saved in 5 ns time intervals are visualized. The ligands of the proteins are shown in ball and stick models (grey carbons), whereas the GlcNAc present in ADAMTS-5 is shown with green carbons. The ribbons for A, B, C chains of the collagen fragments are visualized grey; the ribbons of D, E, F chains are shown in orange. The water molecules/ions present in the solvation box are not visualized.

3. Discussion

The ability to treat early stages of osteoarthritis with minimal side effects is a prime consideration in any treatment. Our study was focused on candidate dogs with early onset osteoarthritis.

Symptoms of pain noted during palpation by the attending veterinarian, mobility and agility marks evaluated by the patient-holders as well as an independent video-based assessment of the mobility of all the dogs in the study are displayed in Figures 1–3. As revealed by the data in the glucosamine group and even more clearly in the collagen hydrolysate group: the lameness of dogs with mild symptoms clearly improved, Figure 3. Intermolecular interactions of the glucosamine entity present on the ADAMTS-5 protein surface (as presented in Figure 9B) can influence the triple-helical structure of collagen present in the cartilage. Beside the administration of glucosamine sulfate the interactions of collagen fragments with matrix metalloprotease–carbohydrate complexes underline the importantance of glycobiological aspects of cartilage health.

A visible difference in the thigh musculature between healthy and diseased legs clearly decreased in all three groups. Additionally, there was a striking reduction in pain during palpation of the knee joint in both the collagen group and glucosamine groups. During the study period, this was accompanied by a significant reduction in symptoms while standing, climbing stairs, jumping and after prolonged strain. An obvious reduction in touch sensitivity of the affected joint and the spinal cord, respectively, as well as an obvious increase in running pleasure was also found in these two groups. Similarly, a clear reduction in the symptoms while standing and a reduced touch sensitivity of the affected joint and an increase in running pleasure was found in the joint diet group. This group displayed minimal improvement in the other four parameters. The HCPI (Helsinki Chronic Pain Index; Table 2) and the QOL (Quality of Live score) improved in all three groups. The observed clinical improvements, particularly through the administration of glucosamine sulfate and collagen hydrolysate, indicate a positive effect for these two compounds.

It was impossible to detect the effect of the standard dog food in this study. In order to observe the effect of standard food a placebo group has to be created, comprising dogs fed in an ordinary way. This was forbidden due the fact that the animals were sick and needed to be treated. Consequently, group 3 was entitled as commercial joint diet group. It was the fatty acid-related group where we expected healing success as well. The food in group 3 was changed completely (no collagen or glucosamine enrichment) and the dogs were administered with power food only. The food for this group can be entitled as power food because it was designed to contain valuable fatty acids. The feeding in group 1 and 2 was different. The dogs obtained standard dog food but enriched with collagen hydrolysate (Group 1) or sulfated glucosamine (Group 2). While the feeding within Group 2 or Group 3 matched standard feeding protocols, fish-oil-enriched collagen hydrolysate feeding is more or less a novel protocol. Independently of the therapeutic options used for Groups 1 to 3, the beneficial effect of treatment (but slightly different) was monitored in all three groups of the dogs.

Our combined clinical, cell biological, biochemical, biophysical and molecular modeling approach on canine and equine patients is a feasible strategy to answer a number of questions related to collagen hydrolysates, sulfated glycans and lipids as chondroprotective food supplements. Articular cartilage destruction is mediated by the loss of collagen type II and proteoglycans and this loss is a characteristic feature of osteoarthritic (OA) symptoms. Our results show that it is possible to correlate the influence of collagen hydrolysates on cartilage tissue [32–34] through specific biochemical pathways and cell–biological processes [4,7,8]. We found that collagen hydrolysates were able to alter the levels of MMP-3 without changing the level of TIMP-1 (Tissue Inhibitors of MetalloProteinases-1; data not shown). In addition, we recognized the involvement of collagen hydrolysates and sulfated glucosamine in several key biochemical processes which are directly correlated with cartilage health. As noted, collagen hydrolysates contain mixtures of collagen fragments of various length. We show here that modeling is a useful tool in evaluating specific interactions in protein binding sites and interactions between these proteins and collagen fragments. The impact of sulfation in the case of glucosamine is discussed here in detail. In comparison to sulfated GlcNAc, we analyzed the interactions of sulfated Neu5Ac, which is an interesting member of the sialic acid family with bio-medical relevance [24,25,27,28,30,57]. In addition, the effect of chondroprotective collagen hydrolysate of fish or jellyfish origin on cell cultures is similar to the effect of collagen hydrolysate of bovine origin used in the present dog study. We note that the EU Community approval/registration of fish or jellyfish originated collagen hydrolysate is not completed yet. No doubt further investigation on the impact of these interactions on protein activity in relation to targeting diseases will be crucial in further evaluating their effect on the extracellular matrix and therapeutic value.

Cartilage markers (MMP-3 and TIMP-1, Figure 5A,B) were analyzed over a time period of 8 weeks from a homogenous group of 23 German Shephard dogs of nearly the same weight. This was important in order to determine a daily dose of 20 g. One could argue that a dose for smaller dogs with a lower body weight has to be adapted to these patients. Since collagen hydrolysate and sulfated glucosamine are nutrition supplements without any toxic effect, overdosing in smaller dogs theoretically could have led to increased positive effects. This, however, was not observed during our study. Cell assays, molecular modeling studies, examination of eight horses and one dog in a long-time study were necessary in order to find out in which way our results can be extended to different species (including humans) and to collagen hydrolysates from other resources (e.g., fish skin and jellyfish). Therefore, Figure 4A,B is not shown in order to document a state before and after a treatment with collagen hydrolysate. The effects of collagen hydrolysates on equine cells have been documented in detail in the literature (Raabe et al., 2010). It is also feasible to analyze the impact of collagen hydrolysate on the migration of nerve cells (Zhang et al., 2016). In this context Figure 4B demonstrates that it was possible to observe the differentiation of stem cells treated with collage hydrolysate by staining with polysialic acid.

To figure out whether the positive effects of collagen hydrolysate may be detectable or useful in other species that display osteoarthritis related problems in their movements, we also treated selected horses (50 g/day for a normal-sized horse and 25 g/day for a smaller horse e.g., a Shetland pony) In the case of a Holstein horse, a Hanoverian horse, an Arabian horse, an American Quarter horse, a Trotter, an English Blood horse, a Shetland pony and a Trakehner horse positive responses were detectable with corresponding methods as discussed here for the dog patients.

Overall, all three therapies have a positive effect on dogs' health, justifying their individual use. However, the data presented here along with the supplementary data indicated that sulfated glucosamine and collagen hydrolysate used as supplementary nutraceuticals are more effective than high-quality dog food alone, with collagen hydrolysate and sulfated glucosamine having similar positive effects on cartilage health. However, importantly the data indicate that supplementing a dog's diet with collagen has the greatest effect on reducing lameness, thus suggesting that the goal of increasing collagen levels should be incorporated into a treatment regime that targets the OA symptom of lameness.

4. Materials and Methods

4.1. Dog Osteoarthritis and Drug Administration

Dogs were chosen based on a thorough anamnestic workup, a general and an orthopedic examination (including an X-ray examination) as well as a blood draw. Subsequently, 52 dogs were randomized into three groups. 20 dogs received collagen hydrolysate, 21 dogs received glucosamine sulfate and 11 dogs received the special diet. The animals in all three groups were fed with the supplements or the special diet over a period of 16 weeks. During this time, follow up examinations were carried out after 4, 8 and 16 weeks. Data from a separate study of 23 German Shepard dogs were used in our study to analyze the MMP-3 data over a time-period of 8 weeks. Furthermore, 8 horses (including a pony) were examined in order to determine the efficacy of this treatment design in other species.

Various dogs with early osteoarthritis (OA) were examined in a randomized clinical study examining the therapeutic effect of nutraceuticals. Specifically, the impact of (A) a collagen hydrolysate, (B) tablets of sulfated glucosamine and (C) a high-quality dog-food, i.e., Hills-JD (containing vitamins and enriched with fatty acids, especially EPA) on joint health was evaluated. The dogs were fed Hills-JD instead of a placebo, since the dogs already displayed osteoarthritis symptoms and were therefore already being treated accordingly. The main lipid-component of HillsJD is eicosapentaenoic acid (EPA) which is enriched in sea-fishes such as salmon and herring. The administered peptides, carbohydrates and lipids were delivered via the gastro-intestinal tract into the blood-stream and administered in this way to the crucial target tissues in the organism. A dose of 20 g collagen hydrolysate was administered per day and dog patient (based on the daily collagen requirements in food for wolves). The dose was not reduced for smaller dogs since a higher amount of this nutraceutical is completely harmless (as tested in a cell biological assays).

Sulfated GlcNAc in the form of tablets, collagen hydrolysate from Gelita dry powder, Hills JD high quality dog-food were used to target dogs' osteoarthritis. Fish collagen hydrolysate is produced by the skin of deep water ocean fish (cod, haddock and pollock). The fish collagen (Norland Products Inc., Cranbury, NJ, USA) consisted primarily of alpha 1 and alpha 2 chains in a 2:1 ratio with a MW between 4.5 and 21 kDa [7,10].

The QOL-score (Quality of life) combines the mood of the animal, its mobility and agility, joy of playing, sounds of pain and problems with climbing stairs. Dog-patient handlers were provided with a questionnaire which evaluated the QOL score. In addition, to remove any perceived bias, a veterinary doctor, not involved in the study in any other capacity, assessed video footage of the treated animals to provide an independent QOL estimate.

4.2. Cell Biology Tests and Blood Parameters Determination

The cell biology tests used are the same as those described in our former publications Raabe et al. [10], Zhang et al. [26] and Petridis et al. [53]. We focused on the impact of collagen hydrolysates on the differentiation of chondrocytes as well as on the role of sialic acids as contact structures of the cell surface as differentiation markers.

Blood samples were obtained from all dogs and horses under study in order to clarify any existing medical condition. The blood samples were taken after stasis and disinfection with 70% alcohol on the anterior vein cephalic with a 7.5 mL S-Monovette (Sarstedt) and an attached cannula (Sarstedt). An amount of 16 IU served as anticoagulant Heparin. The blood was centrifuged at 3000 rpm for 10 min after collection. A large blood count (hematology), an organ profile and an IgG/IgM borreliosis antibody titer were created for each dog in the Synlab Augsburg laboratory. Blood was drawn as part of the treatment.

The samples obtained were labelled and stored in a deep freezer until evaluation.

MMP-3: A mouse anti-dog stromelysin-1 monoclonal antibody MAC-084 (UCB Celltech, Slough, UK) was used to coat the ELISA plates (Greiner Bio-One GmbH, Kremsmünster, Austria) by incubation of 10 g/50 mL PBS buffer. After overnight incubation at 4 °C., the blood plasma samples were applied undiluted to the ELISA plates and incubated at 4 °C for two hours. The second antibody, a rabbit anti-dog stromelysin-1 polyclonal antibody (Biotrend Chemikalien GmbH, Köln, Germany) was added at a 1:8000 dilution and incubated again for two hours at 4 °C. The last two-hour incubation at 4 °C was carried out with a peroxidase-labeled goat anti-rabbit antibody (Sigma Aldricks, Saint Louis, MO, USA) at a 1:20,000 dilution. The amount of bound peroxidase as a measure of the concentration of MMP-3 present in the sample was determined using tetramethylbenzidine as the peroxidase substrate. Three washing steps are carried out between each new antibody coating in order to separate unbound antigens from the sample. The enzyme reaction was stopped by the addition of sulfuric acid. Prostromelysin (UCB Celltech, Slough, UK) in a concentration of 126 ng/mL was used as the standard. The resulting yellow color change was measured at 450 nm in a Spectra Photometer (Tecan, Männedorf, Switzerland).

TIMP-1: The ELISA plates (Greiner) were treated with an anti-dog TIMP-1 monoclonal antibody MAC-080 (Celltech) in a concentration of 5.7 g/50 mL PBS buffer with incubation overnight at 4 °C. The blood plasma samples were applied to the ELISA plates at a 1:7 dilution. After a two-hour incubation at room temperature on the Thermostar (13MG), a rabbit anti-human TIMP-1 polyclonal antibody (Biotrend) in a 1:2000 dilution was used as the second antibody. After a further incubation of two hours at room temperature on the Thermostar, coating was carried out with a peroxidase-labeled goat anti-rabbit antibody (Sigma) at a 1:4000 dilution. The amount of bound peroxidase as a measure of the concentration of TIMP-1 present in the sample was determined using tetramethylbenzidine as the peroxidase substrate. Several washing steps were carried out between each new antibody coating in order to separate unbound antigens from the sample. The enzyme reaction was stopped by the addition of sulfuric acid. Recombinant dog TIMP-1 was used to generate a standard curve with a concentration range of 27.5 ng/mL. The resulting yellow color complex was measured at 450 nm in a Spectra Photometer (Tecan) [49].

4.3. *Statistical Analysis*

Preliminary data processing started with Microsoft Excel (Office 2000 package, Microsoft, Redmond, WA, USA). The biomedical data of animals under study were evaluated on the computers in the local computer network (LAN) of the Biomathematics and Data Processing unit of the Veterinary Medicine Department of the Justus Liebig University in Gießen. The statistical evaluations were carried out using the BMDP/Dynamic, Release 8.1 (Statistical Solutions Ltd., Cork, Ireland) [58] program package. Missing data in Tables are marked with *. Consequently, the given entry is treated as a missing value by the BMDP program. To describe the data, arithmetic means (x^-), standard deviations (s), minima (x_{min}), maxima (x_{max}) and sample sizes (n) were calculated and presented in a table for quantitative, approximately normally distributed characteristics. The qualitative characteristics were counted separately according to groups and presented in the form of frequency tables. To statistically test the group and time influence for significance, a two-factor analysis of variance with repeated measurements with regard to time was carried out with the program BMDP2V in groups 1 and 2 with approximately normally distributed characteristics. If the values were missing, this was conducted using the BMDP5V (so-called "forest test"). With regard to the quantitative characteristics, the group comparison of these two groups with normal distribution used the t-test and otherwise the Wilcoxon-Mann–Whitney test (BMDP3D). For the semiquantitative characteristics, the exact Wilcoxon-Mann–Whitney test using the "StatXact" program (V1, Cytel, Waltham, MA, USA) was applied to compare the two groups. For the comparison of qualitative characteristics, frequency tables were generated for all three groups with the program BMDP4F. The qualitative characteristics were checked in the case of two expressions regarding significant correlations for each point in time only for groups 1 and 2 with the exact test by Fisher. The Fisher–Freeman–Halton test was used for more than two values. The "StatXact" program was used here (Cytel, 2010 [59]). The evaluation of the statistical significance was based on the significance level $\alpha = 0.05$; this means results with $p \leq 0.05$ were given as statistically significant. In addition, the exact p-value was given, if possible. Group 3, as a trailing group, was not included in the significance calculation.

4.4. *Nuclear Magnetic Resonance (NMR) Spectroscopy*

Proton NMR was applied to analyze the Fortigel collagen hydrolysate in terms of its fragment size distribution (DOSY [7]) and possible identification of certain amino acid types (TOCSY/NOESY). Mass-spectrometry and NMR previously provided a detailed molecular analysis of the collagen hydrolysates under study [4,7–9]. In the NMR tubes, collagen hydrolysates were dissolved at an amount of 3 mg in 0.5 mL water (90% H_2O/10% D_2O). The NMR experiments were performed on a 600 MHz Bruker Avance III spectrometer (Bruker, Karlsruhe, Germany) at 298 K. 2D-TOCSY experiments (DIPSI-2; mixing time 80 ms) and 2D-NOESY (mixing times 200 or 400 ms) were recorded with 512 (F1) $\times$ 1024 (F2) complex data points and a spectral widths of 7212 Hz (12 ppm). Water suppression was performed using excitation sculpting and, per increment, 16 scans were accumulated with an inter-scan recovery delay of 1.5 s. For processing we used zero-filling to 1024 (F1) × 2048 (F2) data points prior to Fourier transformation, followed by baseline correction in both dimensions. Spectra were calibrated on internal water.

4.5. Molecular Modeling

The structures of glucosamines, i.e., *N*-Acetyl Glucosamine (GlcNAc) and *N*-Acetyl Neuraminic acid (Neu5Ac; also sialic acid) were downloaded from PUBCHEM (https://pubchem.ncbi.nlm.nih.gov/, accessed on 12 July 2019) in SDF format and imported into the Maestro V. 12.3.013 (Schrödinger LLC, New York, NY, USA) [60] project table. Both molecules were then sulfated using the Maestro molecular builder option. Their molecular structures are presented in Scheme 1. An advanced conformational search for carbohydrate side chain orientations were then carried out maintaining their $^4C_1$ forms for GlcNAc and GlcNAc-sulf and $^1C_4$ for Neu5Ac and Neu5Ac-sulf ring conformations. The geometries of five selected low-energy conformations of the four carbohydrates were ab initio (DFT B3LYP 6-31G**) optimized (releasing all geometric parameters) with the Gaussian [61] program (G09 version, Wallingford, CT, USA) and were then used as input ligands for molecular docking into matrix proteins like MMP-3 and aggrecanases (e.g., ADAMTS-5), present in the dog and horses organisms.

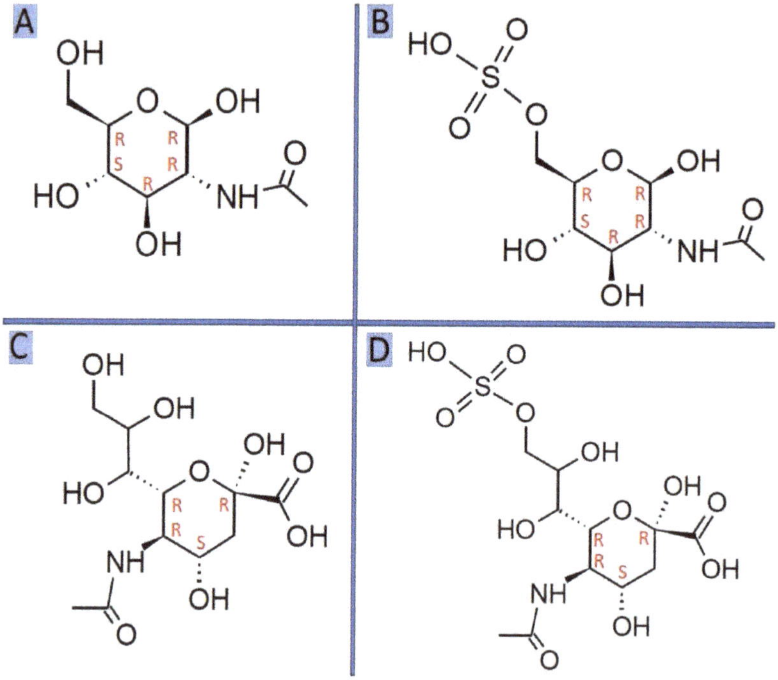

Scheme 1. Molecular structures of the carbohydrates in standard and sulfated forms. (**A**) 2-Acetamido-2-deoxy-D-glucopyranoside (GlcNAc); (**B**) 6-O-Sulfoxy-2-Acetamido-2-deoxy-D-glucopyranoside (GlcNAc-sulf); (**C**) *N*-Acetyl-Neuraminic Acid (Neu5Ac); (**D**) 9-O-Sulfoxy-*N*-Acetyl-Neuraminic Acid (Neu5Ac-sulf).

The atomic coordinates of MMP-3 (2JT6.pdb [13]), ADAMTS-5 (2RJQ.pdb [12]) and a collagen fragment (1EI8.pdb [62]) structures were downloaded from the protein database and imported into Maestro. All protein geometries were processed (adding missing atoms, fixing bond orders, assign partial charges) by "Protein Preparation Wizard" of the Maestro program (V12.3.013, Schrödinger LLC, New York, NY, USA) [60].

The possible binding sites of MMP-3 and ADAMTS-5 were evaluated using the SiteMap program (V3.9, Schrödinger LLC, New York, NY, USA) [63,64] of Schrödinger LLC. The G09-optimized conformations of four ligands (Scheme 1) were docked into all SiteMap predicted binding sites of MMP-3 and ADAMTS-5 using the GLIDE program [65–68]. While flexible docking was considered for all side chains of the carbohydrates, the pyranose rings were fixed in 4C1 for 1C4 forms as stated above. All protein–ligand complexes resulting from GLIDE flexible were optimized (OPLS-2005 force field) and were tableted/ordered according their GLIDE docking scores.

The HEX program [69] was used to generate and preoptimize the geometries of the MMP-3/collagen and ADAMTS-5/collagen supramolecular complexes. From around 100 generated complexes the lowest-energy ones were selected for further molecular dynamics (MD) studies.

These HEX-output files were imported into Maestro and were processed by standard methods (as indicated above by "Protein Preparation Wizard") to obtained the structures prepared for MD runs using the Desmond [60,70] program The OPLS-2005 force field (the up-to-date version of the OPLS force field family [71,72]) was used to carry out the simulation studies. The protein–collagen complexes were initially solvated in Maestro (SPC water model [73] with the water molecules added within a 1 nm buffer around the proteins) and the resulting structures were then minimized and equilibrated for 5ns. The final structures after equilibration were submitted for 50 ns NPT (pressure at 1.01325 bar) molecular dynamics (MD) simulations with the Desmond program at 300 K. Molecular geometries resulting from simulations were saved at 10 ps intervals and were used for further analysis. These geometries (5000 altogether) from each simulation were exported into pdb format and were used for analysis of interaction profiles using the PLIP program [74]. The xml files resulted from the PLIP calculation were imported into Microsoft Access for analysis and data mining.

Schrödinger's Maestro [60] was used for visualization of molecular structures, their complexes and protein–carbohydrate ligand interaction profiles.

5. Conclusions

The experimental and computational methods applied were found to be useful tools in providing valuable information on the relationship between therapeutic value and mechanism. Such approaches will be key prior to these or other similar compounds being adopted further as potential medical therapies.

Collagen hydrolysate and sulfated glucosamine and potentially the fatty acid and vitamin rich food diet in the control group show similar benefits with respect to a treatment of early osteoarthritis symptoms. The positive effects in all three groups seems to be comparable, however, in contrast to sulfated glucosamine, collagen-hydrolysate provides more options for an improved therapy. Collagen hydrolysates are defined mixtures of short, long and medium-sized collagen fragments. Fortigel, used here, is a well-defined collagen hydrolysate that can be considered the gold-standard. Our NMR and molecular modeling techniques in combination with cell assays described here were essential in better defining possible mechanisms contributing to the improvement of the dog-patients. Furthermore, they provide a foundation for follow-up studies. These follow-up studies would include further examining the effect of this treatment in other species (e. g. horses) and a comparable analysis of various collagen hydrolysate compositions (e.g., fish skin, jellyfish). We note that even if the collagen-hydrolysates are from one species their compositions can be different depending on the formulation used by the supplier [8].

The positive effects we observed in the glucosamine (group 2) and the trailing group (group 3) were not surprising given their known use in the treatment of osteoarthritis. However, the clear and positive results in the collagen hydrolysate group (group 1) were not predictable at the beginning of the study. During the 16 weeks study period muscle and leg circumferences increased and pain symptoms were significantly reduced with this treatment. The study also clearly shows that there is variability among individual dogs, with some reacting well while others react weakly to the nutraceuticals under study. Since this may be based on the individual genetic makeup of the dog and subtle differences in the stage of disease having a third option becomes a desirable option that may provide added benefit to some animals. Additionally, sulfated glucosamine belongs to the standard therapies in the treatment of early osteoarthritic symptoms while only limited information exists about the molecular background of its beneficial effect, especially with respect to the impact of the sulfate group. Additionally, in the case of collagen hydrolysate, which is not part of a standard therapy, a number of structural questions which are related to its therapeutic functions are still open. Therefore, we combined the feeding study with intense molecular modeling calculations describing the stability of, e.g., complexes of MMP-3 with the nutraceuticals of group 1 and group 2. These data have provided us with an initial insight into unravelling key mechanisms of action for these compounds and avenues for future study and for treatment.

Supplementary Materials: The following are available online at https://www.mdpi.com/article/10.3390/md19100542/s1: Figure S1. Assessment of Complaints after invalidation/ burden. Figure S2. Jumping study of the dog patients. Figure S3. Back pain touch sensitivity of the dog patients. Figure S4. Joint pain sensitivity of the dog patients. Figure S5. Joy of running marks of the dog patients as revealed by the patient-holders. Figure S6. X-ray data of the left and right femoral joints (A left; B right) obtained from each dog at the beginning of the study. Figure S7. Canine dog patients with beginning OA symptoms were examined at the different time frames. Figure S8. Agility and mobility of dogs with beginning OA symptoms. Figure S9. Lameness of dogs with beginning OA symptoms. Video S1: Mp4 video file illustrating the behaviour of the dogs.

Author Contributions: H.-C.S., N.Z., M.J.-B., T.E. planed the study; M.J.-B. performed the clinical part of the dog study; T.E., T.K. worked on molecular modeling and MD-simulations; M.B.-R., K.H., H.L., M.J.-B. and A.K.P. evaluation of the blood and cell probes; R.S. evaluated the links between sialic acids and cartilage health; A.K., H.-C.S., J.S., N.Z., P.E., R.Z. were involved in data analysis and processing and wrote selected parts of the manuscripts; H.-C.S., J.W.H., T.K. contributed to data analysis, graphical presentation of the results and prepared the final version of the manuscript. All authors have read and agreed to the published version of the manuscript.

Funding: Elements of the project are financed by the European Commission's Framework Program 7 (Bio-NMR; project number 261863). This publication is the result of the project implementation: Open Scientific Community for Modern Interdisciplinary Research in Medicine (OPENMED), ITMS2014+: 313011V455 supported by the Operational Programme Integrated Infrastructure, funded by the ERDF. Parts of the presented reseach were also supported by National Natural Science Foundation of China (Project No. 82001286) and Natural Science Foundation of Shandong province (Project No. ZR2020QH112).

Institutional Review Board Statement: This study was initiated at the Jusus-Liebig-University Gießen (Germany) as an animal observation study in the framework of a thesis about therapeutic improvements against early osteoarthritis symptoms of dogs and horses. The study was conducted by experienced veterinarians. All patient-holders were provided with the details of the study prior to signing the declaration of consent. All patients participating in the study were treated according to the guidelines in veterinary medicine. Instead of a placebo group a diet with fish oil and vitamins was applied which is to a standard therapy in veterinary medicine.

Informed Consent Statement: Not applicable.

Data Availability Statement: The data presented in this study are available on request from the corresponding authors.

Acknowledgments: We thank Ralf Boelens, Hans Wienk (University Utrecht (NL)), Steffen Oesser (CRI Kiel), Martin Kramer, Lutz-F. Litzke, Klaus Failing, Uschi Siebler (FB 10 University Gießen) and Eckhard Wolf (Faculty of Veterinary Medicine, Gene Center and Department of Biochemistry, Ludwig-Maximilians University, Munich, Germany) for scientific support and Philipp Siebert (RI-B-NT) for technical assistance. Werner Jahn from the horse clinic in Bargteheide (Schleswig-Holstein,

Germany) is thanked for valuable discussions concerning arthritic therapies on horses as well as Shaida von Berenberg-Gossler (Hamburg, Germany) for her important hints about the behavior of dressage horses as well as Götz Dreismann (Practice for small animals and horses, Tornesch, Schleswig-Holstein, Germany) for fruitful discussions about sulfated glucosamines. Ivano Bertini who unfortunately passed away in 2012 was over the years at many scientific meetings an inspiring discussion partner concerning his pioneering NMR work in the field of matrix metalloproteinases and paramagnetic molecules. We also thank the company Gelita for collagen hydrolysates and the Carl-Friedrich-von-Weizsäcker Gesellschaft e. V.-Wissen und Verantwortung for multiple support.

Conflicts of Interest: The authors declare that they have no conflict of interest.

References

1. Tacke, S.; Gollwitzer, A.; Grammel, L.; Henke, J. Pain therapy in small pets. *Tierarztliche Praxis. Ausgabe K Kleintiere/Heimtiere* **2017**, *45*, 53–60. [CrossRef]
2. Bockstahler, B.; Levine, D.; Millis, D.L.; Wandrey, S.O.N. *Essential Facts of Physiotherapy in Dogs and Cats*; BE VetVerlag: Babenhausen, Germany, 2004.
3. Benavente, M.; Arias, S.; Moreno, L.; Martínez, J. Production of Glucosamine Hydrochloride from Crustacean Shell. *J. Pharm. Pharmacol.* **2015**, *3*, 20–26. [CrossRef]
4. Siebert, H.C.; Burg-Roderfeld, M.; Eckert, T.; Stötzel, S.; Kirch, U.; Diercks, T.; Humphries, M.J.; Frank, M.; Wechselberger, R.; Tajkhorshid, E.; et al. Interaction of the alpha2A domain of integrin with small collagen fragments. *Protein Cell* **2010**, *1*, 393–405. [CrossRef]
5. Krylov, V.B.; Grachev, A.A.; Ustyuzhanina, N.E.; Ushakova, N.A.; Preobrazhenskaya, M.E.; Kozlova, N.I.; Portsel, M.N.; Konovalova, I.N.; Novikov, V.Y.; Siebert, H.C.; et al. Preliminary structural characterization, anti-inflammatory and anticoagulant activities of chondroitin sulfates from marine fish cartilage. *Russian Chem. Bull.* **2011**, *60*, 746–753. [CrossRef]
6. Burg-Roderfeld, M.; Eckert, T.; Siebert, H.C. Bioaktive Kollagenfragmente. Neue struktur-biologische Studien an Kollagen-Integrin-Komplexen belegen Justus Liebigs wegweisende Ideen. *Spiegel der Forschung* **2011**, *28*, 36–43.
7. Stötzel, S.; Schurink, M.; Wienk, H.; Siebler, U.; Burg-Roderfeld, M.; Eckert, T.; Kulik, B.; Wechselberger, R.; Sewing, J.; Steinmeyer, J.; et al. Molecular organization of various collagen fragments as revealed by atomic force microscopy and diffusion-ordered NMR spectroscopy. *ChemPhysChem* **2012**, *13*, 3117–3125. [CrossRef]
8. Schadow, S.; Simons, V.S.; Lochnit, G.; Kordelle, J.; Gazova, Z.; Siebert, H.C.; Steinmeyer, J. Metabolic Response of Human Osteoarthritic Cartilage to Biochemically Characterized Collagen Hydrolysates. *Int. J. Mol. Sci.* **2017**, *18*, 207. [CrossRef]
9. Schadow, S.; Siebert, H.C.; Lochnit, G.; Kordelle, J.; Rickert, M.; Steinmeyer, J. Collagen metabolism of human osteoarthritic articular cartilage as modulated by bovine collagen hydrolysates. *PLoS ONE* **2013**, *8*, e53955. [CrossRef]
10. Raabe, O.; Reich, C.; Wenisch, S.; Hild, A.; Burg-Roderfeld, M.; Siebert, H.C.; Arnhold, S. Hydrolyzed fish collagen induced chondrogenic differentiation of equine adipose tissue-derived stromal cells. *Histochem Cell Biol.* **2010**, *134*, 545–554. [CrossRef]
11. Bertini, I.; Calderone, V.; Cosenza, M.; Fragai, M.; Lee, Y.M.; Luchinat, C.; Mangani, S.; Terni, B.; Turano, P. Conformational variability of matrix metalloproteinases: Beyond a single 3D structure. *Proc. Natl. Acad. Sci. USA* **2005**, *102*, 5334–5339. [CrossRef]
12. Mosyak, L.; Georgiadis, K.; Shane, T.; Svenson, K.; Hebert, T.; McDonagh, T.; Mackie, S.; Olland, S.; Lin, L.; Zhong, X.; et al. Crystal structures of the two major aggrecan degrading enzymes, ADAMTS4 and ADAMTS-5. *Protein Sci. Publ. Protein Soc.* **2008**, *17*, 16–21. [CrossRef] [PubMed]
13. Alcaraz, L.A.; Banci, L.; Bertini, I.; Cantini, F.; Donaire, A.; Gonnelli, L. Matrix metalloproteinase-inhibitor interaction: The solution structure of the catalytic domain of human matrix metalloproteinase-3 with different inhibitors. *J. Biol. Inorg. Chem. JBIC Publ. Soc. Biol. Inorg. Chem.* **2007**, *12*, 1197–1206. [CrossRef] [PubMed]
14. Sadowski, T.; Steinmeyer, J. Effects of tetracyclines on the production of matrix metalloproteinases and plasminogen activators as well as of their natural inhibitors, tissue inhibitor of metalloproteinases-1 and plasminogen activator inhibitor-1. *Inflamm. Res.* **2001**, *50*, 175–182. [CrossRef] [PubMed]
15. Masuyer, G.; Schwager, S.L.; Sturrock, E.D.; Isaac, R.E.; Acharya, K.R. Molecular recognition and regulation of human angiotensin-I converting enzyme (ACE) activity by natural inhibitory peptides. *Sci. Rep.* **2012**, *2*, 717. [CrossRef]
16. Kawakami, Y.; Matsuo, K.; Murata, M.; Yudoh, K.; Nakamura, H.; Shimizu, H.; Beppu, M.; Inaba, Y.; Saito, T.; Kato, T.; et al. Expression of Angiotensin II Receptor-1 in Human Articular Chondrocytes. *Arthritis* **2012**, *2012*, 648537. [CrossRef] [PubMed]
17. Nakamura, F.; Tsukamoto, I.; Inoue, S.; Hashimoto, K.; Akagi, M. Cyclic compressive loading activates angiotensin II type 1 receptor in articular chondrocytes and stimulates hypertrophic differentiation through a G-protein-dependent pathway. *FEBS Open Bio* **2018**, *8*, 962–973. [CrossRef]
18. Kouguchi, T.; Ohmori, T.; Shimizu, M.; Takahata, Y.; Maeyama, Y.; Suzuki, T.; Morimatsu, F.; Tanabe, S. Effects of a chicken collagen hydrolysate on the circulation system in subjects with mild hypertension or high-normal blood pressure. *Biosci. Biotechnol. Biochem.* **2013**, *77*, 691–696. [CrossRef]
19. Kosinska, M.K.; Ludwig, T.E.; Liebisch, G.; Zhang, R.; Siebert, H.C.; Wilhelm, J.; Kaesser, U.; Dettmeyer, R.B.; Klein, H.; Ishaque, B.; et al. Articular Joint Lubricants during Osteoarthritis and Rheumatoid Arthritis Display Altered Levels and Molecular Species. *PLoS ONE* **2015**, *10*, e0125192. [CrossRef]

20. Oke, S.; Aghazadeh-Habashi, A.; Weese, J.S.; Jamali, F. Evaluation of glucosamine levels in commercial equine oral supplements for joints. *Equine Vet. J.* **2006**, *38*, 93–95. [CrossRef]
21. Eckert, T.; Stötzel, S.; Burg-Roderfeld, M.; Sewing, J.; Lütteke, T.; Nifantiev, N.E.; Vliegenthart, J.F.G.; Siebert, H.-C. In silico Study on Sulfated and Non-Sulfated Carbohydrate Chains from Proteoglycans in Cnidaria and Interaction with Collagen. *Open J. Phys. Chem.* **2012**, *2*, 123–133. [CrossRef]
22. Bhunia, A.; Vivekanandan, S.; Eckert, T.; Burg-Roderfeld, M.; Wechselberger, R.; Romanuka, J.; Bächle, D.; Kornilov, A.V.; von der Lieth, C.-W.; Jiménez-Barbero, J.S.; et al. Why Structurally Different Cyclic Peptides Can Be Glycomimetics of the HNK-1 Carbohydrate Antigen. *J. Am. Chem. Soc.* **2010**, *132*, 96–105. [CrossRef]
23. Tsvetkov, Y.E.; Burg-Roderfeld, M.; Loers, G.; Arda, A.; Sukhova, E.V.; Khatuntseva, E.A.; Grachev, A.A.; Chizhov, A.O.; Siebert, H.C.; Schachner, M.; et al. Synthesis and molecular recognition studies of the HNK-1 trisaccharide and related oligosaccharides. The specificity of monoclonal anti-HNK-1 antibodies as assessed by surface plasmon resonance and STD NMR. *J. Am. Chem. Soc.* **2012**, *134*, 426–435. [CrossRef] [PubMed]
24. Toegel, S.; Pabst, M.; Wu, S.Q.; Grass, J.; Goldring, M.B.; Chiari, C.; Kolb, A.; Altmann, F.; Viernstein, H.; Unger, F.M. Phenotype-related differential alpha-2,6- or alpha-2,3-sialylation of glycoprotein N-glycans in human chondrocytes. *Osteoarthr. Cartil.* **2010**, *18*, 240–248. [CrossRef] [PubMed]
25. Schauer, R.; Kamerling, J.P. Exploration of the Sialic Acid World. *Adv. Carb. Chem. Biochem.* **2018**, *75*, 1–213. [CrossRef]
26. Zhang, R.; Loers, G.; Schachner, M.; Boelens, R.; Wienk, H.; Siebert, S.; Eckert, T.; Kraan, S.; Rojas-Macias, M.A.; Lütteke, T.; et al. Molecular Basis of the Receptor Interactions of Polysialic Acid (polySia), polySia Mimetics, and Sulfated Polysaccharides. *ChemMedChem* **2016**, *11*, 990–1002. [CrossRef]
27. Siebert, H.-C.; Scheidig, A.; Eckert, T.; Wienk, H.; Boelens, R.; Mahvash, M.; Petridis, A.K.; Schauer, R. Interaction studies of sialic acids with model receptors contribute to nanomedical therapies. *J. Neurol. Disord.* **2015**, *3*, 1–6. [CrossRef]
28. Siebert, H.-C.; Lu, S.-Y.; Wechselberger, R.; Born, K.; Eckert, T.; Liang, S.; Lieth, C.-W.v.d.; Jiménez-Barbero, J.; Schauer, R.; Vliegenthart, J.F.G.; et al. A lectin from the Chinese bird-hunting spider binds sialic acids. *Carbohydr. Res.* **2010**, *344*, 1515–1525. [CrossRef]
29. Zhang, R.; Wu, L.; Eckert, T.; Burg-Roderfeld, M.; Rojas-Macias, M.A.; Lütteke, T.; Krylov, V.B.; Argunov, D.A.; Datta, A.; Markart, P.; et al. Lysozyme's lectin-like characteristics facilitates its immune defense function. *Q. Rev. Biophys.* **2017**, *50*, e9. [CrossRef]
30. Zhang, R.; Eckert, T.; Lütteke, T.; Hanstein, S.; Scheidig, A.; Bonvin, A.M.; Nifantiev, N.E.; Kozar, T.; Schauer, R.; Enani, M.A.; et al. Structure-Function Relationships of Antimicrobial Peptides and Proteins with Respect to Contact Molecules on Pathogen Surfaces. *Curr. Top. Med. Chem.* **2016**, *16*, 89–98. [CrossRef]
31. Kar, R.K.; Gazova, Z.; Bednarikova, Z.; Mroue, K.H.; Ghosh, A.; Zhang, R.; Ulicna, K.; Siebert, H.C.; Nifantiev, N.E.; Bhunia, A. Evidence for Inhibition of Lysozyme Amyloid Fibrillization by Peptide Fragments from Human Lysozyme: A Combined Spectroscopy, Microscopy, and Docking Study. *Biomacromolecules* **2016**, *17*, 1998–2009. [CrossRef]
32. Oesser, S.; Adam, M.; Babel, W.; Seifert, J. Oral administration of (14)C labeled gelatin hydrolysate leads to an accumulation of radioactivity in cartilage of mice (C57/BL). *J. Nutr.* **1999**, *129*, 1891–1895. [CrossRef] [PubMed]
33. Oesser, S.; Seifert, J. Stimulation of type II collagen biosynthesis and secretion in bovine chondrocytes cultured with degraded collagen. *Cell Tissue Res.* **2003**, *311*, 393–399. [CrossRef] [PubMed]
34. Schunck, M.; Louton, H.; Oesser, S. The Effectiveness of Specific Collagen Peptides on Osteoarthritis in Dogs-Impact on Metabolic Processes in Canine Chondrocytes. *Open J. Anim. Sci.* **2017**, *07*, 254–266. [CrossRef]
35. Dobenecker, B.; Reese, S.; Jahn, W.; Schunck, M.; Hugenberg, J.; Louton, H.; Oesser, S. Specific bioactive collagen peptides (PETAGILE((R))) as supplement for horses with osteoarthritis: A two-centred study. *J. Anim. Physiol. Anim. Nutr.* **2018**, *102* (Suppl. 1), 16–23. [CrossRef]
36. Simons, V.S.; Lochnit, G.; Wilhelm, J.; Ishaque, B.; Rickert, M.; Steinmeyer, J. Comparative Analysis of Peptide Composition and Bioactivity of Different Collagen Hydrolysate Batches on Human Osteoarthritic Synoviocytes. *Sci. Rep.* **2018**, *8*, 17733. [CrossRef]
37. Porfírio, E.; Fanaro, G.B. Collagen supplementation as a complementary therapy for the prevention and treatment of osteoporosis and osteoarthritis: A systematic review. *Revista Brasileira de Geriatria e Gerontologia* **2016**, *19*, 153–164. [CrossRef]
38. Li, R.; Qiao, S.; Zhang, G. Analysis of angiotensin-converting enzyme 2 (ACE2) from different species sheds some light on cross-species receptor usage of a novel coronavirus 2019-nCoV. *J. Infect.* **2020**, *80*, 469–496. [CrossRef]
39. Saponaro, F.; Rutigliano, G.; Sestito, S.; Bandini, L.; Storti, B.; Bizzarri, R.; Zucchi, R. ACE2 in the Era of SARS-CoV-2: Controversies and Novel Perspectives. *Front. Mol. Biosci.* **2020**, *7*. [CrossRef]
40. Lam, S.D.; Bordin, N.; Waman, V.P.; Scholes, H.M.; Ashford, P.; Sen, N.; van Dorp, L.; Rauer, C.; Dawson, N.L.; Pang, C.S.M.; et al. SARS-CoV-2 spike protein predicted to form complexes with host receptor protein orthologues from a broad range of mammals. *Sci. Rep.* **2020**, *10*, 16471. [CrossRef]
41. Zhang, N.; Liu, C.; Zhang, R.; Jin, L.; Yin, X.; Zheng, X.; Siebert, H.C.; Li, Y.; Wang, Z.; Loers, G.; et al. Amelioration of clinical course and demyelination in the cuprizone mouse model in relation to ketogenic diet. *Food Funct.* **2020**, *11*, 5647–5663. [CrossRef] [PubMed]
42. Zhang, N.; Liu, C.; Jin, L.; Zhang, R.; Siebert, H.C.; Wang, Z.; Prakash, S.; Yin, X.; Li, J.; Hou, D.; et al. Influence of Long-Chain/Medium-Chain Triglycerides and Whey Protein/Tween 80 Ratio on the Stability of Phosphatidylserine Emulsions (O/W). *ACS Omega* **2020**, *5*, 7792–7801. [CrossRef]

43. Zhang, R.; Jin, L.; Zhang, N.; Petridis, A.K.; Eckert, T.; Scheiner-Bobis, G.; Bergmann, M.; Scheidig, A.; Schauer, R.; Yan, M.; et al. The Sialic Acid-Dependent Nematocyst Discharge Process in Relation to Its Physical-Chemical Properties Is A Role Model for Nanomedical Diagnostic and Therapeutic Tools. *Mar. Drugs* **2019**, *17*, 469. [CrossRef]
44. Zhang, R.; Zhang, N.; Mohri, M.; Wu, L.; Eckert, T.; Krylov, V.B.; Antosova, A.; Ponikova, S.; Bednarikova, Z.; Markart, P.; et al. Nanomedical Relevance of the Intermolecular Interaction Dynamics-Examples from Lysozymes and Insulins. *ACS Omega* **2019**, *4*, 4206–4220. [CrossRef]
45. Mele, E. Epidemiologie der Osteoarthritis-Osteoarthrose(OA). *Vet. Focus* **2007**, *17*, 4–10. [CrossRef]
46. Belshaw, Z.; Asher, L.; Harvey, N.D.; Dean, R.S. Quality of life assessment in domestic dogs: An evidence-based rapid review. *Vet. J.* **2015**, *206*, 203–212. [CrossRef]
47. Hansen, B.D. Assessment of pain in dogs: Veterinary clinical studies. *ILAR J.* **2003**, *44*, 197–205. [CrossRef] [PubMed]
48. Hielm-Björkman, A.K.; Kuusela, E.; Liman, A.; Markkola, A.; Saarto, E.; Huttunen, P.; Leppäluoto, J.; Tulamo, R.-M.; Raekallio, M. Evaluation of methods for assessment of painassociated with chronic osteoarthritis in dogs. *JAVMA* **2003**, *11*, 1552–1558. [CrossRef] [PubMed]
49. Weide, N. *The Application of Gelatinehydrolysate in Clinical Orthopedic Healthy Dogs and Dogs with Chronic Defects on the Locomotor System*; Tierärztliche Hochschule: Hannover, Germany, 2004.
50. Hielm-Björkman, A. *Assessment of Chronic Pain and Evaluation of Three Complementary Therapies (Gold Implants, Green Lipped Mussel and a Homeopathic Combination Preparation) for Canine Osteoarthritis, Using Ran Domized, Controlled, Double-Blind Study Designs*; Ubiversity of Helsinki: Helsinki, Finland, 2007.
51. Sastravaha, A.; Suwanna, N.; Sinthusingha, C.; Noosud, J.; Roongsitthicha, A. Ameliorative Effects of Omega-3 Concentrate in Managing Coxofemoral Osteoarthritic Pain in Dogs. *Thai. J. Vet. Med.* **2016**, *46*, 305–311.
52. Seales, E.C.; Jurado, G.A.; Singhal, A.; Bellis, S.L. Ras oncogene directs expression of a differentially sialylated, functionally altered beta1 integrin. *Oncogene* **2003**, *22*, 7137–7145. [CrossRef] [PubMed]
53. Petridis, A.K.; Nikolopoulos, S.N.; El-Maarouf, A. Physical and functional cooperation of neural cell adhesion molecule and beta1-integrin in neurite outgrowth induction. *J. Clin. Neurosci. Off. J. Neurosurg. Soc. Australas.* **2011**, *18*, 1109–1113. [CrossRef]
54. Luo, Y.; Sinkeviciute, D.; He, Y.; Karsdal, M.; Henrotin, Y.; Mobasheri, A.; Onnerfjord, P.; Bay-Jensen, A. The minor collagens in articular cartilage. *Protein Cell* **2017**, *8*, 560–572. [CrossRef]
55. Kashiwagi, M.; Tortorella, M.; Nagase, H.; Brew, K. TIMP-3 is a potent inhibitor of aggrecanase 1 (ADAM-TS4) and aggrecanase 2 (ADAM-TS5). *J. Biol. Chem.* **2001**, *276*, 12501–12504. [CrossRef]
56. Parkkonen, O.; Nieminen, M.T.; Vesterinen, P.; Tervahartiala, T.; Perola, M.; Salomaa, V.; Jousilahti, P.; Sorsa, T.; Pussinen, P.J.; Sinisalo, J. Low MMP-8/TIMP-1 reflects left ventricle impairment in takotsubo cardiomyopathy and high TIMP-1 may help to differentiate it from acute coronary syndrome. *PLoS ONE* **2017**, *12*, e0173371. [CrossRef] [PubMed]
57. Ertunc, N.; Sato, C.; Kitajima, K. Sialic acid sulfation is induced by the antibiotic treatment in mammalian cells. *Biosci. Biotechnol. Biochem.* **2020**, *84*, 2311–2318. [CrossRef]
58. Dixon, W.J. *BMDP Statistical Software Manual*; University of California Press: Berkeley, CA, USA, 1993.
59. *Cytel Studio StatXact*; Cytel Software Corporation: Cambridge, MA, USA, 2010.
60. Schrödinger. *Maestro, v. 12.3.013*; Schrödinger, LLC: New York, NY, USA, 2020.
61. Frisch, M.J.; Trucks, G.W.; Schlegel, H.B.; Scuseria, G.E.; Robb, M.A.; Cheeseman, J.R.; Scalmani, G.; Barone, V.; Mennucci, B.; Petersson, G.A.; et al. *Gaussian 09*; Gaussian, Inc.: Wallingford, CT, USA, 2009.
62. Bella, J.; Liu, J.; Kramer, R.; Brodsky, B.; Berman, H.M. Conformational effects of Gly-X-Gly interruptions in the collagen triple helix. *J. Mol. Biol.* **2006**, *362*, 298–311. [CrossRef] [PubMed]
63. Halgren, T. New method for fast and accurate binding-site identification and analysis. *Chem. Biol. Drug Des.* **2007**, *69*, 146–148. [CrossRef] [PubMed]
64. Schrödinger. *SiteMap, Version 3.9*; Schrödinger, LLC: New York, NY, USA, 2013.
65. Halgren, T.A.; Murphy, R.B.; Friesner, R.A.; Beard, H.S.; Frye, L.L.; Pollard, W.T.; Banks, J.L. Glide: A new approach for rapid, accurate docking and scoring. 2. Enrichment factors in database screening. *J. Med. Chem.* **2004**, *47*, 1750–1759. [CrossRef]
66. Friesner, R.A.; Banks, J.L.; Murphy, R.B.; Halgren, T.A.; Klicic, J.J.; Mainz, D.T.; Repasky, M.P.; Knoll, E.H.; Shelley, M.; Perry, J.K.; et al. Glide: A new approach for rapid, accurate docking and scoring. 1. Method and assessment of docking accuracy. *J. Med. Chem.* **2004**, *47*, 1739–1749. [CrossRef] [PubMed]
67. Friesner, R.A.; Murphy, R.B.; Repasky, M.P.; Frye, L.L.; Greenwood, J.R.; Halgren, T.A.; Sanschagrin, P.C.; Mainz, D.T. Extra precision glide: Docking and scoring incorporating a model of hydrophobic enclosure for protein-ligand complexes. *J. Med. Chem.* **2006**, *49*, 6177–6196. [CrossRef]
68. Schrödinger. *Glide, Version 6.1*; Schrödinger, LLC: New York, NY, USA, 2013.
69. Ritchie, D.W. Evaluation of protein docking predictions using Hex 3.1 in CAPRI rounds 1 and 2. *Proteins* **2003**, *52*, 98–106. [CrossRef]
70. Bowers, K.J.; Sacerdoti, F.D.; Salmon, J.K.; Shan, Y.; Shaw, D.E.; Chow, E.; Xu, H.; Dror, R.O.; Eastwood, M.P.; Gregersen, B.A.; et al. Molecular dynamics—Scalable algorithms for molecular dynamics simulations on commodity clusters. In Proceedings of the 2006 ACM/IEEE Conference on Supercomputing—SC '06, Tampa, FL, USA, 11–17 November 2006.
71. Jorgensen, W.L.; Tirado-Rives, J. The OPLS [optimized potentials for liquid simulations] potential functions for proteins, energy minimizations for crystals of cyclic peptides and crambin. *J. Am. Chem. Soc.* **1988**, *110*, 1657–1666. [CrossRef]

72. Jorgensen, W.L.; Tirado-Rives, J. Potential energy functions for atomic-level simulations of water and organic and biomolecular systems. *Proc. Natl. Acad. Sci. USA* **2005**, *102*, 6665–6670. [CrossRef] [PubMed]
73. Berendsen, H.J.C.; Grigera, J.R.; Straatsma, T.P. The Missing Term in Effective Pair Potentials. *J. Phys. Chem.* **1987**, *91*, 6269–6271. [CrossRef]
74. Salentin, S.; Schreiber, S.; Haupt, V.J.; Adasme, M.F.; Schroeder, M. PLIP: Fully automated protein-ligand interaction profiler. *Nucleic Acids Res.* **2015**, *43*, W443–W447. [CrossRef] [PubMed]

marine drugs

MDPI

Article

Solid-Phase Extraction Embedded Dialysis (SPEED), an Innovative Procedure for the Investigation of Microbial Specialized Metabolites

Phuong-Y. Mai [1,2], Géraldine Le Goff [1], Erwan Poupon [2], Philippe Lopes [1], Xavier Moppert [3], Bernard Costa [3], Mehdi A. Beniddir [2] and Jamal Ouazzani [1,*]

1 CNRS, Institut de Chimie des Substances Naturelles, UPR 2301, 1, Avenue de la Terrasse, 91190 Gif-sur-Yvette, France; PhuongY.MAI@cnrs.fr (P.-Y.M.); Geraldine.LEGOFF@cnrs.fr (G.L.G.); Philippe.LOPES@cnrs.fr (P.L.)

2 Équipe "Chimie des Substances Naturelles" BioCIS, CNRS, Université Paris-Saclay, 5 Rue J.-B. Clément, 92290 Châtenay-Malabry, France; erwan.poupon@universite-paris-saclay.fr (E.P.); mehdi.beniddir@universite-paris-saclay.fr (M.A.B.)

3 PACIFIC BIOTECH SAS, BP 140 289, 98 701 Arue, Tahiti, French Polynesia; xmoppert@pacific-biotech.pf (X.M.); bcosta@pacific-biotech.pf (B.C.)

* Correspondence: Jamal.Ouazzani@cnrs.fr; Tel.: +33-6-82-81-65-90

Abstract: Solid-phase extraction embedded dialysis (SPEED technology) is an innovative procedure developed to physically separate in-situ, during the cultivation, the mycelium of filament forming microorganisms, such as actinomycetes and fungi, and the XAD-16 resin used to trap the secreted specialized metabolites. SPEED consists of an external nylon cloth and an internal dialysis tube containing the XAD resin. The dialysis barrier selects the molecular weight of the trapped compounds, and prevents the aggregation of biomass or macromolecules on the XAD beads. The external nylon promotes the formation of a microbial biofilm, making SPEED a biofilm supported cultivation process. SPEED technology was applied to the marine *Streptomyces albidoflavus* 19-S21, isolated from a core of a submerged Kopara sampled at 20 m from the border of a saltwater pond. The chemical space of this strain was investigated effectively using a dereplication strategy based on molecular networking and in-depth chemical analysis. The results highlight the impact of culture support on the molecular profile of *Streptomyces albidoflavus* 19-S21 secondary metabolites.

Keywords: solid-phase extraction SPE; XAD resin; molecular networking; *Streptomyces*; specialized metabolites; dereplication

Citation: Mai, P.-Y.; Le Goff, G.; Poupon, E.; Lopes, P.; Moppert, X.; Costa, B.; Beniddir, M.A.; Ouazzani, J. Solid-Phase Extraction Embedded Dialysis (SPEED), an Innovative Procedure for the Investigation of Microbial Specialized Metabolites. *Mar. Drugs* **2021**, *19*, 371. https://doi.org/10.3390/md19070371

Academic Editors: Florbela Pereira and Susana P. Gaudencio

Received: 15 June 2021
Accepted: 23 June 2021
Published: 26 June 2021

1. Introduction

Specialized metabolites (also known as secondary metabolites) produced by living organisms represent an inexhaustible source of molecules of biological interest to solve current and future public health challenges. This area of research, especially in the field of metabolites from micro-organisms, was accelerated by the development of genome-based technologies [1,2]. The era of drug lead discovery from culturable bacteria is not nearing its end, however its success relies on researchers' ability to innovate in strategies used to collect samples from the environment [3] and methods used to trap specialized metabolites from culture media [4]. Nevertheless, one of the major persisting drawbacks is the isolation of sufficient quantities of compounds to carry out chemical and biological investigations.

Among various concentration techniques, Amberlite XAD resin trapping of organic compounds gained recent interest and finds application in plant [5,6] marine invertebrate [7,8], and microbial [9–18] specialized metabolite extraction.

We have recently extended the exploitation of in-situ XAD-16 extraction of mycelium forming microorganisms, actinomycetes and fungi [9–18], known as the major providers of valuable bioactive compounds [19,20]. Compared to submerged cultivation, we showed that in-situ XAD-16 extraction significantly impacts the diversity and the yields of target compounds [9,18].

Although this approach strongly facilitates the extraction of target products with considerable savings in the use of organic solvents, application of in-situ XAD-16 extraction to mycelium forming micro-organisms leads to significant entrapment of the resin beads into the filamentous network, and complicates the separation of these two compartments. As a consequence, during the elution step of the resin/mycelium mixture by appropriate solvents, the analytical profile is often contaminated with undesired compounds, which compromises the purification steps. The solid-phase extraction embedded dialysis (SPEED technology) is based on a physical separation between the microbial biomass and the resin used for in-situ solid phase extraction. It includes a two-layer barrier consisting of an external nylon filter cloth (NFC) and an internal dialysis tube (DT) containing the resin beads. According to the molecular cut of the DT, only molecules with appropriate molecular weight can flow from the cultivation broth to the resin. This selectivity added to the ease of recovering clean resin beads and eluate, makes SPEED technology an indisputable added value to the study of microbial specialized metabolites. The SPEED technology is reported in this paper for the first time and summarized in Figure 1.

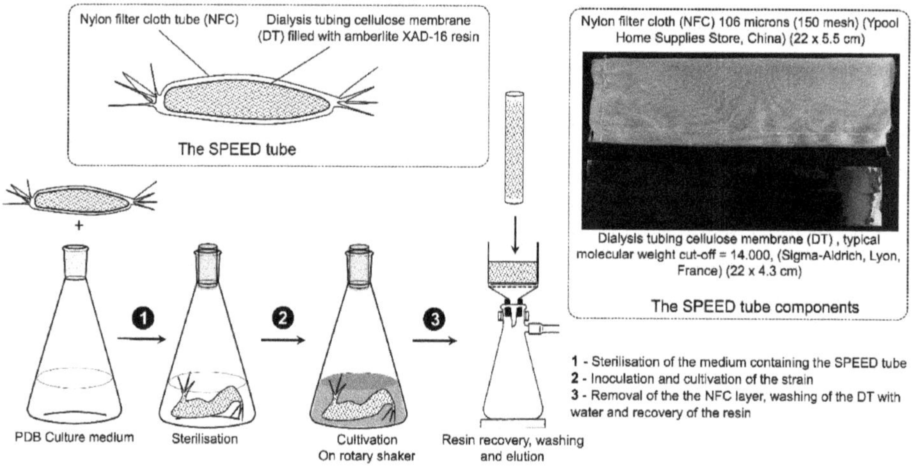

Figure 1. Schematic representation of SPEED technology.

In order to develop and optimize SPEED technique, a case-study was needed. An ongoing project from our consortium appeared to provide an ideal framework towards this end. In our efforts to isolate and investigate micro-organisms from underexplored ecosystems, samples from microbial mats called 'Kopara' were collected from Rangiroa atoll, in French Polynesia. Kopara mats were previously described as vertically organized cyanobacteria strata of 20 to 50 cm thickness. The Kopara geomorphology, physico-chemistry and microbial diversity were previously reported [21–23], however only bacterial pigments and exopolymers (exopolysaccharides and poly-β-hydroxyalkanoates) were studied and were shown to be secreted by some Kopara microbial isolates [24,25]. Our running program is dedicated to the isolation, for the first time, of filament-forming microorganisms, actinomycetes and fungi, from Kopara samples. To do so, 56 Kopara samples and 37 other materials (water, animals) from different locations of Rangiroa atoll at different depth from surface to −20 cm or more were collected (Figure 2).

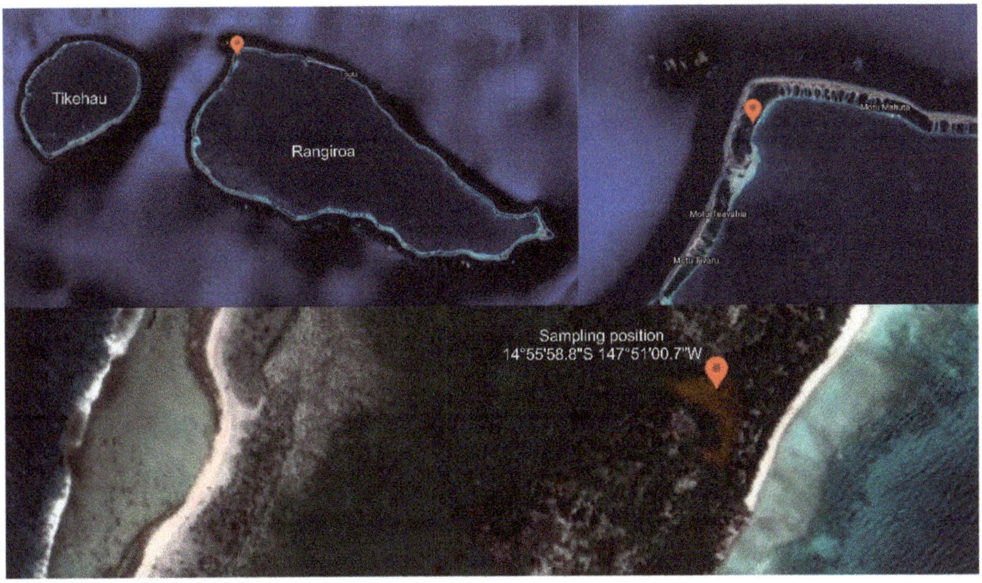

Figure 2. Kopara sampling location reported in this work.

Facing a large number of samples and to avoid the rediscovery of known compounds, which is the major issue in natural product chemistry, the immediate identification of known compounds and prioritization of interesting strains that produce potential new compounds deserve intense effort. To meet this challenge, the dereplication strategy using metabolomics profiling based on mass spectrometry has been employed to perform the potential interesting strain screening program. Indeed, molecular networking approach allows the organization of untargeted tandem mass spectrum datasets according to their spectral similarity and generates clusters of structurally related metabolites. This approach has become a powerful tool for navigating the chemical space of complex biological systems and can be used to view the chemical constituents of a wide variety of extracts in a single map [26].

2. Results and Discussions

2.1. Collection Site and Strain Identification

Starting from the Kopara sample (see Section 4), the stain *Streptomyces albidoflavus* 19-S21 was isolated and purified by serial inoculation on Potatoes Dextrose Agar slants. From the phylogenetic analysis based on the 16S rRNA sequence, the isolate was found in the *albidoflavus* group (Figure 3). Since all of the species in this clade (*S. canescens*, *S. champvatii*, *S. coelicolor*, *S. felleus*, *S. globisporus* ssp *caucasicus*, *S. griseus* ssp. *solvifaciens*, *S. limosus*, *S. odorifer*, *S. sampsonii*) were previously classified as heterotypic synonyms of *S. albidoflavus* [27], we have named the isolate *Streptomyces albidoflavus* 19-S21 with the GenBank® accession number MW446171.

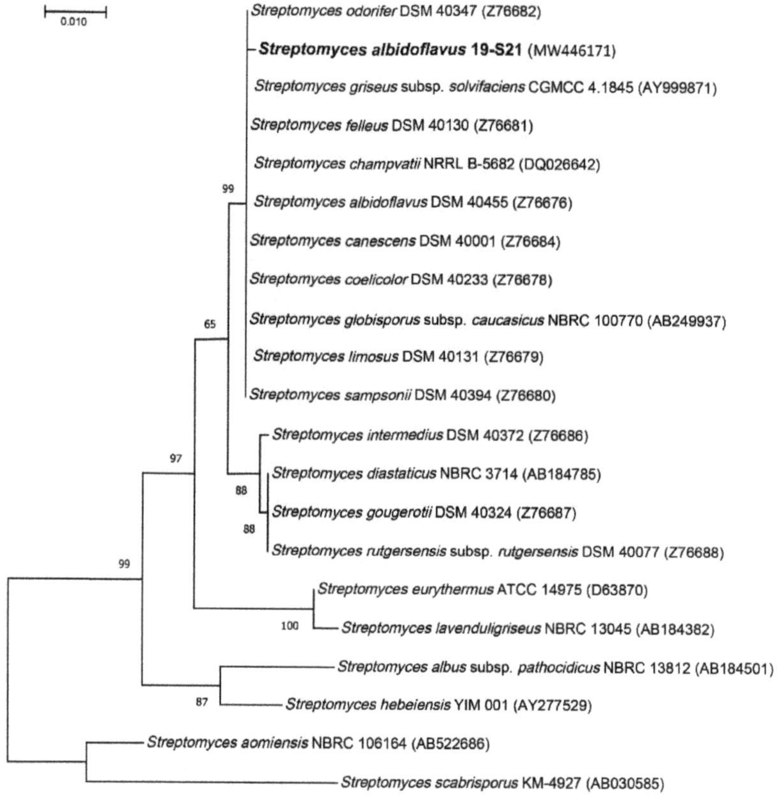

Figure 3. Maximum-likelihood tree obtained from 16S rRNA sequence alignment of the isolate and *Streptomyces* spp. of the *albidoflavus* group of species and close relatives selected from [28]. Bootstrap values are reported as percentages (1000 replicates). GenBank® accessions are mentioned between brackets.

2.2. *S. albidoflavus* 19-S21 Cultivation according to SPEED Technology

As described above, the main advantage of SPEED technology is the physical separation of the strain mycelium and the XAD-16 resin beads, used for in-situ SPE. The DT barrier is a second advantage as it discriminates between large biomolecules and secondary metabolites. The 1.4 kD cut-off of the dialysis membrane guarantees permeability to all families of specialized metabolites [29].

Beyond these substantial improvements, we made an unexpected and intriguing observation which was not only reproducible for the strain *S. albidoflavus* 19-S21, but also for other actinomycetes and fungi (S11). Thus, compared to the submerged cultivation in which the mycelium/resin mixture is homogenously spread in the medium (Figure 4A), under SPEED condition, the mycelium formed a dense and stable biofilm attached to the external nylon filter cloth (NFC), with almost no mycelium floating in the medium (Figure 4B). When the SPEED tube was recovered, the biofilm remained sticking to the NFC (Figure 4D,E), and was removed by gentle scraping under running water, before removing the dialysis tube (DT). Therefore, SPEED technology cannot be assimilated to a classical submerged cultivation as the biomass adopts a biofilm type organization.

At the end of the SPEED cultivation period and the removal of the NFC, the DTs were recovered easily and cleanly (Figure 5). The subsequent steps consist of the classical recovery of the resin and metabolite elution as reported in Section 4.

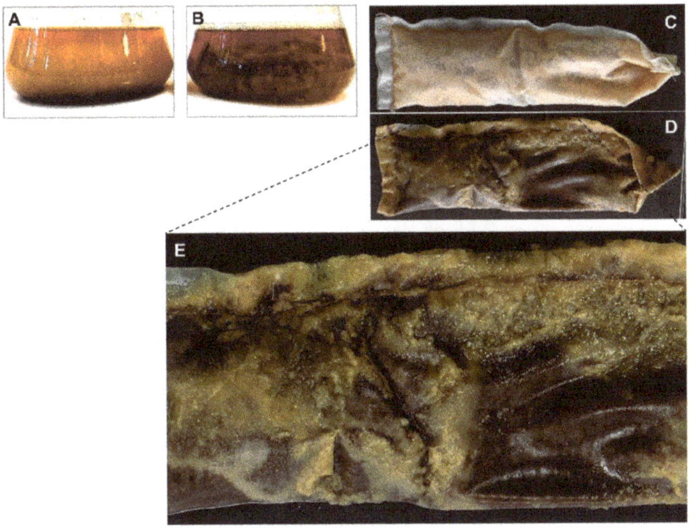

Figure 4. Difference between submerged and SPEED cultivation of *S. albidoflavus* 19-S21 in PDB medium: (**A**) 11 days submerged cultivation with in-situ SPE with XAD-16 resin; (**B**) 11 days SPEED cultivation; (**C**) SPEED tube after removal of the biofilm layer; (**D**) SPEED tube with the biofilm layer; (**E**) Focus on D showing the biofilm layer attached to the NFC.

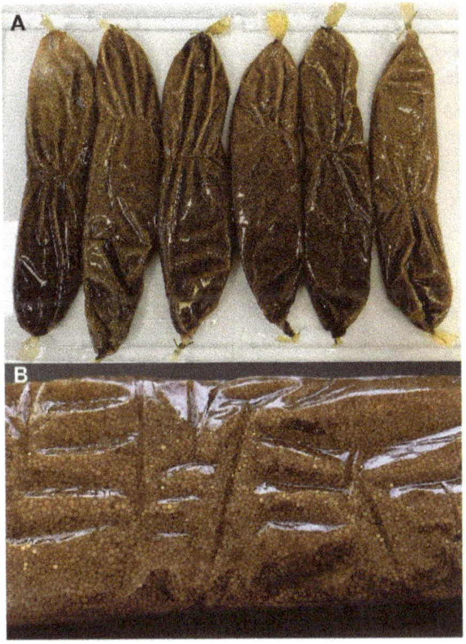

Figure 5. Dialysis tubes (DT) recovery: (**A**) after SPEED cultivation of *S. albidoflavus* 19-S21 in PDB medium; (**B**) Focus showing colored resin inside the DT.

Microbial biofilm association to nylon nets and cloth is well documented, mainly in the aquaculture context [30] and treatment of polluted water [31]. Nylon was also used to support and promote algal biofilm growth [32].

2.3. Molecular Networking-Based Chemical Exploration of S. albidoflavus 19-S21 Specialized Metabolites

The strain was cultivated in different conditions (see Section 4). Resins and media were extracted with ethyl acetate and methanol consequently. In LSF, insignificant quantity and diversity of metabolites were observed. This was also the case for all methanol extracts. On the other hand, the ethyl acetate extracts of the resins showed various metabolic HPLC profiles. In order not to miss any compound, all ethyl acetate and methanol extracts of the resins were analyzed.

SPEED extracts were submitted to UPLC-MS/MS profiling and the resulting data were processed following the feature-based molecular networking workflow [33]. The global molecular network was color-tagged according to multiple culture conditions and the solvents used for the extraction. The MS/MS data were annotated using the GNPS spectral library (Figure S1) [34]. The network consists of 2714 nodes, consisting of 136 clusters and regrouping nodes with related structures.

All library hits resulting from GNPS dereplication are listed in Table S1 in Supporting Information. The nodes with annotation are also visualized in Cytoscape® 3.7.2 [35] and filled by different color codes to easily distinguish the dereplicated nodes from the non-dereplicated ones (Figure S2).

According to the global molecular network, the strain specialized metabolites varied according to the different culture conditions. One cluster of surugamides (Figure 6A) has been found to be produced only in solid culture Surugamides belonging to a known family of cyclic octapeptides, initially isolated from a Marine *Streptomyces* sp. JAMM992 and has also been proved to possess anticancer and antifungal properties [36]. One cluster of desferioxamines (Figure 6B), which are siderophores produced by bacteria, has been found mainly in methanol extracts and produced by the strain in liquid culture condition. Antimycin A1 along with three other antimycins (antimycins A2, A3, and A4) were annotated and produced by the strain in different culture conditions (Figure 6C). Antimycins include various scaffolds due to the differences in the size of the lactone and its substitution patterns. These compounds have been described for many *Streptomyces* sp. and exhibited interesting biological activities, such as antifungal, insecticidal, nematocidal, and piscicidal activities, because of their ability to block the electron transport in mitochondria. Several antimycin classes have also been reported to possess potent anti-inflammatory and antitumoral activities [37,38].

One unannotated cluster (D in Figure 6) has been detected on the global molecular network. A compound in this cluster at $m/z = 335.1459$, attracted our attention because of its salient production in SPEED culture condition (node encircled in red color in Figure 6). As a way to dereplicate this node, the molecular formula related to its exact mass was generated and then searched against the AntiBase® database (Wiley) and the Dictionary of Natural Products®. The database search yielded 125 hits with only one molecule, tetrodecamycin, being reported from the species *Streptomyces nashvillensis* MJ885-mF8 [39]. All the 125 hit compounds and their biological source are listed in Table S2.

2.4. Isolation of Representative Compounds

In order to confirm HRMS-based dereplication of the compounds at $m/z = 335.1459$ along with the annotations provided by the GNPS, we used the resin extract to purify the representative compounds of major molecular node. *S. albidoflavus* 19-S21 was cultivated according to two procedures involving XAD-16 in-situ extraction during the culture; LSF-SPE [9] and SPEED technology. The resins were extracted by ethyl acetate followed by methanol, and the aqueous filtrated medium was concentrated under vacuum. These three fractions were analyzed by thin layer chromatography (TLC) and HPLC confirming that almost all the formed metabolites were recovered in the ethyl acetate extract. Figure 7 represents a superposition of the ELSD chromatograms of LSF-SPE (dashed line) and SPEED extracts (continuous line). One of the major compounds at 20.2 min is produced only in SPEED condition (Figure 7A,B). The molecular formula was established as $C_{18}H_{23}O_6$ based on its HR-ESIMS data ($[M + H]^+$ at 335.1496) (Figure S5). The compound was identified as tetrodecamycin by comparison of its ^1H and ^{13}C NMR data with those reported in literature (Figures S6 and S7) [39]. The other major non-polar compounds eluted after 40 min were also investigated. These compounds were characterized as fatty acids by comparison with literature [40]. The experimental data of 14-methylpentadecanoic acid, which is one of the fatty acids, were mentioned in the Supplementary Information (Figures S8–S10). The compounds between 22 and 40 min belong to the antimycin-type depsipeptides. To demonstrate the performance of the dereplication approach based on molecular networking, compound with *m/z* 507.2339 (Figures 6C and 7A) was further isolated (Figure 6C) and fully characterized. The structural data are reported in the experimental section and compared to literature as actinomycin A4a (Figures S3 and S4) [41,42].

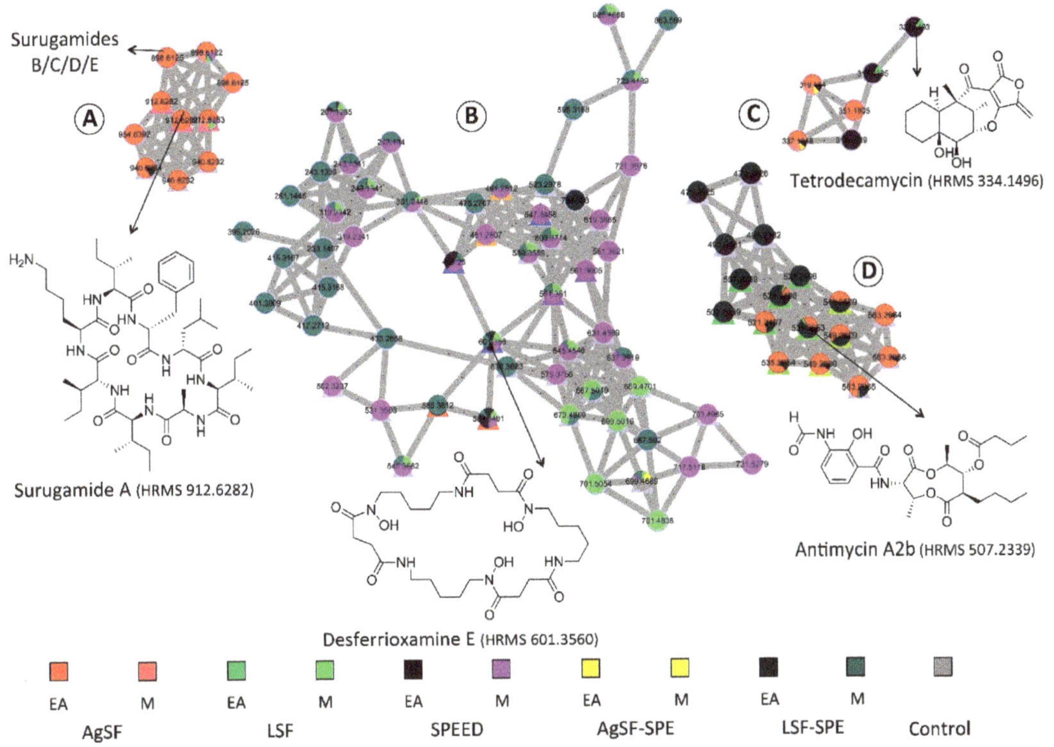

Figure 6. The molecular network built from different crude extracts of the strain *Streptomyces albidoflavus*. Some clusters with annotation are highlighted in this figure: (**A**) Cluster of surugamide family; (**B**) Cluster related to desferrioxamines; (**C**) Antimycin-type depsipeptide clusters; and (**D**) Unannotated cluster mainly produced in SPEED culture condition. In this figure, EA stands for ethyl acetate and M stands for methanol. The control condition represents different ethyl acetate and methanol extracts of resin XAD from different culture conditions and also those of PDB agar, which were not inoculated by the strains.

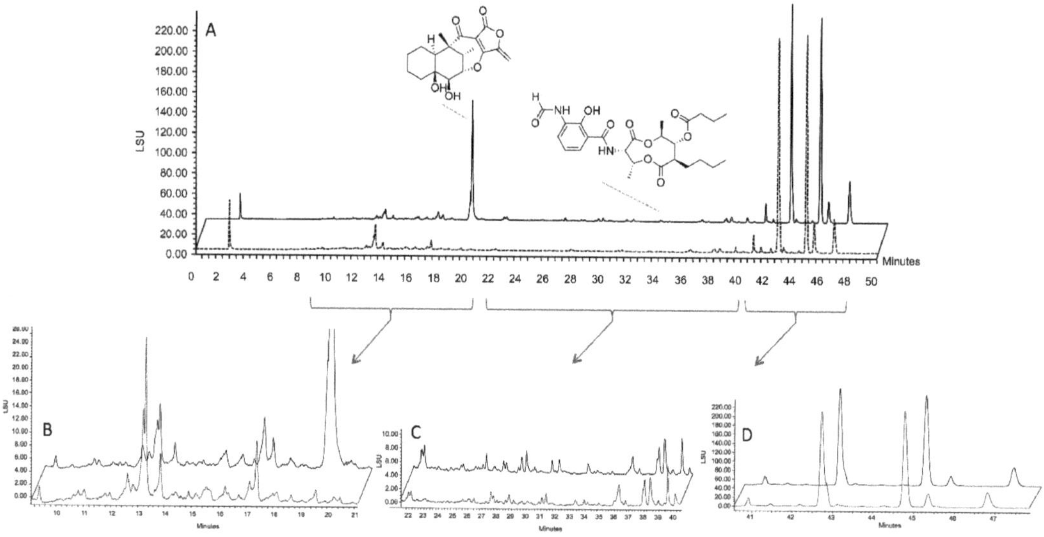

Figure 7. Comparison of HPLC profiles under SPEED and LSF-SPE culture conditions: (**A**) HPLC-ELSD analysis of the SPEED (continuous line) and LSF-SPE (dashed line). According to the UV spectrum of compounds we can delimit three zones: (**B**) containing mainly tetrodecamycin; (**C**) zone containing mainly antimycin-type depsipeptides; and (**D**) fatty acid zone.

3. Discussion

Molecular networking offers the possibility to map additional information, such as biological, analytical, and taxonomic details over networks [43]. Hence, the strain *Streptomyces albidoflavus* 19-S21 was prioritized for further study based on its chemical originality after examination of a multi-informative annotated global molecular network. This strain was isolated from a core of a submerged Kopara, sampled at 20 m from the border of a saltwater pond. The strain was cultivated in Potatoes Dextrose Broth (PDB) under different conditions including SPEED technology.

SPEED technology, as disclosed in this paper, opens a new area in microbial cultivation. The biofilm formed could be assimilated to a solid culture which may explain the difference in the formed metabolites compared to LSF-SPE liquid culture. It is well documented that the life cycle of filamentous micro-organisms, actinomycetes and fungi, is drastically impacted by the cultivation support; and that the regulators of cell cycle phases impacts in parallel the expression of specialized metabolites clusters [44,45]. The life cycle including filament, sexual organs, and fructifications production takes place naturally on living supports like roots, bark, and leaves in plants, or on rocks, soil, or dead wood. In the marine ecosystem, these microorganisms are mainly associated to sponges and corals [46,47].

In plants, the formation of biofilm provides major advantages to symbionts and impacts the strain metabolome [48,49]. Recent attempts have been reported in the literature, aiming at culturing marine microorganisms on a cotton scaffold [50]. Microbial colonies were formed on the cotton fibers and the metabolites profile was significantly impacted. In SPEED procedure, the molecular cut-off discrimination of the internal dialysis tube, and the biofilm-like growth on the external nylon cloth are the main advantages. The XAD resin inside the dialysis tube allows the solid phase extraction of metabolites below the dialysis molecular cut, and the nylon tissue pores separate physically the mycelium from the resin, which made in-situ SPE very easy to handle and the biomass to grow as this sticky and dense biofilm. The next step is to convert this proof of concept to a technological device, allowing the scale-up and automation of the experiments.

4. Materials and Methods

4.1. Strain Isolation

In September 2018, a Kopara sample was collected from a core of a submerged Kopara mat located at 20 m from the border of a saltwater pond at the Rangiroa atoll, French Polynesia (Sampling coordinates 14°55′58.8″ S 147°51′00.7″ W). The Kopara sample was ground and homogenized in sterile water and decanted. The suspension was serially diluted, plated on PDB agar slants, and incubated at 28 °C for 1 to 6 weeks. The strain was cultivated in Potatoes Dextrose Broth (PDB Difco, Fisher Scientific, Illkirch, France). The stain *Streptomyces albidoflavus* 19-S21 was isolated and purified by serial inoculations on Potatoes Dextrose agar slants.

4.2. Phylogeny Investigation

Genomic DNA isolation and amplification of the ITS region was performed as described previously [51]. Amplicons were sequenced by Sanger sequencing and the sequences were aligned against the 16S ribosomal RNA database of the Targeted Loci project of NCBI using MUSCLE. The alignment was manually inspected and gaps were removed. The evolutionary history was inferred by using the maximum likelihood method and Tamura-Nei model [52] with 1000 replicates. The initial tree for the heuristic search was obtained automatically by applying Neighbor-Join and BioNJ algorithms to a matrix of pairwise distances estimated using the maximum composite likelihood (MCL) approach, and then selecting the topology with superior log likelihood value. Evolutionary analyses were conducted in MEGA X version 10.1.7 [53].

4.3. Strain Cultivation with In-Situ SPEED Technology

Streptomyces albidoflavus 19-S21 mycelium was conserved at −20 °C in 20% glycerol and was revived for 5 days on a 3 × 15 cm Petri plates (NUNC DISH 150 × 10, Thermo Fisher Scientific, Les Ulis, France) containing PDB agar (Difco, Thermo Fisher Scientific). For liquid cultivation, sterile water was poured onto the plates (16 mL per plate), and the mycelium recovered by gentle scratching of the surface with a scalpel. Then, 10 × 2 L Erlenmeyer containing 1 L of PDB medium and a SPEED tube before sterilization (Figure 1) were inoculated. Each DT tube was filled with 40 g of XAD-16 resin (AMBERLITE® XAD®16HP N, DOW France SAS, Saint-Denis, France). The mycelium suspension was then introduced in each Erlenmeyer (4 mL) and the strain cultivated for 13 days under stirring (130 rpm, 28 °C). After cultivation, the SPEED tubes were taken out from the Erlenmeyer, rinsed thoroughly under running water to remove the sticking biomass. The external NFC tube was removed and the DT recovered and washed back under running water. The XAD resin was then recovered from the DT, placed in a Büchner funnel, washed extensively with water, then dried under vacuum to remove the residual water. Then, 425 g of XAD-16 resin was recovered from the 10 L cultivation and was submitted to the extraction steps. The strain was cultivated in 5 conditions:

- Agar-state fermentation (AgSF);
- Liquid-state fermentation (LSF);
- SPEED cultivation;
- Agar-state fermentation coupled to SPE (AgSF-SPE) [11];
- Liquid-state fermentation coupled to SPE (LSF-SPE).

4.4. Extraction/Purification Procedures

The 425 g of XAD-16 resin were transferred in a 2 L glass bottle (Duran) and the trapped compounds gently eluted with 3 × 1 L of ethyl acetate (4 h per extraction). The extracts were pooled, dried on anhydrous sodium sulfate, and evaporated under reduced pressure to offer 577 mg of extract. The resin is extracted back with 2 × 1 L of methanol (4 h per extraction) and the methanol evaporated leading to 1.15 g of extract.

The classical purification procedure involves a flash chromatography step followed by semi-preparative HPLC purification of the flash chromatography fractions.

4.5. Characterization, Isolation, and Structural Elucidation Experiments

The analytical HPLC system consisted of an Alliance Waters 2695 controller coupled with a PhotoDiode Array detector Waters 2996 (UV), an evaporative light-scattering detector (ELSD) Waters 2424 detector and a mass detector Waters QDa (MS) (Waters SAS, Saint-Quentin-en-Yvelines, France). A Sunfire C18 column (4.6 × 150 mm, 3.5 µm) was used with a flow rate of 0.7 mL/min. The elution gradient consisted of a linear gradient from 100% solvent A to 100% solvent B in 40 min, then 10 min at 100% B (Solvent A: H_2O + 0.1% HCOOH, Solvent B: ACN + 0.1% HCOOH). Preparative HPLC was performed using the same gradient on a semi-preparative Sunfire C_{18} column (10 × 250 mm, 5 µm) using a Waters autosampler 717, a pump 600, a photodiode array detector 2996, and an ELSD detector 2420 (Waters SAS, Saint-Quentin-en-Yvelines, France). Pre-packed silica gel Redisep columns were used for flash chromatography using a Combiflash-Companion chromatogram (Serlabo, Entraigues-sur-la-Sorgue, France). All other chemicals and solvents were purchased from SDS (SDS, Peypen, France). NMR experiments were performed using a Bruker Avance III 600 MHz spectrometer equipped with a TCI cryo-probe head, and a Bruker Avance 500 MHz spectrometer (Bruker, Vienna, Austria). The spectra were acquired in CD_3OD (δ_H 3.31 ppm and δ_C 49.15 ppm), in $CDCl_3$ (δ_H 7.26 ppm and δ_C 77.16 ppm).

4.6. Data Dependent LC-ESI-HRMS2 Analysis

UPLC-ESI-HRMS^2 analyses were achieved by coupling the UPLC system to a hybrid quadrupole time of-flight mass spectrometer Agilent 6546 (Agilent Technologies, Massy, France) equipped with an ESI source, operating in both positive and negative ion mode.

A ZORBAX® Eclipse Plus C18 UPLC column (2.1 × 50 mm; i.d. 1.8 µm, Agilent) was used, with a flow rate of 0.5 mL·min^{-1} and a linear gradient from 5% B (A: H_2O + 0.1% formic acid, B: Acetonitrile + 0.1% formic acid) to 100% B over 15 min. Source parameters were set as followed: capillary temperature at 320 °C, source voltage at 3500 V, sheath gas flow rate at 11 L·min^{-1}. The divert valve was set to waste for the first 3 min. MS scans were operated in full-scan mode from *m/z* 100 to 1200 (0.1 s scan time) with a mass resolution of 67,000 at *m/z* 922. A MS^1 scan was followed by MS2 scans of the five most intense ions above an absolute threshold of 3000 counts. Selected parent ions were fragmented at a collision energy fixed at 35 eV and an isolation window of 1.3 amu. In the positive-ion mode, purine $C_5H_4N_4$ $[M + H]^+$ ion (*m/z* 121.050873) and the hexakis (1H,1H,3H-tetrafluoropropoxy)-phosphazene $C_{18}H_{18}F_{24}N_3O_6P_3$ $[M + H]^+$ ion (*m/z* 922.009 798) were used as internal lock masses. In the negative-ion mode, trifluoroacetic acid (CF_3CO_2H, *m/z* 112.98559) and the trifluoroacetate adduct with *m/z* 1033.988109 were used. A permanent MS/MS exclusion list criterion was set to prevent oversampling of the internal calibrant. LC-UV and MS data acquisition and processing were performed using MassHunter® Workstation software (Agilent Technologies, Massy, France).

4.7. MS Data Processing and Feature-Based Molecular Networking—GNPS

The MS2 data files, related to the 21 extracts were converted from the .d (Agilent) standard data-format to .mzML format using the MSConvert software, part of the ProteoWizard package [54]. All .mzML were then processed using MZmine 2v53 [55]. The mass detection was realized keeping the noise level at 10,000 at MS1 level and at 1000 at MS2. The ADAP chromatogram builder was used using a minimum group size of scans of 2, a group intensity threshold of 3000, a minimum highest intensity of 3.0E3 and *m/z* tolerance of 0.005 *m/z* or 50 ppm. The chromatogram deconvolution was performed using the Wavelets (ADAP) with the following settings: *m/z* range for MS2 scan pairing (Da) = 0.06, RT range for

MS2 scan pairing (min) = 1, S/N threshold = 5, S/N estimator = Intensity window SN, min feature height = 3000, coefficient/area threshold = 2, Peak duration range = 0.00–0.90 and RT wavelet range = 0.00–0.09 [56]. Isotopes were grouped using the isotopic peaks grouper algorithm with an *m/z* tolerance of 5 ppm and a RT tolerance of 0.2 min with the most intense peak. The peak alignment algorithm was used with the following settings: *m/z* tolerance of 0.004 or 5 ppm, weight for *m/z* of 1, retention time tolerance of 0.1, and weight for RT of 1. The resulted peak list was filtered to keep only rows with MS2 features. The .mgf and .csv (for RT, *m/z*, peak areas) files were exported using the dedicated "Export/Submit to GNPS/FBMN" option. The raw data files related to the LC-MS/MS analysis of the fractions were deposited on the public MassIVE repository under the accession number: MSV000087546. The MS/MS spectrum of tetrodecamycin was deposited in the GNPS spectral library under the identifier: CCMSLIB00006581621.

4.8. Molecular Networking Parameters

A molecular network was created using the online FBMN workflow (version release_27) at GNPS (http://gnps.ucsd.edu, accessed on 7 March 2021) with a parent mass tolerance of 0.02 Da and an MS/MS fragment ion tolerance of 0.02 Da. A network was then created where edges were filtered to have a cosine score above 0.6 and more than 3 matched peaks. Further edges between two nodes were kept in the network if and only if each of the nodes appeared in each other's respective top 10 most similar nodes. The spectra in the network were then searched against GNPS spectral libraries. All matches kept between network spectra and library spectra were required to have a score above 0.6 and at least 4 matched peaks. The analog search has also performed. The molecular networking data were analyzed and visualized using Cytoscape® (ver. 3.7.2) [36].

Supplementary Materials: The following are available online at https://www.mdpi.com/article/10.3390/md19070371/s1.

Author Contributions: Conceptualization, J.O. and M.A.B.; Methodology, J.O., M.A.B., G.L.G.; investigation, P.-Y.M., G.L.G., P.L., and M.A.B.; Resources, X.M. and B.C.; Data curation, P.-Y.M., G.L.G., and M.A.B.; ; Writing—original draft preparation, P.-Y.M., J.O., and M.A.B.; Writing—review and editing, E.P., X.M., and B.C.; Visualization, P.-Y.M., G.L.G., J.O., and M.A.B.; Supervision, J.O., G.L.G., M.A.B., and E.P.; Project administration and funding acquisition, M.A.B. and E.P. All authors have read and agreed to the published version of the manuscript.

Funding: This study was supported by a Ph.D. grant (P.-Y.M.) from the "Ministère de l'Enseignement Supérieur, de la Recherche et de l'Innovation, France" through Doctoral School "Innovation thérapeutique: du fondamental à l'appliqué" and sponsorship from "Université Paris-Saclay".

Data Availability Statement: Data are available from the corresponding author.

Acknowledgments: Kopara samples were collected by Pacific Biotech Partner.

Conflicts of Interest: The authors declare no conflict of interest.

Abbreviations

GNPS: Global Natural Product Social Molecular Networking; FBMN: Feature-Based Molecular Networking; ADAP: Automated Data Analysis Pipeline; MassIVE: Mass Spectrometry Interactive Virtual Environment; PDA: Photo-diode detector; LSD: light scattering detector; RT: retention time; S/N: signal/noise.

References

1. Romano, J.D.; Tatonetti, N.P. Informatics and Computational Methods in Natural Product Drug Discovery: A Review and Perspectives. *Front. Genet.* **2019**, *10*, 368. [CrossRef] [PubMed]
2. Harvey, A.L.; Edrada-Ebel, R.; Quinn, R.J. The re-emergence of natural products for drug discovery in the genomics era. *Nat. Rev. Drug Discov.* **2015**, *14*, 111–129. [CrossRef] [PubMed]

3. Kaeberlein, T.; Lewis, K.; Epstein, S.S. Isolating "Uncultivable" Microorganisms in Pure Culture in a Simulated Natural Environment. *Science* **2002**, *296*, 1127–1129. [CrossRef]
4. Hernandez, A.; Nguyen, L.T.; Dhakal, R.; Murphy, B.T. The need to innovate sample collection and library generation in microbial drug discovery: A focus on academia. *Nat. Prod. Rep.* **2021**, *38*, 292–300. [CrossRef] [PubMed]
5. Komaraiah, P.; Ramakrishna, S.V.; Reddanna, P.; Kavi Kishor, P.B. Enhanced production of plumbagin in immobilized cells of Plumbago rosea by elicitation and in situ adsorption. *J. Biotechnol.* **2003**, *101*, 181–187. [CrossRef]
6. Klvana, M.; Legros, R.; Jolicoeur, M. In situ extraction strategy affects benzophenanthridine alkaloid production fluxes in suspension cultures of Eschscholtzia californica. *Biotechnol. Bioeng.* **2005**, *89*, 280–289. [CrossRef]
7. Vlachou, P.; Le Goff, G.; Alonso, C.; Alvarez, P.A.; Gallard, J.F.; Fokialakis, N.; Ouazzani, J. Innovative Approach to Sustainable Marine Invertebrate Chemistry and a Scale-Up Technology for Open Marine Ecosystems. *Mar. Drugs* **2018**, *16*, 152. [CrossRef]
8. Bojko, B.; Onat, B.; Boyaci, E.; Psillakis, E.; Dailianis, T.; Pawliszyn, J. Application of in situ Solid-Phase Microextraction on Mediterranean Sponges for Untargeted Exometabolome Screening and Environmental Monitoring. *Front. Mar. Sci.* **2019**, *6*. [CrossRef]
9. Le Goff, G.; Martin, M.T.; Iorga, B.I.; Adelin, E.; Servy, C.; Cortial, S.; Ouazzani, J. Isolation and characterization of unusual hydrazides from Streptomyces sp. impact of the cultivation support and extraction procedure. *J. Nat. Prod.* **2013**, *76*, 142–149. [CrossRef] [PubMed]
10. Le Goff, G.; Martin, M.T.; Servy, C.; Cortial, S.; Lopes, P.; Bialecki, A.; Smadja, J.; Ouazzani, J. Isolation and characterization of alpha,beta-unsaturated gamma-lactono-hydrazides from *Streptomyces* sp. *J. Nat. Prod.* **2012**, *75*, 915–919. [CrossRef]
11. Le Goff, G.; Adelin, E.; Cortial, S.; Servy, C.; Ouazzani, J. Application of solid-phase extraction to agar-supported fermentation. *Bioprocess. Biosyst. Eng.* **2013**, *36*, 1285–1290. [CrossRef]
12. Adelin, E.; Servy, C.; Martin, M.T.; Arcile, G.; Iorga, B.I.; Retailleau, P.; Bonfill, M.; Ouazzani, J. Bicyclic and tetracyclic diterpenes from a Trichoderma symbiont of *Taxus baccata*. *Phytochemistry* **2014**, *97*, 55–61. [CrossRef] [PubMed]
13. Dallery, J.F.; Le Goff, G.; Adelin, E.; Iorga, B.I.; Pigne, S.; O'Connell, R.J.; Ouazzani, J. Deleting a Chromatin Remodeling Gene Increases the Diversity of Secondary Metabolites Produced by *Colletotrichum higginsianum*. *J. Nat. Prod.* **2019**, *82*, 813–822. [CrossRef] [PubMed]
14. Adelin, E.; le Goff, G.; Retailleau, P.; Bonfill, M.; Ouazzani, J. Isolation of the antibiotic methyl (R,E)-3-(1-hydroxy-4-oxocyclopent-2-en-1-yl)-acrylate EA-2801 from *Trichoderma atroviridae*. *J. Antibiot.* **2017**, *70*, 1053–1056. [CrossRef]
15. Le Goff, G.; Lopes, P.; Arcile, G.; Vlachou, P.; van Elslande, E.; Retailleau, P.; Gallard, J.F.; Weis, M.; Benayahu, Y.; Fokialakis, N.; et al. Impact of the Cultivation Technique on the Production of Secondary Metabolites by *Chrysosporium lobatum* TM-237-S5, Isolated from the Sponge *Acanthella cavernosa*. *Mar. Drugs* **2019**, *17*, 678. [CrossRef]
16. Samy, M.N.; Le Goff, G.; Lopes, P.; Georgousaki, K.; Gumeni, S.; Almeida, C.; Gonzalez, I.; Genilloud, O.; Trougakos, I.; Fokialakis, N.; et al. Osmanicin, a Polyketide Alkaloid Isolated from Streptomyces osmaniensis CA-244599 Inhibits Elastase in Human Fibroblasts. *Molecules* **2019**, *24*, 2239. [CrossRef] [PubMed]
17. Gonzalez-Menendez, V.; Crespo, G.; Toro, C.; Martin, J.; de Pedro, N.; Tormo, J.R.; Genilloud, O. Extending the Metabolite Diversity of the Endophyte *Dimorphosporicola tragani*. *Metabolites* **2019**, *9*, 197. [CrossRef]
18. Gonzalez-Menendez, V.; Asensio, F.; Moreno, C.; de Pedro, N.; Monteiro, M.C.; de la Cruz, M.; Vicente, F.; Bills, G.F.; Reyes, F.; Genilloud, O.; et al. Assessing the effects of adsorptive polymeric resin additions on fungal secondary metabolite chemical diversity. *Mycology* **2014**, *5*, 179–191. [CrossRef] [PubMed]
19. Lee, N.; Hwang, S.; Kim, J.; Cho, S.; Palsson, B.; Cho, B.K. Mini review: Genome mining approaches for the identification of secondary metabolite biosynthetic gene clusters in Streptomyces. *Comput. Struct. Biotechnol. J.* **2020**, *18*, 1548–1556. [CrossRef] [PubMed]
20. Keller, N.P. Fungal secondary metabolism: Regulation, function and drug discovery. *Nat. Rev. Microbiol.* **2019**, *17*, 167–180. [CrossRef]
21. Defarge, C.; Trichet, J.; Maurin, A.; Hucher, M. Kopara in Polynesian atolls: Early stages of formation of calcareous stromatolites. *Sediment. Geol.* **1994**, *89*, 9–23. [CrossRef]
22. Richert, L.; Roland, L.; Annie, H.; Claude, P. Cyanobacterial populations that build 'kopara' microbial mats in Rangiroa, Tuamotu Archipelago, French Polynesia. *Eur. J. Phycol.* **2006**, *41*, 259–279. [CrossRef]
23. Che, L.M.; Andréfouet, S.; Bothorel, V.; Guezennec, M.; Rougeaux, H.; Guezennec, J.; Deslandes, E.; Trichet, J.; Matheron, R.; Campion, T.L.; et al. Physical, chemical, and microbiological characteristics of microbial mats (KOPARA) in the South Pacific atolls of French Polynesia. *Can. J. Microbiol.* **2001**, *47*, 994–1012. [CrossRef] [PubMed]
24. Simon-Colin, C.; Raguénès, G.; Crassous, P.; Moppert, X.; Guezennec, J. A novel mcl-PHA produced on coprah oil by Pseudomonas guezennei biovar. tikehau, isolated from a "kopara" mat of French Polynesia. *Int. J. Biol. Macromol.* **2008**, *43*, 176–181. [CrossRef]
25. Guézennec, J.; Moppert, X.; Raguenes, G.; Richert, L.; Costa, B.; Simon-Colin, C. Microbial mats in French Polynesia and their biotechnological applications. *Process. Biochem.* **2011**, *46*, 16–22. [CrossRef]
26. Fox Ramos, A.E.; Evanno, L.; Poupon, E.; Champy, P.; Beniddir, M.A. Natural products targeting strategies involving molecular networking: Different manners, one goal. *Nat. Prod. Rep.* **2019**, *36*, 960–980. [CrossRef]
27. Rong, X.; Guo, Y.; Huang, Y. Proposal to reclassify the *Streptomyces albidoflavus* clade on the basis of multilocus sequence analysis and DNA-DNA hybridization, and taxonomic elucidation of *Streptomyces griseus* subsp. solvifaciens. *Syst. Appl. Microbiol.* **2009**, *32*, 314–322. [CrossRef] [PubMed]

28. Labeda, D.P.; Goodfellow, M.; Brown, R.; Ward, A.C.; Lanoot, B.; Vanncanneyt, M.; Swings, J.; Kim, S.B.; Liu, Z.; Chun, J.; et al. Phylogenetic study of the species within the family Streptomycetaceae. *Antonie Van Leeuwenhoek* **2012**, *101*, 73–104. [CrossRef]
29. Lamichhane, S.; Sen, P.; Dickens, A.M.; Hyötyläinen, T.; Orešič, M. An Overview of Metabolomics Data Analysis: Current Tools and Future Perspectives. *Compr. Anal. Chem.* **2018**, *82*, 387–413. [CrossRef]
30. Canada, P.; Pereira, A.; Nogueira, N.; Png-Gonzalez, L.; Andrade, C.; Xavier, R. Analysis of bacterial microbiome associated with nylon and copper nets in an aquaculture context. *Aquaculture* **2020**, *516*, 734540. [CrossRef]
31. Zhong, H.; Wang, H.; Tian, Y.; Liu, X.; Yang, Y.; Zhu, L.; Yan, S.; Liu, G. Treatment of polluted surface water with nylon silk carrier-aerated biofilm reactor (CABR). *Bioresour. Technol.* **2019**, *289*, 121617. [CrossRef] [PubMed]
32. Venable, M.E.; Podbielski, M.R. Impact of substrate material on algal biofilm biomass growth. *Environ. Sci. Pollut. Res.* **2019**, *26*, 7256–7262. [CrossRef] [PubMed]
33. Nothias, L.F.; Petras, D.; Schmid, R.; Duhrkop, K.; Rainer, J.; Sarvepalli, A.; Protsyuk, I.; Ernst, M.; Tsugawa, H.; Fleischauer, M.; et al. Feature-based molecular networking in the GNPS analysis environment. *Nat. Methods* **2020**, *17*, 905–908. [CrossRef]
34. Wang, M.; Carver, J.J.; Phelan, V.V.; Sanchez, L.M.; Garg, N.; Peng, Y.; Nguyen, D.D.; Watrous, J.; Kapono, C.A.; Luzzatto-Knaan, T.; et al. Sharing and community curation of mass spectrometry data with Global Natural Products Social Molecular Networking. *Nat. Biotechnol.* **2016**, *34*, 828–837. [CrossRef]
35. Shannon, P.; Markiel, A.; Ozier, O.; Baliga, N.S.; Wang, J.T.; Ramage, D.; Amin, N.; Schwikowski, B.; Ideker, T. Cytoscape: A software environment for integrated models of biomolecular interaction networks. *Genome Res.* **2003**, *13*, 2498–2504. [CrossRef]
36. Almeida, E.L.; Kaur, N.; Jennings, L.K.; Carrillo Rincon, A.F.; Jackson, S.A.; Thomas, O.P.; Dobson, A.D.W. Genome Mining Coupled with OSMAC-Based Cultivation Reveal Differential Production of Surugamide A by the Marine Sponge Isolate Streptomyces sp. SM17 When Compared to Its Terrestrial Relative *S. albidoflavus* J1074. *Microorganisms* **2019**, *7*, 394. [CrossRef] [PubMed]
37. Liu, J.; Zhu, X.; Kim, S.J.; Zhang, W. Antimycin-type depsipeptides: Discovery, biosynthesis, chemical synthesis, and bioactivities. *Nat. Prod. Rep.* **2016**, *33*, 1146–1165. [CrossRef]
38. Li, H.; Huang, H.; Hou, L.; Ju, J.; Li, W. Discovery of Antimycin-Type Depsipeptides from a wbl Gene Mutant Strain of Deepsea-Derived *Streptomyces somaliensis* SCSIO ZH66 and Their Effects on Pro-inflammatory Cytokine Production. *Front. Microbiol.* **2017**, *8*, 678. [CrossRef]
39. Tsuchida, T.; Iinuma, H.; Nishida, C.; Kinoshita, N.; Sawa, T.; Hamada, M.; Takeuchi, T. Tetrodecamycin and dihydrotetrodecamycin, new antimicrobial antibiotics against *Pasteurella piscicida* produced by *Streptomyces nashvillensis* MJ885-mF8. I. Taxonomy, fermentation, isolation, characterization and biological activities. *J. Antibiot.* **1995**, *48*, 1104–1109. [CrossRef]
40. Richardson, M.B.; Williams, S.J. A practical synthesis of long-chain iso-fatty acids (iso-C12-C19) and related natural products. *Beilstein J. Org. Chem.* **2013**, *9*, 1807–1812. [CrossRef]
41. Barrow, C.J.; Oleynek, J.J.; Marinelli, V.; Sun, H.H.; Kaplita, P.; Sedlock, D.M.; Gillum, A.M.; Chadwick, C.C.; Cooper, R. Antimycins, inhibitors of ATP-citrate lyase, from a Streptomyces sp. *J. Antibiot.* **1997**, *50*, 729–733. [CrossRef] [PubMed]
42. Inai, M.; Nishii, T.; Tanaka, A.; Kaku, H.; Horikawa, M.; Tsunoda, T. Total Synthesis of the (+)-Antimycin A Family. *Eur. J. Org. Chem.* **2011**, *2011*, 2719–2729. [CrossRef]
43. Mai, P.Y.; Levasseur, M.; Buisson, D.; Touboul, D.; Eparvier, V. Identification of Antimicrobial Compounds from *Sandwithia guyanensis*-Associated Endophyte Using Molecular Network Approach. *Plants* **2019**, *9*, 47. [CrossRef]
44. Flardh, K.; Buttner, M.J. Streptomyces morphogenetics: Dissecting differentiation in a filamentous bacterium. *Nat. Rev. Microbiol.* **2009**, *7*, 36–49. [CrossRef] [PubMed]
45. Calvo, A.M.; Cary, J.W. Association of fungal secondary metabolism and sclerotial biology. *Front. Microbiol.* **2015**, *6*, 62. [CrossRef] [PubMed]
46. Abd El-Rahman, T.M.A.; Tharwat, N.A.; Abo El-Souad, S.M.S.; El-Beih, A.A.; El-Diwany, A.I. Biological activities and variation of symbiotic fungi isolated from Coral reefs collected from Red Sea in Egypt. *Mycology* **2020**, *11*, 243–255. [CrossRef]
47. Calabon, M.S.; Sadaba, R.B.; Campos, W.L. Fungal diversity of mangrove-associated sponges from New Washington, Aklan, Philippines. *Mycology* **2019**, *10*, 6–21. [CrossRef]
48. Brescia, F.; Marchetti-Deschmann, M.; Musetti, R.; Perazzolli, M.; Pertot, I.; Puopolo, G. The rhizosphere signature on the cell motility, biofilm formation and secondary metabolite production of a plant-associated Lysobacter strain. *Microbiol. Res.* **2020**, *234*, 126424. [CrossRef]
49. Rieusset, L.; Rey, M.; Muller, D.; Vacheron, J.; Gerin, F.; Dubost, A.; Comte, G.; Prigent-Combaret, C. Secondary metabolites from plant-associated Pseudomonas are overproduced in biofilm. *Microb. Biotechnol.* **2020**, *13*, 1562–1580. [CrossRef]
50. Timmermans, M.L.; Picott, K.J.; Ucciferri, L.; Ross, A.C. Culturing marine bacteria from the genus Pseudoalteromonas on a cotton scaffold alters secondary metabolite production. *MicrobiologyOpen* **2019**, *8*, e00724. [CrossRef]
51. Letsiou, S.; Bakea, A.; Le Goff, G.; Lopes, P.; Gardikis, K.; Alonso, C.; Alvarez, P.A.; Ouazzani, J. In vitro protective effects of marine-derived Aspergillus puulaauensis TM124-S4 extract on H2O2-stressed primary human fibroblasts. *Toxicol. Vitr. Int. J. Publ. Assoc. BIBRA* **2020**, *66*, 104869. [CrossRef] [PubMed]
52. Tamura, K.; Nei, M. Estimation of the number of nucleotide substitutions in the control region of mitochondrial DNA in humans and chimpanzees. *Mol. Biol. Evol.* **1993**, *10*, 512–526. [CrossRef] [PubMed]
53. Kumar, S.; Stecher, G.; Li, M.; Knyaz, C.; Tamura, K. MEGA X: Molecular Evolutionary Genetics Analysis across Computing Platforms. *Mol. Biol. Evol.* **2018**, *35*, 1547–1549. [CrossRef]

54. Chambers, M.C.; Maclean, B.; Burke, R.; Amodei, D.; Ruderman, D.L.; Neumann, S.; Gatto, L.; Fischer, B.; Pratt, B.; Egertson, J.; et al. A cross-platform toolkit for mass spectrometry and proteomics. *Nat. Biotechnol.* **2012**, *30*, 918–920. [CrossRef]
55. Pluskal, T.; Castillo, S.; Villar-Briones, A.; Orešič, M. MZmine 2: Modular framework for processing, visualizing, and analyzing mass spectrometry-based molecular profile data. *BMC Bioinform.* **2010**, *11*, 395. [CrossRef]
56. Myers, O.D.; Sumner, S.J.; Li, S.; Barnes, S.; Du, X. One Step Forward for Reducing False Positive and False Negative Compound Identifications from Mass Spectrometry Metabolomics Data: New Algorithms for Constructing Extracted Ion Chromatograms and Detecting Chromatographic Peaks. *Anal. Chem.* **2017**, *89*, 8696–8703. [CrossRef]

marine drugs

Article

Potency- and Selectivity-Enhancing Mutations of Conotoxins for Nicotinic Acetylcholine Receptors Can Be Predicted Using Accurate Free-Energy Calculations

Dana Katz [1], Michael A. DiMattia [1], Dan Sindhikara [1,†], Hubert Li [1], Nikita Abraham [2] and Abba E. Leffler [1,*]

1 Schrödinger, Inc., 120 West 45th St., New York, NY 10036, USA; dana.katz@schrodinger.com (D.K.); michael.dimattia@schrodinger.com (M.A.D.); dan.sindhikara@merck.com (D.S.); hubert.li@schrodinger.com (H.L.)
2 D.E. Shaw India Private Ltd., Hyderabad 500096, India; nikita.abraham@schrodinger.com
* Correspondence: abba.leffler@schrodinger.com
† Current address: Merck and Co., Inc., Kenilworth, NJ 07033, USA.

Abstract: Nicotinic acetylcholine receptor (nAChR) subtypes are key drug targets, but it is challenging to pharmacologically differentiate between them because of their highly similar sequence identities. Furthermore, α-conotoxins (α-CTXs) are naturally selective and competitive antagonists for nAChRs and hold great potential for treating nAChR disorders. Identifying selectivity-enhancing mutations is the chief aim of most α-CTX mutagenesis studies, although doing so with traditional docking methods is difficult due to the lack of α-CTX/nAChR crystal structures. Here, we use homology modeling to predict the structures of α-CTXs bound to two nearly identical nAChR subtypes, α3β2 and α3β4, and use free-energy perturbation (FEP) to re-predict the relative potency and selectivity of α-CTX mutants at these subtypes. First, we use three available crystal structures of the nAChR homologue, acetylcholine-binding protein (AChBP), and re-predict the relative affinities of twenty point mutations made to the α-CTXs LvIA, LsIA, and GIC, with an overall root mean square error (RMSE) of 1.08 ± 0.15 kcal/mol and an R^2 of 0.62, equivalent to experimental uncertainty. We then use AChBP as a template for α3β2 and α3β4 nAChR homology models bound to the α-CTX LvIA and re-predict the potencies of eleven point mutations at both subtypes, with an overall RMSE of 0.85 ± 0.08 kcal/mol and an R^2 of 0.49. This is significantly better than the widely used molecular mechanics—generalized born/surface area (MM-GB/SA) method, which gives an RMSE of 1.96 ± 0.24 kcal/mol and an R^2 of 0.06 on the same test set. Next, we demonstrate that FEP accurately classifies α3β2 nAChR selective LvIA mutants while MM-GB/SA does not. Finally, we use FEP to perform an exhaustive amino acid mutational scan of LvIA and predict fifty-two mutations of LvIA to have greater than 100X selectivity for the α3β2 nAChR. Our results demonstrate the FEP is well-suited to accurately predict potency- and selectivity-enhancing mutations of α-CTXs for nAChRs and to identify alternative strategies for developing selective α-CTXs.

Keywords: conotoxin; nicotinic acetylcholine receptor; selectivity; free-energy perturbation

Citation: Katz, D.; DiMattia, M.A.; Sindhikara, D.; Li, H.; Abraham, N.; Leffler, A.E. Potency- and Selectivity-Enhancing Mutations of Conotoxins for Nicotinic Acetylcholine Receptors Can Be Predicted Using Accurate Free-Energy Calculations. *Mar. Drugs* **2021**, *19*, 367. https://doi.org/10.3390/md19070367

Academic Editors: Susana P Gaudencio and Florbela Pereira

Received: 27 May 2021
Accepted: 22 June 2021
Published: 25 June 2021

1. Introduction

Nicotinic acetylcholine receptors (nAChRs), members of the pentameric ligand-gated ion channel family and commonly referred to as Cys-loop receptors [1], are divided into muscle-type and neuronal-type. Neuronal-type receptors are homopentamers or heteropentamers of various subunit compositions. Each interface is made up of the principal side (+) of an α subunit (α2–α10) and the complementary side (−) of an α subunit (α7, α9) or β subunits (β2–β4) in homo and heteropentamers, respectively, which have distinct biophysical and pharmacological properties [2,3]. Subunits are composed of an extracellular domain (ECD), a transmembrane domain (TMD), and an intracellular domain arranged similarly to barrel staves to form a cation-conducting central pore. The binding pocket for acetylcholine lies in the "orthosteric site" at the interface of adjacent principal and complementary subunits in the extracellular domain. The nAChRs play important roles in vital physiological processes (α3β2 nAChR) and in diseases, including schizophrenia (α7 nAChR), addiction (α3β4 nAChR, α4β2 nAChR), and pain (α9α10 nAChR) [4–6]. The high degree of sequence identity between interchangeable nAChRs subunits (57–70%) makes selective inhibition of a specific nAChR difficult and increases the risk of unwanted side effects due to activity at off-target nAChRs [1].

α-Conotoxins (α-CTXs) are small, disulfide-rich peptides (usually ~12 to 20 amino acids in length) that are isolated from the venom of predatory marine cone snails, which have attracted special interest as possible nAChR therapeutics and tool compounds due to their ability to discriminate between similar nAChRs [7–9]. These conotoxins bind to orthosteric sites on nAChRs and function as competitive antagonists by inhibiting activity of the channel [7]. The so-called "4/7" α-CTXs have been proven to be particularly adept at discerning differences between closely related nAChRs [10]. NMR structures have revealed that these conotoxins contain two disulfide bonds with four residues in the first intercysteine loop (loop 1) and seven residues in the second intercysteine loop (loop 2), as well as a variable number of N-terminal residues and often C-terminal post-translational modifications. Some principles for improving the selectivity of these conotoxins via mutagenesis have begun to emerge [11], such as focusing efforts on loop 2 vs. loop 1. In addition, the locations and thermodynamics of water sites in the peptide toxin binding pockets of ion channels, as computed by inhomogeneous solvation theory implemented in the WaterMap algorithm, have recently been shown to explain structure–activity relationships (SAR) for bungarotoxin and the muscle-subtype nAChR [12]; however, accurately predicting selectivity-enhancing mutations is still an arduous process with much uncertainty that would benefit from new approaches [13].

Free-energy perturbation (FEP) is a rigorous computational method for estimating relative binding free energies (RBFE) that has been used to successfully predict the selectivity profiles of small molecules for kinases and phosphodiesterases [14,15]. For peptides, FEP can compute the RBFE between a wild-type and point mutant ($\Delta\Delta G_{FEP}$) via an "alchemical transformation" that "mutates" the wild-type (WT) sidechain to the mutant sidechain through a series of intermediates known as λ windows (Figure 1) [16,17]. Notably, FEP incorporates sampling of all degrees of freedom via molecular dynamics (MD) simulations to account for conformational variations in ligand–receptor interactions and permits the displacement and introduction of explicit waters during the simulation [18]. This contrasts with the widely used molecular mechanics–generalized born/surface area (MM-GB/SA) method, in which no alchemical transformation is performed, a static structure is used, and an implicit representation of the solvent is employed [19]. In principle, using FEP to predict the selectivity of conotoxin mutants at nAChRs is straightforward—FEP simulations of the conotoxin mutation of interest are run at the target and off-target nAChRs and then selectivity is calculated through the differences in the resulting ΔΔGs; however, to date no crystal or cryoelectron microscopy (Cryo-EM) structure of the pentameric nicotinic receptor ECD in complex with an α-conotoxin has been obtained [20]. As a result, low-resolution homology models of α-CTXs bound to nAChRs based on soluble homologues of the ECD of nAChRs [21,22], acetylcholine-binding protein (AChBP) from the mollusks *Aplysia californica* (Ac-AChBP) or *Lymnaea stagnalis* (Ls-AChBP), must be employed instead (Figure 2A,B). Ac-AChBP has low sequence identity to nAChR subtypes (<30%), but shares an overall architecture and key binding site residues with nAChRs and is highly amenable to co-crystallization with α-CTXs [23]. While such nAChR homology models can be successful at qualitatively rationalizing the selectivity profiles of α-CTX mutants [24,25], the ability to use them to quantitatively predict potency and selectivity is undetermined.

$$\Delta G_{complex} = \sum_{i=0}^{N} \Delta G(\lambda_i \rightarrow \lambda_{i+1})$$

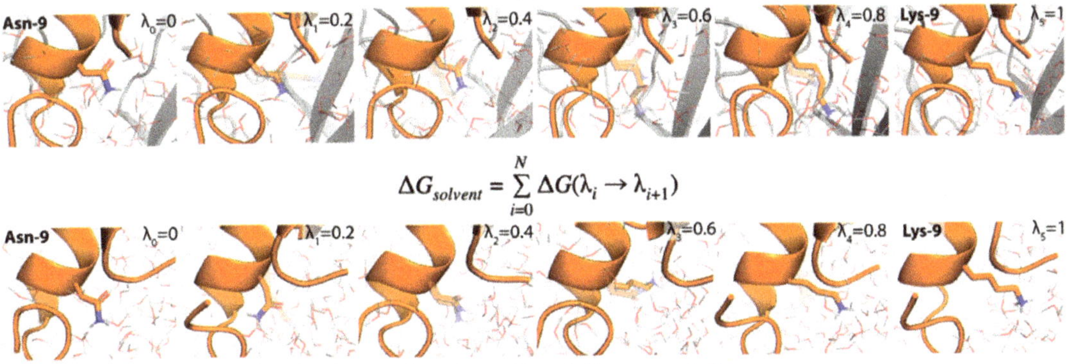

$$\Delta\Delta G(Asn\text{-}9 \rightarrow Lys\text{-}9) = \Delta G_{complex} - \Delta G_{solvent}$$

Figure 1. FEP calculation of the relative binding free energy due to a mutation. The peptide being mutated is represented in orange and the receptor to which it is bound is depicted in gray. Water molecules are shown as lines, with oxygens colored red and hydrogens colored white. The λ window is shown in the upper right-hand corner of each frame. In particular, λ = 0 represents the unmutated sidechain (Asn-9, leftmost frame) and λ = 1 represents the fully mutated sidechain (Lys-9, rightmost frame). For clarity, only six λ windows are shown, although significantly more are used in a typical FEP calculation.

In this study, we use FEP to retrospectively predict potency and selectivity data for an archetypical system, the α-CTX LvIA from *Conus lividus*, which is naturally 18-fold more selective for the α3β2 nAChR than the highly similar α3β4 nAChR [26] (Figure 2C,D). The α3β2 nAChR is involved in a variety of physiological processes and the α3β4 nAChR is implicated in nicotine addiction [11]. This conotoxin and nAChR pair serves as a rigorous test for FEP selectivity calculations because the ECDs of the α3β2 and α3β4 nAChRs are 68% identical and point mutants of LvIA with a wide range of selectivity levels, some of which are counterintuitive, have been identified [26]. For example, LvIA[N9A] is >2000-fold more selective for the α3β2 nAChR than the α3β4 nAChR, although this mutant does not make significantly different contacts between the subtypes [26] (Figure 2C,D). We begin by examining the suitability of AChBP/α-CTX complexes as templates for nAChR/α-CTX homology models by using FEP and MM-GB/SA to retrospectively predict radioligand binding data for the conotoxins LvIA and GIC at Ac-AChBP and the conotoxin LsIA at Ls-AChBP [13,26,27] (Figure 2E). Second, we build homology models of the α3β2 and α3β4 nAChRs and retrospectively test the accuracy of FEP and MM-GB/SA in predicting the potency and selectivity of a set of point mutations of LvIA at these subtypes [26]. Third, in silico we mutate each non-cysteine position on LvIA to every genetically encoded amino acid (except cysteine) and use cloud-based FEP simulations to predict the selectivity levels of the resulting 225 mutants. Taken together, this study expands the domain of applicability of FEP to include selectivity calculations for α-CTXs and nAChRs, illustrates in principle how such an approach could be employed in a biologics drug discovery program devoted to this ion channel target and peptide modality, and identifies approaches for engineering selectivity into α-CTXs.

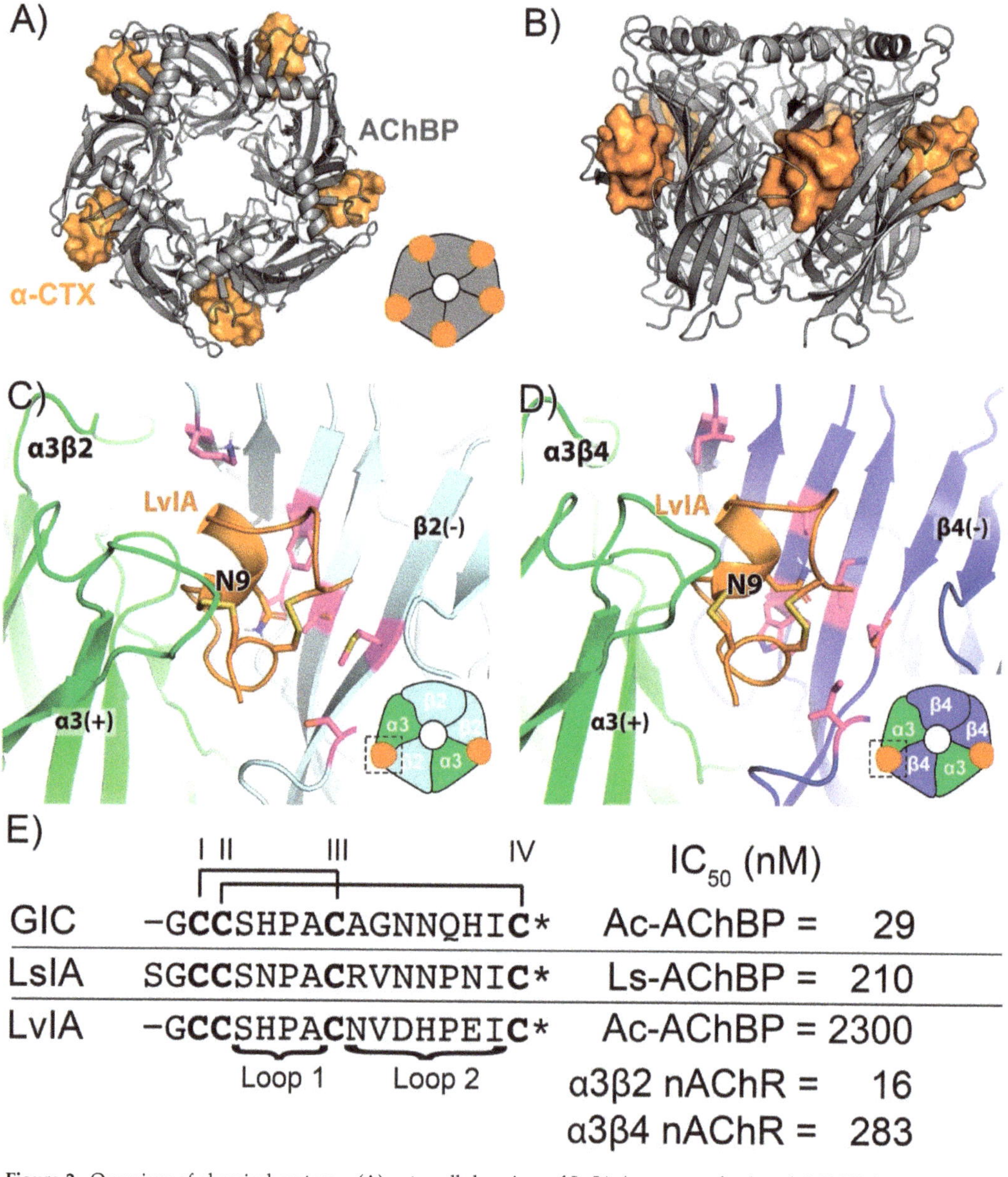

Figure 2. Overview of chemical systems: (**A**) extracellular view of LvIA (orange surface) and AChBP (gray cartoon); (**B**) transmembrane view of LvIA (orange surface) and AChBP (gray cartoon); (**C**) binding interface of LvIA and α3β2 nAChR; (**D**) binding interface of LvIA and α3β4 nAChR. LvIA (orange), AChBP (gray), α3 (green), β2 (pale cyan), and β4 (blue) are depicted in above images. Residues shown in pink differ between β subunits, lie within the binding interface of LvIA, and have a sidechain pointing towards the binding pocket (**E**) sequences of LvIA, LsIA, and GIC and their respective IC_{50}s for different receptors. An asterisk (*) indicates an amidated C-terminus. Lines connecting cysteines labeled with Roman numerals indicate disulfide bonds.

2. Results

2.1. Performance of FEP and MM-GB/SA on Mutagenesis Data

2.1.1. Performance for AChBP

First, we sought to examine the suitability of AChBP/α-CTX complexes as templates for nAChR/α-CTX homology models. Using a test set of twenty mutants for three different α-CTXs bound to AChBP receptors, we were able to re-predict the experimental affinities of the mutants relative to the WT (converted into $\Delta\Delta G_{EXP}$), with an overall root mean square error (RMSE) of 1.08 ± 0.15 kcal/mol and an R^2 of 0.62 (Table 1 and Figure 3A) using FEP. MM-GB/SA was also used but performed worse, with an RMSE of 2.77 ± 0.54 kcal/mol and R^2 of 0.18 (Table 1 and Figure 3B). The reported prime MM-GB/SA energies were rescaled by a factor of three in accordance with previous publications [19,28]. The performance by α-CTX is broken down in Table 2. LvIA bound to Ac-AChBP had comparable performance for FEP and MM-GB/SA, with RMSE values of 1.03 ± 0.19 kcal/mol and 1.83 ± 0.37 kcal/mol and R^2 values of 0.76 and 0.60, respectively. GIC bound to Ac-AChBP had a lower RMSE value with FEP as compared to MM-GB/SA, with values of 1.27 ± 0.42 and 2.98 ± 1.03, respectively; however, for both methods, there were no correlations. For LsIA, MM-GB/SA predictions had an RMSE of 4.58 ± 1.62 kcal/mol and an R^2 of 0.93, but an inverse correlation. For FEP, the RMSE was 0.75 ± 0.26 kcal/mol with an R^2 of 0.80 when run using the OPLS3e force field. Interestingly, when the same mutations for LsIA were run with OPLS4, as performed for all other systems, the performance degraded, with a higher RMSE value of 2.34 ± 0.65 kcal/mol (Table S1).

Table 1. Performance by receptor.

Receptor	Number of Mutations	Potency Range (kcal/mol)	FEP		MM-GB/SA	
			R^2	RMSE	R^2	RMSE
AChBP	20	−1.90–3.66	0.62	1.08 ± 0.15	0.18	2.77 ± 0.54
nAChR	22	−1.19–2.51	0.49	0.85 ± 0.08	0.06 *	1.96 ± 0.24
Total	42	−1.90–3.66	0.58	0.96 ± 0.09	0.07	2.37 ± 0.31

* Negative correlation coefficient.

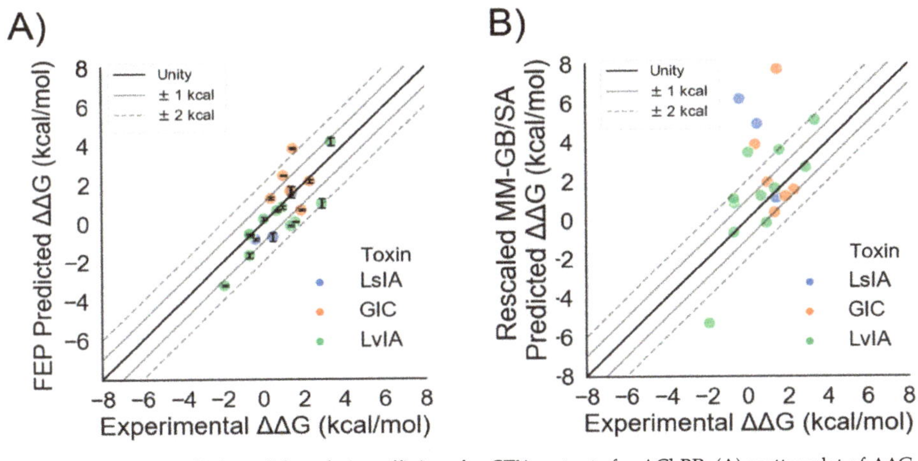

Figure 3. Quantitative prediction of the relative affinity of α-CTX mutants for AChBP: (**A**) scatter plot of $\Delta\Delta G_{FEP}$ vs. $\Delta\Delta G_{EXP}$; (**B**) scatter plot of $\Delta\Delta G_{MM\text{-}GB/SA}$ vs. $\Delta\Delta G_{EXP}$ with unity (solid, black line), ±1 kcal/mol error bands (solid gray lines), and ±2 kcal/mol error bands (dashed, gray lines) superimposed. The error bars show the standard error of the mean (SEM) from three independent FEP simulations.

Table 2. Performance by conotoxin.

Toxin	Receptor	Number of Mutations	Potency Range (kcal/mol)	FEP		MM-GB/SA	
				R^2	RMSE	R^2	RMSE
LvIA	Ac-AChBP	11	−1.90–3.36	0.76	1.03 ± 0.19	0.60	1.83 ± 0.37
	α3β2 nAChR	11	−1.19–2.51	0.82	0.93 ± 0.11	0.03 *	2.04 ± 0.26
	α3β4 nAChR	11	−0.85–1.77	0.12	0.77 ± 0.10	0.11 *	1.88 ± 0.47
GIC	Ac-AChBP	6	0.41–2.32	0.00	1.27 ± 0.42	0.05 *	2.98 ± 1.03
LsIA	Ls-AChBP	3	−0.38–1.45	0.80	0.75 ± 0.26	0.93 *	4.58 ± 1.62

* Negative correlation coefficient.

2.1.2. Performance for α3β2 and α3β4 nAChRs

With the AChBP/α-CTX complexes validated by FEP, we proceeded to use these structures to build homology models of the α3β2 and α3β4 nAChRs in order to retrospectively test the ability of FEP to predict the potency and selectivity levels of various α-CTX point mutants bound to these nAChR subtypes. FEP was able to accurately predict the relative potencies of twenty-two mutations using homology models of the two subtypes, with an RMSE of 0.85 ± 0.08 kcal/mol and an R^2 of 0.49 (Table 1 and Figure 4A). MM-GB/SA performed worse than FEP, with an RMSE of 1.96 ± 0.24 kcal/mol and an R^2 of 0.06 (Table 1 and Figure 4B). For the α3β2 and α3β4 nAChRs, FEP re-predicted the experimental ΔΔGs, with RMSE values of 0.93 ± 0.11 kcal/mol and 0.77 ± 0.10 kcal/mol and R^2 values of 0.82 and 0.12, respectively (Table 2). MM-GB/SA performed significantly worse, with an RMSE of 2.04 ± 0.26 kcal/mol and an R^2 of 0.03 for the α3β2 nAChR and with an RMSE of 1.88 ± 0.47 kcal/mol and an R^2 of 0.11 for the α3β4 nAChR.

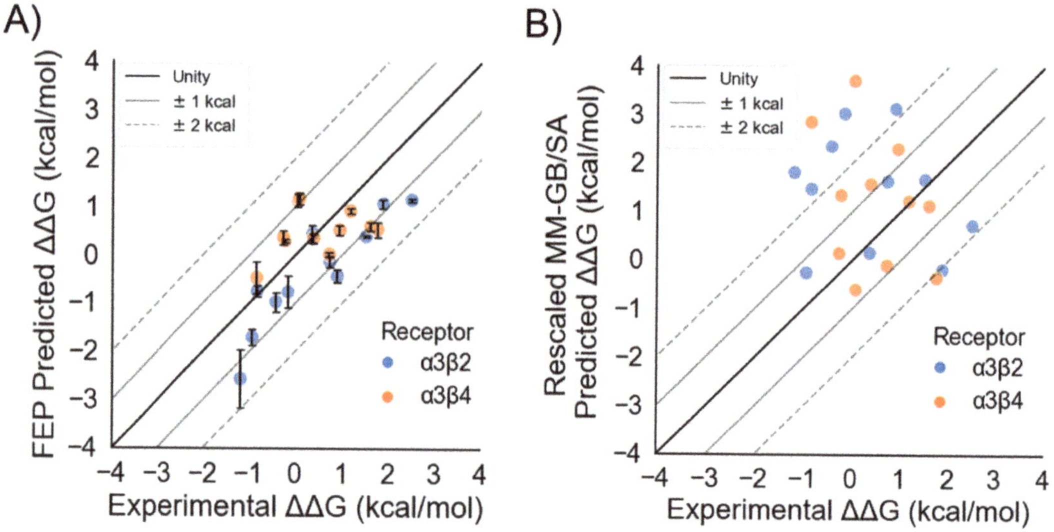

Figure 4. Quantitative prediction of the relative potency levels of LvIA mutants at the α3β2 and α3β4 nAChRs: (**A**) scatter plot of $\Delta\Delta G_{FEP}$ vs. $\Delta\Delta G_{EXP}$; (**B**) scatter plot of $\Delta\Delta G_{MM\text{-}GB/SA}$ vs. $\Delta\Delta G_{EXP}$ with unity (solid, black line), ±1 kcal/mol error bands (solid gray lines), and ±2 kcal/mol error bands (dashed, gray lines) superimposed. The error bars show the standard error of the mean (SEM) from three independent FEP simulations.

2.1.3. Performance of FEP by Type of Mutation

The performance of FEP and MM-GB/SA was also broken down by the type of mutation (Table 3). Charge-change mutations, which are typically difficult for FEP to predict [29], showed an RMSE of 0.82 ± 0.22 kcal/mol with FEP, performing better than

MM-GB/SA that had an RMSE of 2.87 ± 0.67 kcal/mol. The correlation for charge-change mutations was higher than the overall R^2 values for both FEP and MM-GB/SA, with R^2 values of 0.79 and 0.22, respectively. Neutral mutations were also comparable to the overall FEP and MM-GB/SA performance, with RMSE values of 1.02 ± 0.10 kcal/mol and 2.11 ± 0.35 kcal/mol and an R^2 values of 0.39 and 0.00, respectively. We also categorized the mutations by the differences between heavy atoms in the WT and mutant residue. When mutating a bigger residue to a smaller one, FEP and MM-GB/SA had RMSE values of 0.95 ± 0.09 kcal/mol and 2.06 ± 0.22 kcal/mol, respectively. Small residues that were mutated to bigger residues had a higher RMSE for FEP, with a value of 1.41 ± 0.40 kcal/mol. The RMSE for MM-GB/SA was also higher, with a value of 3.00 ± 1.04 kcal/mol. Mutations that had no difference in heavy atoms had an RMSE of 0.87 ± 0.14 kcal/mol for FEP but a value of 3.36 ± 1.16 kcal/mol for MM-GB/SA.

Table 3. Performance by charge and size change.

Type of Mutation	Number of Mutations	Potency Range (kcal/mol)	FEP		MM-GB/SA	
			R^2	RMSE	R^2	RMSE
		By charge				
Charge-Change	13	−1.90–3.36	0.79	0.82 ± 0.22	0.22	2.87 ± 0.67
Neutral	29	−1.19–2.51	0.39	1.02 ± 0.10	0.00	2.11 ± 0.35
		By size				
Big-to-Small	32	−1.90–3.36	0.60	0.95 ± 0.09	0.16	2.06 ± 0.22
Small-to-Big	5	0.73–1.89	0.24	1.41 ± 0.40	0.07	3.00 ± 1.04
No change in heavy atoms	5	−0.94–1.77	0.48	0.87 ± 0.14	0.11 *	3.36 ± 1.16

* Negative correlation coefficient.

FEP also performed better than MM-GB/SA in classifying mutations as having a gain in potency or affinity (ΔΔG < 0 kcal/mol) versus a loss in potency or affinity (ΔΔG > 0 kcal/mol). The area under the curve (AUC) of a receiver operating characteristic (ROC) plot for FEP was 0.94, with a statistically significant *p*-value of <0.01 and a 95% confidence interval (CI) of 0.88 to 1.0 (Table 4), whereas MM-GB/SA performed worse, with an AUC of 0.66 with a p-value of 0.09 (Table 4). FEP had an accuracy of 88%, while MM-GB/SA had an accuracy of 71%. For twenty-four mutations at AChBP, FEP had an AUC of 0.98, as compared to MM-GB/SA with an AUC of 0.76 (Figure 5A). For mutations at nAChRs, FEP performed significantly better than MM-GB/SA, with AUC values of 0.92 and 0.60, respectively (Figure 5B).

Table 4. Performance in classifying gain of potency mutations.

Receptor	Number of Mutations	Potency Range (kcal/mol)	FEP AUC	MM-GB/SA AUC
AChBP	24	−1.90–3.66	0.98 (0.93 to 1.0)	0.76 (0.47 to 1.0)
nAChR	32	−1.19–3.83	0.92 (0.82 to 1.0)	0.60 (0.40 to 0.80)
Total	56	−1.90–3.83	0.94 (0.88 to 1.0)	0.66 (0.49 to 0.82)

2.2. Performance in Classifying Selective LvIA Mutants

We next assessed the ability of FEP and MM-GB/SA to accurately classify LvIA mutants >100X selective for the α3β2 nAChR over the α3β4 nAChR. FEP was able to correctly classify all four selective mutants, namely LvIA[N9L], LvIA[N9K], LvIA[N9I], and LvIA[N9A] (Figure 5C), with only one mutation, Lv1A[V10A], being incorrectly classified as selective. In contrast, MM-GB/SA predicted all four selective mutants as unselective (Figure 5D). The most notable mutation is LvIA[N9A], which has an experimentally measured 2032-fold selectivity [26], with experimental ΔΔG values of −1.19 kcal/mol and 1.61 kcal/mol at the α3β2 and α3β4 nAChRs, respectively. FEP correctly predicted this selectivity, with a predicted ΔΔG of −2.56 ± 0.61 kcal/mol at the α3β2 nAChR and

0.60 ± 0.08 kcal/mol at the α3β4 nAChR, equivalent to a predicted 3690-fold selectivity. In contrast, MM-GB/SA predicted LvIA[N9A] to have a ΔΔG of 1.81 kcal/mol at the α3β2 nAChR and ΔΔG of 1.13 kcal/mol at the α3β4 nAChR, equivalent to a predicted 6-fold selectivity, which is an underestimate by about three orders of magnitude. Overall, FEP had an accuracy of 91% in classifying mutations as being selective or non-selective, with a significant *p*-value of 0.015, as calculated by Fisher's exact test, whereas MM-GB/SA had an accuracy of 55%, which was not statistically significant. We also tested how sensitive the MM-GB/SA accuracy was to the specific protein conformation employed by repeating the calculations with poses of the α3β2 and α3β4 nAChRs extracted from three different points along the homology modeling and simulation workflows (Figure S1). In all cases, the accuracy was less than 65%, and at most half of the selective mutations were correctly identified. Performing the MM/GB-SA calculations using an ensemble of ten poses did lead to the correct classification of LvIA[N9K] as selective, but overall did not result in a statistically significant improvement in accuracy (Figure S2).

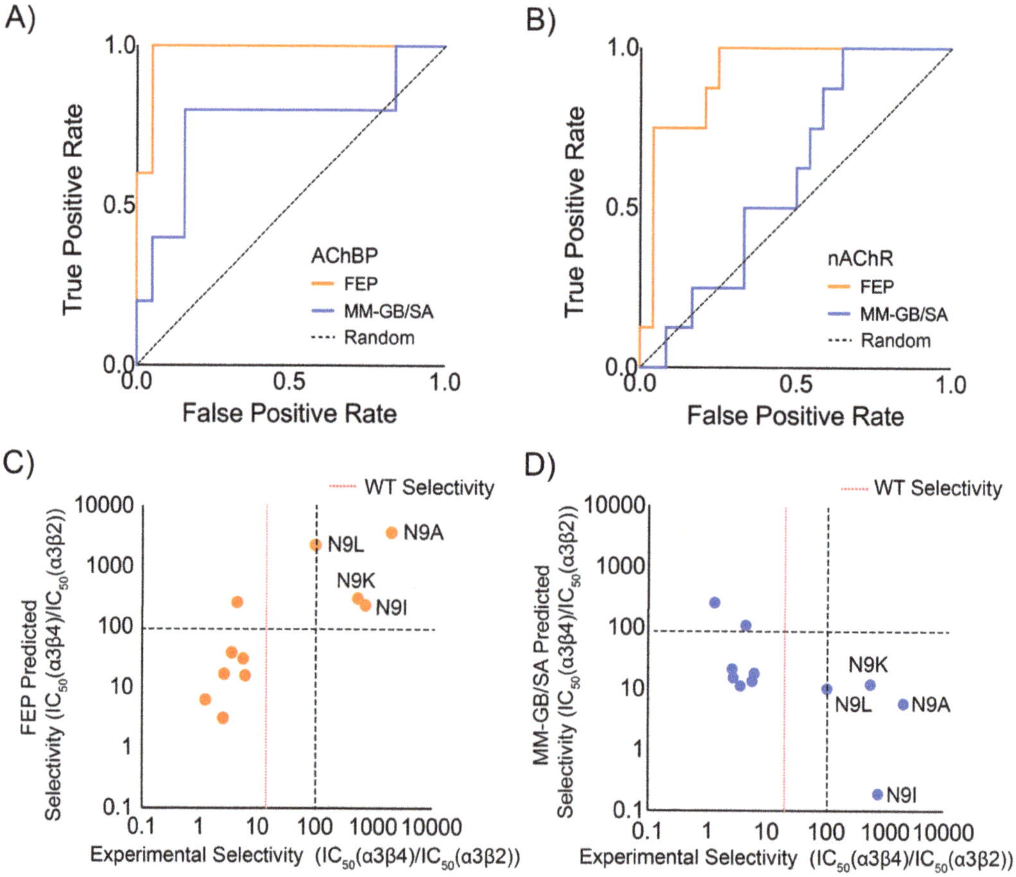

Figure 5. Classification of potency- and selectivity-enhancing LvIA mutants: (**A**) ROC plot comparing the ability of FEP and MM-GB/SA to classify mutations to LvIA, GIC, and LsIA that gain affinity for AChBP relative to WT; (**B**) ROC plot comparing the ability of FEP and MM-GB/SA to classify LvIA mutations that gain potency for the α3β2 or α3β4 nAChR relative to WT; (**C**) classification of the selectivity of LvIA mutants by FEP; (**D**) classification of the selectivity of LvIA mutants by MM-GB/SA.

Although FEP can correctly classify selective mutations, understanding the structural basis for the selectivity of LvIA for the α3β2 nAChR over the α3β4 nAChR could provide insight for future mutagenesis studies. Because the 18-fold selectivity of LvIA for the α3β2 nAChR cannot be readily explained by the differential interactions it makes between the two subtypes (Figure 2C,D), we hypothesized that computing and visualizing the water thermodynamic maps in the binding sites of the two subtypes could explain the selectivity of LvIA. To test this hypothesis, "apo" WaterMap simulations (conotoxin not present) were run for both the α3β2 nAChR and α3β4 nAChR and the locations of the unstable water sites (medium-energy or high-energy) were compared to the pose of LvIA. WaterMap placed a total of 61 water sites within 3 Å of LvIA at α3β2 nAChR and a total of 66 water sites within 3 Å of LvIA at the α3β4 nAChR, allowing us to compare the two WaterMaps further and investigate differences in the water site energetics. At the α3β2 nAChR, thirty-three of these unstable water sites overlapped with the binding mode of LvIA (overlap factor greater than 0.1) (Figure 6A,C) versus seventeen at the α3β4 nAChR (Figure 6B,D). Taken together, these results suggest that LvIA displaces more and higher-energy unstable waters when binding to the α3β2 nAChR than the α3β4 nAChR, which could account for why it is more potent in the former subtype. These findings are consistent with a previous study in which water thermodynamics was used to explain mutagenesis data for a variety of peptide toxins for different ion channels [12].

2.3. *In Silico Scan for Putative Selectivity-Enhancing Mutations with FEP*

Although an alanine scan of LvIA succeeded in identifying a mutation such as LvIA[N9A] that is ~2000X selective [26], we were curious to see if mutations with an even greater degree of selectivity could be identified in silico. To address this question, an exhaustive amino acid scan of LvIA was performed. Each non-cysteine position on LvIA was mutated to every amino acid (except cysteine). We then predicted the $\Delta\Delta G_{FEP}$ values of these 225 point mutations at both the α3β2 and α3β4 nAChRs and the resulting selectivity ratios (Figure 7). Our scan predicted selective mutations at nine different residues, including all four residues in loop 1 and five in loop 2. No mutations were predicted to be selective at the N-terminal LvIA[G1]. In loop 1, 6% of mutations at LvIA[S4], 21% of mutations at LvIA[H5], 78% of mutations at LvIA[P6], and 6% of mutations at LvIA[A7] were predicted to be selective. In loop 2, 67% of mutations at LvIA[N9], 39% of mutations at LvIA[V10], 53% of mutations at LvIA[D11], no mutations at LvIA[H12], 11% of mutations at both LvIA[P13] and LvIA[E14], and no mutations at LvIA[I15] were predicted to be selective (Figure 7A). Overall, out of 225 mutations, fifty-two were predicted to be >100X selective, with four predicted to be >10,000X selective. Of the mutations predicted to be selective, 38% were located on loop 1 and 62% were located on loop 2 (Figure 7B, left panel). We also examined the $\Delta\Delta G_{FEP}$ at the two receptors to understand why these mutations were predicted to be selective (Figure 7B, right panel). Overall, 65% were predicted to be selective due to an increase in potency at the α3β2 nAChR ($\Delta\Delta G_{FEP} < 0$) and decrease in potency at the α3β4 nAChR ($\Delta\Delta G_{FEP} > 0$). Interestingly, nine mutations predicted to be selective had a gain of potency at both receptors, but the magnitude of the gain was much larger at the α3β2 nAChR than at the α3β4 nAChR ($\Delta\Delta G_{FEP}(\alpha3\beta2) << 0$, $\Delta\Delta G_{FEP}(\alpha3\beta4) < 0$). For example, a charge-change mutation at position ten on LvIA had a predicted ΔΔG of −2.12 kcal/mol at the α3β2 nAChR and a predicted ΔΔG of −0.84 kcal/mol at the α3β4 nAChR. Finally, nine mutations were predicted to be selective due to a loss in potency at both receptors, but with a much greater loss in potency at the α3β4 nAChR than at the α3β2 nAChR ($\Delta\Delta G_{FEP}(\alpha3\beta2) > 0$, $\Delta\Delta G_{FEP}(\alpha3\beta4) >> 0$) (Figure 7B, right panel). For example, a mutation at position five on LvIA had predicted ΔΔG values of 1.02 kcal/mol and 3.3 kcal/mol at the α3β2 and α3β4 nAChRs, respectively. Although these findings remain to be experimentally validated, taken together they suggest that additional highly selective mutations for LvIA may exist.

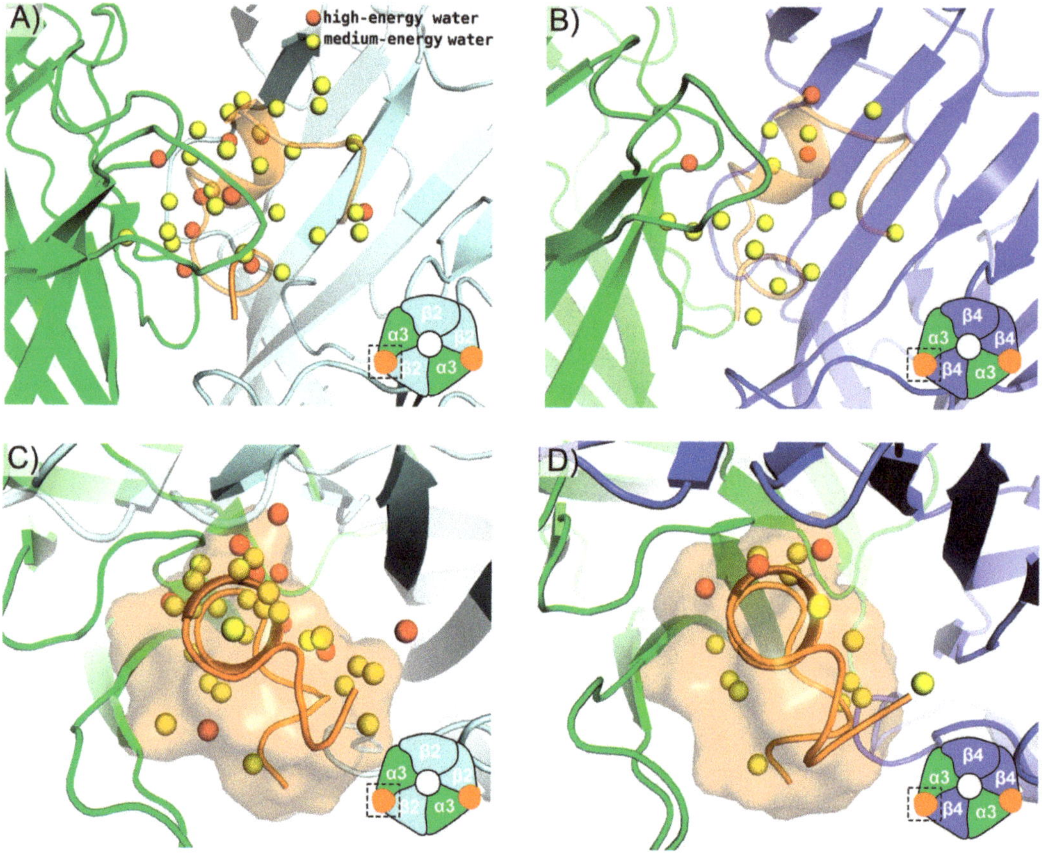

Figure 6. WaterMaps of nAChR subtypes. The apo (**A**) α3β2 nAChR binding site and (**B**) α3β4 nAChR binding site are shown with their respective WaterMaps. LvIA is shown as an orange, semi-transparent cartoon for reference but is not present during the WaterMap simulations. (**C**) Extracellular view of α3β2 nAChR binding site and WaterMap (**D**) Extracellular view of α3β4 nAChR binding site and WaterMap. A semi-transparent orange surface is shown around LvIA. Medium-energy water sites with predicted ΔG > 1.5 kcal/mol are colored yellow and high-energy water sites with predicted ΔG > 3.5 kcal/mol are colored red. For clarity, only medium-energy or high-energy water sites that overlap with the position of LvIA in the bound state are shown.

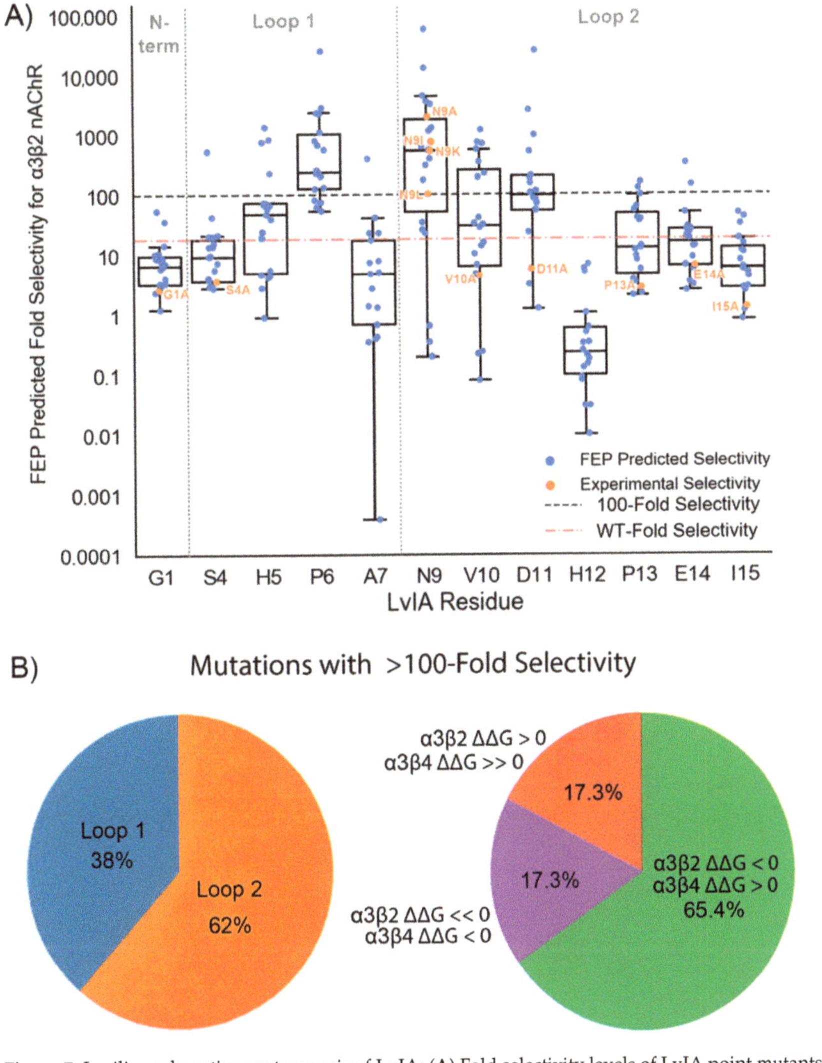

Figure 7. In silico exhaustive mutagenesis of LvIA: (**A**) Fold selectivity levels of LvIA point mutants predicted by FEP (blue points) and measured experimentally (orange points) are plotted by residue, with box plots overlaid. The black dashed line denotes the cutoff for a mutation to be considered selective (100X), while the red dot-dashed line denotes the fold selectivity of the WT LvIA (18X); (**B**) Pie charts show the compositions of point mutations predicted to be selective by the loop they are on (left panel) and by their predicted ΔΔGs at each nAChR subtype (right panel).

3. Discussion

The ability to accurately predict how a mutation to an α-CTX will affect its potency and selectivity for nAChRs is a "grand challenge" in the field [30]. Computational methods have the potential to help meet this challenge, but their ability to recapitulate known data must be rigorously assessed using challenging test cases before they can be used prospectively [12,31]. Here, we performed such a study by examining the ability of FEP to retrospectively predict a wide range of potency and selectivity levels of LvIA mutants for the highly similar α3β2 and α3β4 nAChRs.

3.1. FEP Quantitatively Predicts the Relative Changes in Free Energy of Conotoxin Mutants for AChBPs and nAChRs with Accuracy

We sought to build on the previous success in finding a correlation between measured and predicted potency levels [32,33] of α-CTX mutants for nAChRs by quantitatively predicting the magnitudes and signs of the ΔΔGs due to the mutations. For the two nAChRs, FEP gave an overall RMSE of 0.85 ± 0.08 kcal/mol and an R^2 of 0.49, suggesting this aim was achieved (Table 1 and Figure 4). In contrast, the more widely used MM-GB/SA method gave an RMSE of 1.96 ± 0.24 kcal/mol and R^2 of 0.06 (Table 1 and Figure 4). These results are consistent with the emerging view that accounting for the dynamics of α-CTX/nAChR interactions, as is the case in FEP, is necessary to accurately model them [30,34,35]. They are also consistent with the results of a similar study in which FEP was retrospectively applied to homology models of small molecules bound to proteins [36].

Of the five systems modeled in this study, LsIA/Ls-AChBP required additional effort to be modeled accurately. The LsIA/Ls-AChBP system was purposefully included, despite only having three mutational data points, because it is the sole example of an α-CTX crystallized in complex with Ls-AChBP. From a structural biology perspective, the LsIA[R10F] and LsIA[R10M] mutations involve altering a complex network of contacts between WT LsIA[R10] and Ls-AChBP that include a cation-π interaction with Ls-AChBP[Y164] and a salt bridge interaction with Ls-AChBP[D160], the latter of which may be influenced by crystal contacts [27]. FEP predictions on these mutations were degraded with the OPLS4 force field [37] compared to the OPL3e forcefield [38] (Table S1). This was likely caused by a reduction in the salt bridge strength in the updated parameterization and the absence of an explicit cation-π term in the forcefield [39].

Finally, two specific sets of mutations also proved difficult for FEP. The first was the GIC/Ac-AChBP system, for which the R^2 value was 0 and the RMSE was 1.27 ± 0.42 kcal/mol. Although this RMSE is within the error range of the 1 kcal/mol RMSE considered desirable for FEP models, the R^2 value may be low due to the small sample size and dynamic range of the data [40]. FEP also performed less well for the 'small-to-big' group of mutations, with an R^2 value of 0.24 and an RMSE of 1.41 ± 0.40 kcal/mol. This could reflect the fact that mutations that gain size can lead to protein reorganization, which is difficult to sample on the timescale of FEP simulations [17]. Nonetheless, these caveats should not obscure the main finding of this study, which is that overall FEP can accurately retrospectively predict the free-energy changes of α-CTX mutants for nAChRs.

3.2. FEP Accurately Classifies Conotoxin Mutations That Enhance Selectivity for an nAChR

Overall, FEP was able to correctly classify conotoxin mutations that gain selectivity for one nAChR subtype over another. We found that FEP classified all four LvIA mutants with >100X fold selectivity for the α3β2 nAChR over the α3β4 nAChR as true positives at the cost of only one false positive prediction, with an overall accuracy of 91% (Figure 5). In contrast, MM-GB/SA did not identify any selective mutations correctly and had an overall accuracy of 55%. The ability of FEP to classify selectivity-enhancing mutations is an indication of the method's predictive power and suggests it might be complementary to experimental methods, such as alanine scanning, which are expensive and time-consuming. Future studies may focus on going beyond the classification of selectivity to quantitatively predicting its magnitude. However, this is an intrinsically more difficult problem due to the propagation of uncertainty in the final selectivity prediction (i.e., the difference between two predictions with 1 kcal/mol error each will have a propagated error of 1.4 kcal/mol if they are uncorrelated) [14]. Higher-resolution α-CTX structures complexed with different nAChR ECD subtypes may enable such calculations. More broadly, our dynamics-based approach in FEP for computing selectivity is in line with a similar study that found that inclusion of multiple frames in MM-GB/SA calculations could be an important factor in prospectively identifying selective mutations of the conotoxin RegIIA for the α3β2 nAChR over the α3β4 nAChR [41].

3.3. An Exhaustive In Silico Scan Predicts Additional Selectivity-Enhancing Point Mutations May Exist for LvIA

We assessed our ability to computationally identify putative selectivity-enhancing mutations by exhaustively mutating LvIA at each position to every (permissible) genetically encoded amino acid, except cysteine, and used FEP to predict the resulting ΔΔGs at both nAChR subtypes. Out of 225 mutations, 23% were predicted to have >100X selectivity for the α3β2 nAChR over the α3β4 nAChR (Figure 7A). In general, our results are in accordance with previous studies and findings. For example, 67% of prospective mutations to LvIA[N9] were predicted >100X selective (Figure 7A), in agreement with the critical role that this residue is known to play in enhancing selectivity for LvIA and other 4/7 α-CTXs [26]. Furthermore, consistent with the hypothesis that residues on loop 2 govern subtype selectivity [42], 62% of the mutations predicted to be selective were present on loop 2 (Figure 7B). One unexpected finding that emerged was that 78% of mutations made to LvIA[P6], which is located on loop 1, were predicted to have some degree of selectivity (Figure 7A). Since proline at this position is highly conserved amongst α-CTXs [10], these predictions are counterintuitive and could be false positives; however, given the excellent retrospective performance of FEP in classifying selective mutations and the fact that proline mutants were not simply indiscriminately predicted to be selective (e.g., those at LvIA[P13] were not), these mutations may warrant future experimental investigation.

Finally, our large-scale in silico scan revealed new strategies for engineering selective α-CTXs. While we found that the majority of the mutations predicted to be selective had the "expected" changes in potencies at the two subtypes (predicted gain in potency for α3β2 nAChR and loss in potency for α3β4 nAChR), two less conventional possibilities emerged as well. In 17% of the cases, predicted selectivity was achieved through loss of potency at both subtypes, although the magnitude of the loss was predicted to be much greater at the α3β4 nAChR. In contrast, a predicted gain in potency for both subtypes, with a larger gain for α3β2 nAChR, was also observed 17% of the time. Taken together, these findings suggest alternate ways to engineer selectivity into conotoxins beyond mutating residues to attempt to "clash" with the off-target nAChR subtype. More generally, computational methods that embrace the dynamics of α-CTX/nAChR interactions [30,41] are increasingly being used to prospectively identify selectivity-enhancing mutations. With the passage of α-CTX antagonists of nAChRs towards clinical trials [43–45], our findings set the stage for the prospective use of FEP to advance such drug discovery efforts.

4. Materials and Methods

4.1. AChBP Protein Preparation

All calculations were performed using the 2021-1 release of Maestro (Schrödinger, Inc., New York, NY, USA), unless otherwise noted. LsIA and Ls-AChBP (PDB: 5T90), LvIA and Ac-AChBP (PDB: 5XGL), and GIC in complex with Ac-AChBP (PDB: 5CO5) were all downloaded from the Protein Data Bank (PDB). For the LsIA/Ls-AChBP structure (PDB: 5T90), the model was manually inspected to adjust sidechain rotamers and rebuild any poorly resolved loops with Coot [46], followed by a round of macromolecular structure refinement with Phenix/OPLS3e (a version of Phenix [47], whereby the OPLS3e force field [38] and VSGB2.1 solvation model [48] are used to calculate energies and gradients; 2020-3 release of Maestro). Each structure was aligned and truncated to include two receptor chains and one toxin bound. The Protein Preparation Wizard was used to cap the N- and C-termini with acetyl and N-methyl amide groups, respectively. Missing sidechains and loops were filled in using Prime. Protonation states were assigned using PROPKA at pH 7.4 and hydrogen bond networks were optimized using the "H-bond assignment" panel. Restrained minimization was carried out using the OPLS4 force field [33], with heavy atoms converged to a root mean square deviation (RMSD) of 0.3 Å.

4.2. nAChR Homology Model Construction

Homology models were built using the 'build homology model' panel in the Multiple Sequence Viewer/Editor Panel in Maestro. The target sequence was imported from Uniprot using the respective ECD sequence for *Rattus norvegicus* β2 (P12390), *Rattus norvegicus* β4 (P12392), or *Rattus norvegicus* α3 (P04757). The template structure used was 5XGL after preparation, as described in the previous section. *Rattus norvegicus* β2 and β4 sequences were each aligned to 5XGL chain A, while the *Rattus norvegicus* α3 sequence was aligned to 5XGL chain B. The LvIA peptide sequence (L8BU87) was used as the target sequence and aligned to 5XGL chain C.

The initial homology model for each subtype was then subject to refinement. Using the 'protein–protein' selection tool, all residues at the binding interface between the conotoxin, principal subunit, and complementary subunit were selected and refined using the 'predict sidechains' panel in Maestro. Once sidechain prediction was completed, the structure underwent the protein preparation protocol described in Section 4.1, except only hydrogens were subjected to restrained minimization. Next, an MD simulation was performed to ensure structural integrity and resolve any remaining steric clashes. Using the 'system builder' panel, an SPC solvent model was placed on the structure. No neutralizing counterions or salt were added. An MD simulation with Desmond (Desmond Molecular Dynamics System, D. E. Shaw Research, New York, NY, USA, 2020. Maestro-Desmond Interoperability Tools, Schrödinger, New York, NY, USA, 2020) was performed for 15 ns on 4 GPUs on a GPU cluster consisting of NVIDIA Pascal-generation GPUs. Following manual inspection, a single representative frame without steric clashes and with low RMSD to the starting model was then selected from the trajectory (the 19th frame for the α3β2 nAChR and the 1st frame for the α3β4 nAChR). These frames were then used as inputs for FEP and MM-GB/SA calculations.

4.3. Selection of Mutants

Forty-two IC_{50}'s due to mutations to LsIA, GIC, and LvIA were gathered from three sources [13,26,27] and all mutations with reported IC_{50} values were used for FEP benchmarking. Fourteen additional IC_{50}'s due to mutations were used to assess classifier performance but not RMSEs, because they were qualified data points at the top of the assay. To convert reported IC_{50} values to $\Delta\Delta G_{EXP}$, the relation $\Delta\Delta G_{EXP} = R \times T \times \ln(IC_{50}(MUT)/IC_{50}(WT))$ was used, in which $IC_{50}(MUT)$ is the IC_{50} of the mutant peptide, $IC_{50}(WT)$ is the IC_{50} of the WT (unmutated) peptide, R is the universal gas constant, and T is the temperature at 298 K with $R \times T = 0.593$ kcal/mol. The specific WT IC_{50} measured in each study was used when converting that study's mutational data into free energies.

4.4. WaterMap Calculations

WaterMap calculations were set up and run using the WaterMap panel in Maestro as previously described [12]. The toxin chain was selected as the ligand and waters within 10 Å of the selected ligand were analyzed. An "apo" (toxin not retained in calculations) WaterMap was run. For the WaterMap analysis, the overlap factor was set to 0.1 to identify water sites that overlap with the coordinates of LvIA. A custom script was then used to categorize water sites based on their free energy. Medium-energy water sites were colored yellow ($1.5 < \Delta G < 3.5$ kcal/mol) and high-energy water sites were colored red ($\Delta G \geq 3.5$ kcal/mol) [12].

4.5. RBFE Calculations with MM-GB/SA

MM-GB/SA calculations were set up in the 'residue scanning' panel. After undergoing the refinement procedure described in Section 4.2, the structure was imported into the 'residue scanning' panel and the 'stability and affinity' calculation type was selected. The toxin chain was chosen to bind to the other two chains in the input structure. Default settings were used for all residue scanning calculations, along with a 0 Å cutoff for sidechain prediction with backbone minimization (only the residue being mutated was permitted to repack). The predicted affinities calculated by MM-GB/SA were then rescaled as described previously by dividing each predicted ΔΔG by a factor of three [19,28]. Additionally, MM-GB/SA calculations were repeated using an ensemble of ten evenly spaced frames selected from the 25 ns MD trajectory of the WT LvIA FEP simulation (described in Section 4.6). The RBFE was then calculated over this ensemble using an in-house script, thermal_mmgbsa.py [49].

4.6. RBFE Calculations with FEP

Retrospective FEP calculations were carried out as follows. The same input structure used for MM-GB/SA calculations was imported into the Protein FEP panel in Maestro and the selectivity calculation type was selected. For each system, the toxin chain was chosen to bind to the two receptor chains. Defaults were used for all parameters other than the simulation time, which was increased to 25 ns, as well as the number of λ windows, which was set to 24 for all perturbation types. The FEP job was run on 4 GPUs on a GPU cluster consisting of NVIDIA Pascal-generation GPUs. Finally, when performing charge-change mutations with FEP, it can be important to perturb to the neutral form of the residue when it is in close proximity to other charged residues and a hydrogen bond network is involved [28]; therefore, for the LsIA[N9D] mutation, N9 was mutated into protonated Asp (ASH), while for the LvIA[N9K] mutation at both the α3β2 nAChR and α3β4 nAChR, N9 was mutated into neutral Lys (LYN). Finally, FEP calculations for LsIA/Ls-AChBP were also performed as described above but using the 2020-3 release of Maestro, which employs the OPLS3e forcefield [38].

4.7. Point Mutation Scan

An amino acid scan was performed at LvIA, in which every non-cysteine residue was mutated into every residue except cysteine, and the resulting RBFEs at the α3β2 nAChR and α3β4 nAChR were computed with FEP. The structure file was imported into the FEP panel and the selectivity calculation was selected. The toxin chain was chosen to bind to the two receptor chains. For each residue, all standard amino acid mutations that were possible for that residue were selected. This resulted in a total of 225 mutations for LvIA at both the α3β2 and α3β4 nAChRs. Mutations to histidine were performed for all three tatuomer and charge forms (HID, HIE, HIP) and the state predicted as being most selective upon mutation was used for plotting and analysis. Default parameters were used with the exception of simulation time, which was set to 20 ns, as well as the number of λ windows, which was set to 24 for all perturbation types. The FEP job ran on FEP+ Web Services, which is a service provided by Schrödinger to run FEP calculations on cloud computing resources using NVIDIA Tesla-generation GPUs.

4.8. Selectivity Calculations

Upon completion of FEP and MM-GB/SA RBFE calculations at the α3β2 nAChR and α3β4 nAChR subtypes, the predicted α3β4/α3β2 selectivity ratio, R, was computed using the relation $R = F \times \exp(\Delta\text{Selectivity}/0.593)$, where $F = IC_{50}(\alpha3\beta4)/IC_{50}(\alpha3\beta2)$ for the WT LvIA and $\Delta\text{Selectivity} = \Delta\Delta G_{MUT}(\alpha3\beta4) - \Delta\Delta G_{MUT}(\alpha3\beta2)$ in kcal/mol.

4.9. Statistics

Statistical analysis of the FEP results and their comparison to experimental data were performed following accepted best practices [50]. To minimize the effects of trial-to-trial variability in $\Delta\Delta G_{FEP}$, every retrospective mutation was run in triplicate with a different random seed and the $\Delta\Delta G_{FEP}$s from each of the three independent simulations were averaged to arrive at a mean $\Delta\Delta G_{FEP}$, which was used in all analyses. Bootstrapped estimates for RMSE and MUE were calculated using the FEP+ panel software in Maestro. For binary classification, the AUC of a ROC plot and its associated CI were computed using Prism 9 with default options (GraphPad Software: San Diego, CA, USA). Mutations with a $\Delta\Delta G_{EXP} < 0$ were classified as having a gain in potency. Mutations with $IC_{50}(\alpha3\beta4)/IC_{50}(\alpha3\beta2) > 100$ were classified as selective.

Supplementary Materials: The following are available online at https://www.mdpi.com/article/10.3390/md19070367/s1, Figure S1: MM-GB/SA selectivity predictions for LvIA mutants using different nAChR conformations, Figure S2: Performance of MM-GB/SA using an ensemble of conformations, Table S1: Comparison of FEP affinity predictions for LsIA mutations using OPLS3e and OPLS4 forcefields.

Author Contributions: Conceptualization, D.K. and A.E.L.; methodology, D.K., D.S. and A.E.L.; software, D.K., D.S. and A.E.L.; validation, D.K., D.S. and A.E.L.; formal analysis, D.K., D.S., M.A.D., H.L., and A.E.L.; investigation, D.K., D.S. and A.E.L.; resources, A.E.L.; data curation, D.K. and A.E.L.; writing—original draft presentation, D.K., D.S., M.A.D., N.A. and A.E.L.; writing—review and editing, D.K., D.S., M.A.D., H.L. and A.E.L.; visualization, D.K, D.S. and A.E.L.; supervision, D.S. and A.E.L.; project administration, A.E.L.; funding acquisition, A.E.L. All authors have read and agreed to the published version of the manuscript.

Funding: This investigation was sponsored and financially supported by the authors' employer, Schrödinger, Inc.

Acknowledgments: The authors thank Robert Abel for his support and guidance, Joe Kaus for expert technical assistance running FEP calculations on the cloud, Dima Lupyan for helpful discussions, and Jon Lindstrom for critical reading of the manuscript.

Conflicts of Interest: The authors declare no conflict of interest.

References

1. Gharpure, A.; Noviello, C.M.; Hibbs, R.E. Progress in nicotinic receptor structural biology. *Neuropharmacology* **2020**, *171*, 108086. [CrossRef]
2. Millar, N.S.; Gotti, C. Diversity of vertebrate nicotinic acetylcholine receptors. *Neuropharmacology* **2009**, *56*, 237–246. [CrossRef] [PubMed]
3. Taly, A.; Corringer, P.-J.; Guedin, D.; Lestage, P.; Changeux, J.-P. Nicotinic receptors: Allosteric transitions and therapeutic targets in the nervous system. *Nat. Rev. Drug Discov.* **2009**, *8*, 733–750. [CrossRef] [PubMed]
4. Dineley, K.T.; Pandya, A.A.; Yakel, J.L. Nicotinic ACh receptors as therapeutic targets in CNS disorders. *Trends Pharm. Sci.* **2015**, *36*, 96–108. [CrossRef] [PubMed]
5. Romero, H.K.; Christensen, S.B.; Di Cesare Mannelli, L.; Gajewiak, J.; Ramachandra, R.; Elmslie, K.S.; Vetter, D.E.; Ghelardini, C.; Iadonato, S.P.; Mercado, J.L.; et al. Inhibition of α9α10 nicotinic acetylcholine receptors prevents chemotherapy-induced neuropathic pain. *Proc. Natl. Acad. Sci. USA* **2017**, *114*, E1825–E1832. [CrossRef]
6. Tregellas, J.R.; Wylie, K.P. Alpha7 Nicotinic Receptors as Therapeutic Targets in Schizophrenia. *Nicotine Tob. Res.* **2018**, *21*, 349–356. [CrossRef]
7. McIntosh, J.M.; Santos, A.D.; Olivera, B.M. Conus peptides targeted to specific nicotinic acetylcholine receptor subtypes. *Annu. Rev. Biochem.* **1999**, *68*, 59–88. [CrossRef]
8. Terlau, H.; Olivera, B.M. Conus venoms: A rich source of novel ion channel-targeted peptides. *Physiol. Rev.* **2004**, *84*, 41–68. [CrossRef]
9. Adams, D.J.; Alewood, P.F.; Craik, D.J.; Drinkwater, R.D.; Lewis, R.J. Conotoxins and their potential pharmaceutical applications. *Drug Dev. Res.* **1999**, *46*, 219–234. [CrossRef]
10. Armishaw, C.J. Synthetic α-Conotoxin Mutants as Probes for Studying Nicotinic Acetylcholine Receptors and in the Development of Novel Drug Leads. *Toxins* **2010**, *2*, 1471–1499. [CrossRef] [PubMed]
11. Lebbe, E.K.M.; Peigneur, S.; Wijesekara, I.; Tytgat, J. Conotoxins Targeting Nicotinic Acetylcholine Receptors: An Overview. *Mar. Drugs* **2014**, *12*, 2970–3004. [CrossRef]
12. Shah, B.; Sindhikara, D.; Borrelli, K.; Leffler, A.E. Water Thermodynamics of Peptide Toxin Binding Sites on Ion Channels. *Toxins* **2020**, *12*, 652. [CrossRef] [PubMed]
13. Lin, B.; Xu, M.; Zhu, X.; Wu, Y.; Liu, X.; Zhangsun, D.; Hu, Y.; Xiang, S.-H.; Kasheverov, I.E.; Tsetlin, V.I.; et al. From crystal structure of α-conotoxin GIC in complex with Ac-AChBP to molecular determinants of its high selectivity for α3β2 nAChR. *Sci. Rep.* **2016**, *6*, 22349. [CrossRef] [PubMed]
14. Albanese, S.K.; Chodera, J.D.; Volkamer, A.; Keng, S.; Abel, R.; Wang, L. Is Structure-Based Drug Design Ready for Selectivity Optimization? *J. Chem. Inf. Model.* **2020**, *60*, 6211–6227. [CrossRef] [PubMed]
15. Moraca, F.; Negri, A.; de Oliveira, C.; Abel, R. Application of Free Energy Perturbation (FEP+) to Understanding Ligand Selectivity: A Case Study to Assess Selectivity between Pairs of Phosphodiesterases (PDE's). *J. Chem. Inf. Model.* **2019**, *59*, 2729–2740. [CrossRef]

16. Hauser, K.; Negron, C.; Albanese, S.K.; Ray, S.; Steinbrecher, T.; Abel, R.; Chodera, J.D.; Wang, L. Predicting resistance of clinical Abl mutations to targeted kinase inhibitors using alchemical free-energy calculations. *Commun. Biol.* **2018**, *1*, 70. [CrossRef]
17. Clark, A.J.; Gindin, T.; Zhang, B.; Wang, L.; Abel, R.; Murret, C.S.; Xu, F.; Bao, A.; Lu, N.J.; Zhou, T.; et al. Free Energy Perturbation Calculation of Relative Binding Free Energy between Broadly Neutralizing Antibodies and the gp120 Glycoprotein of HIV-1. *J. Mol. Biol.* **2017**, *429*, 930–947. [CrossRef]
18. Ross, G.A.; Russell, E.; Deng, Y.; Lu, C.; Harder, E.D.; Abel, R.; Wang, L. Enhancing Water Sampling in Free Energy Calculations with Grand Canonical Monte Carlo. *J. Chem. Theory Comput.* **2020**, *16*, 6061–6076. [CrossRef] [PubMed]
19. Beard, H.; Cholleti, A.; Pearlman, D.; Sherman, W.; Loving, K.A. Applying Physics-Based Scoring to Calculate Free Energies of Binding for Single Amino Acid Mutations in Protein-Protein Complexes. *PLoS ONE* **2013**, *8*, e82849. [CrossRef] [PubMed]
20. Zouridakis, M.; Papakyriakou, A.; Ivanov, I.A.; Kasheverov, I.E.; Tsetlin, V.; Tzartos, S.; Giastas, P. Crystal Structure of the Monomeric Extracellular Domain of α9 Nicotinic Receptor Subunit in Complex with α-Conotoxin RgIA: Molecular Dynamics Insights Into RgIA Binding to α9α10 Nicotinic Receptors. *Front. Pharmacol.* **2019**, *10*, 474. [CrossRef] [PubMed]
21. Brejc, K.A.; van Dijk, W.J.; Klaassen, R.V.; Schuurmans, M.; van der Oost, J.; Smit, A.B.; Sixma, T.K. Crystal structure of an ACh-binding protein reveals the ligand-binding domain of nicotinic receptors. *Nature* **2001**, *411*, 269–276. [CrossRef]
22. Giastas, P.; Zouridakis, M.; Tzartos, S.J. Understanding structure-function relationships of the human neuronal acetylcholine receptor: Insights from the first crystal structures of neuronal subunits. *Br. J. Pharmacol.* **2018**, *175*, 1880–1891. [CrossRef]
23. Celie, P.H.; Kasheverov, I.E.; Mordvintsev, D.Y.; Hogg, R.C.; van Nierop, P.; van Elk, R.; van Rossum-Fikkert, S.E.; Zhmak, M.N.; Bertrand, D.; Tsetlin, V.; et al. Crystal structure of nicotinic acetylcholine receptor homolog AChBP in complex with an alpha-conotoxin PnIA variant. *Nat. Struct. Mol. Biol.* **2005**, *12*, 582–588. [CrossRef] [PubMed]
24. Hopping, G.; Wang, C.I.; Hogg, R.C.; Nevin, S.T.; Lewis, R.J.; Adams, D.J.; Alewood, P.F. Hydrophobic residues at position 10 of α-conotoxin PnIA influence subtype selectivity between α7 and α3β2 neuronal nicotinic acetylcholine receptors. *Biochem. Pharm.* **2014**, *91*, 534–542. [CrossRef]
25. Dutertre, S.; Lewis, R.J. Computational approaches to understand α-conotoxin interactions at neuronal nicotinic receptors. *Eur. J. Biochem.* **2004**, *271*, 2327–2334. [CrossRef]
26. Zhu, X.; Pan, S.; Xu, M.; Zhang, L.; Yu, J.; Yu, J.; Wu, Y.; Fan, Y.; Li, H.; Kasheverov, I.E.; et al. High Selectivity of an α-Conotoxin LvIA Analogue for α3β2 Nicotinic Acetylcholine Receptors Is Mediated by β2 Functionally Important Residues. *J. Med. Chem.* **2020**, *63*, 13656–13668. [CrossRef] [PubMed]
27. Abraham, N.; Healy, M.; Ragnarsson, L.; Brust, A.; Alewood, P.F.; Lewis, R.J. Structural mechanisms for α-conotoxin activity at the human α3β4 nicotinic acetylcholine receptor. *Sci. Rep.* **2017**, *7*, 45466. [CrossRef]
28. Clark, A.J.; Negron, C.; Hauser, K.; Sun, M.; Wang, L.; Abel, R.; Friesner, R.A. Relative Binding Affinity Prediction of Charge-Changing Sequence Mutations with FEP in Protein-Protein Interfaces. *J. Mol. Biol.* **2019**, *431*, 1481–1493. [CrossRef]
29. Rashid, M.H.; Heinzelmann, G.; Kuyucak, S. Calculation of free energy changes due to mutations from alchemical free energy simulations. *J. Theor. Comput. Chem.* **2015**, *14*, 1550023. [CrossRef]
30. Leffler, A.E.; Kuryatov, A.; Zebroski, H.A.; Powell, S.R.; Filipenko, P.; Hussein, A.K.; Gorson, J.; Heizmann, A.; Lyskov, S.; Tsien, R.W.; et al. Discovery of peptide ligands through docking and virtual screening at nicotinic acetylcholine receptor homology models. *Proc. Natl. Acad. Sci. USA* **2017**, *114*, E8100–E8109. [CrossRef] [PubMed]
31. Katz, D.; Sindhikara, D.; DiMattia, M.; Leffler, A.E. Potency-Enhancing Mutations of Gating Modifier Toxins for the Voltage-Gated Sodium Channel NaV1.7 Can Be Predicted Using Accurate Free-Energy Calculations. *Toxins* **2021**, *13*, 193. [CrossRef] [PubMed]
32. Yu, R.; Craik, D.J.; Kaas, Q. Blockade of Neuronal α7-nAChR by α-Conotoxin ImI Explained by Computational Scanning and Energy Calculations. *PLoS Comput. Biol.* **2011**, *7*, e1002011. [CrossRef]
33. Suresh, A.; Hung, A. Molecular simulation study of the unbinding of α-conotoxin [ϒ4E]GID at the α7 and α4β2 neuronal nicotinic acetylcholine receptors. *J. Mol. Graph. Model.* **2016**, *70*, 109–121. [CrossRef]
34. Azam, L.; Papakyriakou, A.; Zouridakis, M.; Giastas, P.; Tzartos, S.J.; McIntosh, J.M. Molecular interaction of α-conotoxin RgIA with the rat α9α10 nicotinic acetylcholine receptor. *Mol. Pharm.* **2015**, *87*, 855–864. [CrossRef]
35. Gulsevin, A.; Papke, R.L.; Stokes, C.; Tran, H.N.T.; Jin, A.-H.; Vetter, I.; Meiler, J. The allosteric activation of α7 nAChR by α-conotoxin MrIC is modified by mutations at the vestibular site. *Biorxiv* **2021**, *10*, 474. [CrossRef]
36. Cappel, D.; Hall, M.L.; Lenselink, E.B.; Beuming, T.; Qi, J.; Bradner, J.; Sherman, W. Relative Binding Free Energy Calculations Applied to Protein Homology Models. *J. Chem. Inf. Model.* **2016**, *56*, 2388–2400. [CrossRef]
37. OPLS4. Available online: https://www.schrodinger.com/products/opls4 (accessed on 24 June 2021).
38. Roos, K.; Wu, C.; Damm, W.; Reboul, M.; Stevenson, J.M.; Lu, C.; Dahlgren, M.K.; Mondal, S.; Chen, W.; Wang, L.; et al. OPLS3e: Extending Force Field Coverage for Drug-Like Small Molecules. *J. Chem. Theory Comput.* **2019**, *15*, 1863–1874. [CrossRef] [PubMed]
39. Turupcu, A.; Tirado-Rives, J.; Jorgensen, W.L. Explicit Representation of Cation−π Interactions in Force Fields with 1/r4 Nonbonded Terms. *J. Chem. Theory Comput.* **2020**, *16*, 7184–7194. [CrossRef] [PubMed]
40. Brown, S.P.; Muchmore, S.W.; Hajduk, P.J. Healthy skepticism: Assessing realistic model performance. *Drug Discov. Today* **2009**, *14*, 420–427. [CrossRef] [PubMed]
41. Xu, Q.; Tae, H.S.; Wang, Z.; Jiang, T.; Adams, D.J.; Yu, R. Rational Design of α-Conotoxin RegIIA Analogues Selectively Inhibiting the Human α3β2 Nicotinic Acetylcholine Receptor through Computational Scanning. *ACS Chem. Neurosci.* **2020**, *11*, 2804–2811. [CrossRef]

42. Dutertre, S.; Nicke, A.; Lewis, R.J. Beta2 subunit contribution to 4/7 alpha-conotoxin binding to the nicotinic acetylcholine receptor. *J. Biol. Chem.* **2005**, *280*, 30460–30468. [CrossRef]
43. Holford, M.; Daly, M.; King, G.F.; Norton, R.S. Venoms to the rescue. *Science* **2018**, *361*, 842–844. [CrossRef]
44. Modica, M.V.; Ahmad, R.; Ainsworth, S.; Anderluh, G.; Antunes, A.; Beis, D.; Caliskan, F.; Serra, M.D.; Dutertre, S.; Moran, Y.; et al. The new COST Action European Venom Network (EUVEN)—Synergy and future perspectives of modern venomics. *GigaScience* **2021**, *10*, 1–5. [CrossRef] [PubMed]
45. Angell, Y.; Holford, M.; Moos, W.H. Peptides 2020: A Clear Therapeutic Vision. *Protein Pept. Lett.* **2018**, *25*, 1042–1043. [CrossRef] [PubMed]
46. Emsley, P.; Lohkamp, B.; Scott, W.G.; Cowtan, K. Features and development of Coot. *Acta Cryst. D Biol. Cryst.* **2010**, *66*, 486–501. [CrossRef] [PubMed]
47. Adams, P.D.; Afonine, P.V.; Bunkóczi, G.; Chen, V.B.; Davis, I.W.; Echols, N.; Headd, J.J.; Hung, L.W.; Kapral, G.J.; Grosse-Kunstleve, R.W.; et al. PHENIX: A comprehensive Python-based system for macromolecular structure solution. *Acta Cryst. D Biol. Cryst.* **2010**, *66*, 213–221. [CrossRef]
48. Li, J.; Abel, R.; Zhu, K.; Cao, Y.; Zhao, S.; Friesner, R.A. The VSGB 2.0 model: A next generation energy model for high resolution protein structure modeling. *Proteins* **2011**, *79*, 2794–2812. [CrossRef] [PubMed]
49. Scriptcenter. Available online: https://www.schrodinger.com/scriptcenter (accessed on 24 June 2021).
50. Mey, A.S.; Allen, B.; Macdonald, H.E.B.; Chodera, J.D.; Kuhn, M.; Michel, J.; Mobley, D.L.; Naden, L.N.; Prasad, S.; Rizzi, A.; et al. Best Practices for Alchemical Free Energy Calculations. *Living J. Comput. Mol. Sci.* **2020**, *2*, 1–48. [CrossRef]

marine drugs

Article

In Vitro and In Silico Characterization of G-Protein Coupled Receptor (GPCR) Targets of Phlorofucofuroeckol-A and Dieckol

Pradeep Paudel [1,2,†], Su Hui Seong [1,3,†], Se Eun Park [1,4], Jong Hoon Ryu [5], Hyun Ah Jung [6,*] and Jae Sue Choi [1,*]

1 Department of Food and Life Science, Pukyong National University, Busan 48513, Korea; ppradeep@olemiss.edu (P.P.); shseong@hnibr.re.kr (S.H.S.); gogo1685@mail.ulsan.ac.kr (S.E.P.)
2 National Center for Natural Products Research, Research Institute of Pharmaceutical Sciences, The University of Mississippi, Oxford, MS 38677, USA
3 Natural Products Research Division, Honam National Institute of Biological Resource, Mokpo 58762, Korea
4 Department of Biomedical Science, Asan Medical Institute of Convergence Science and Technology, Seoul 05505, Korea
5 Department of Life and Nanopharmaceutical Science, Kyung Hee University, Seoul 02447, Korea; jhryu63@khu.ac.kr
6 Department of Food Science and Human Nutrition, Jeonbuk National University, Jeonju 54896, Korea
* Correspondence: jungha@jbnu.ac.kr (H.A.J.); choijs@pknu.ac.kr (J.S.C.); Tel.: +82-63-270-4882 (H.A.J.); +82-51-629-7547 (J.S.C.)
† These authors contributed equally to this work.

Abstract: Phlorotannins are polyphenolic compounds in marine alga, especially the brown algae. Among numerous phlorotannins, dieckol and phlorofucofuroeckol-A (PFF-A) are the major ones and despite a wider biological activity profile, knowledge of the G protein-coupled receptor (GPCR) targets of these phlorotannins is lacking. This study explores prime GPCR targets of the two phlorotannins. In silico proteocheminformatics modeling predicted twenty major protein targets and in vitro functional assays showed a good agonist effect at the α2C adrenergic receptor (α_{2C}AR) and an antagonist effect at the adenosine 2A receptor (A_{2A}R), δ-opioid receptor (δ-OPR), glucagon-like peptide-1 receptor (GLP-1R), and 5-hydroxytryptamine 1A receptor (5-TH_{1A}R) of both phlorotannins. Besides, dieckol showed an antagonist effect at the vasopressin 1A receptor (V_{1A}R) and PFF-A showed a promising agonist effect at the cannabinoid 1 receptor and an antagonist effect at V_{1A}R. In silico molecular docking simulation enabled us to investigate and identify distinct binding features of these phlorotannins to the target proteins. The docking results suggested that dieckol and PFF-A bind to the crystal structures of the proteins with good affinity involving key interacting amino acid residues comparable to reference ligands. Overall, the present study suggests α_{2C}AR, A_{2A}R, δ-OPR, GLP-1R, 5-TH_{1A}R, CB_1R, and V_{1A}R as prime receptor targets of dieckol and PFF-A.

Keywords: phhlorotannins; GPCRs; agonist; antagonist; dieckol; PFF-A; molecular docking

Citation: Paudel, P.; Seong, S.H.; Park, S.E.; Ryu, J.H.; Jung, H.A.; Choi, J.S. In Vitro and In Silico Characterization of G-Protein Coupled Receptor (GPCR) Targets of Phlorofucofuroeckol-A and Dieckol. *Mar. Drugs* **2021**, *19*, 326. https://doi.org/10.3390/md19060326

Academic Editors: Susana P. Gaudencio and Florbela Pereira

Received: 10 May 2021
Accepted: 2 June 2021
Published: 4 June 2021

1. Introduction

G protein-coupled receptors (GPCRs) are a family of membrane receptors that regulate human pathophysiology and are the leading target class for pharmaceuticals. At present, GPCRs mediate the effect of approximately one-third of the FDA-approved drugs [1–3]. However, these drugs target mainly biogenic amine receptors, which comprise around 30 members of the GPCR family [3]. There is, therefore, an immense potential within pharmaceuticals/natural products to exploit, considering the remaining family members for which no existing ligands have been identified.

In the traditional drug development process, the high-throughput screening (HTS) approach against drug targets of choice is the very first step to uncover new drugs, which has now been augmented by the in silico method to maximize the probability of novel leads discovery. Traditional Chinese medicine (TCM) is an important research object of network (TCM herbs, targets, diseases, and syndromes) pharmacology, which aims to understand the network-based biological basis of complex diseases [4], and natural polyphenols are abundant in plant-based foods whose network proximity to disease proteins is predictive of the molecule's known therapeutic effects [5].

Secondary metabolites from seaweeds have gained much interest in natural drug discovery, because the marine source is a huge reservoir of natural products with significant biological activities. In addition, secondary metabolites (carotenoids, polyphenols, and polysaccharides) with numerous biological activities make them a potential source of leads. Among marine organisms, marine alga, i.e., green algae (Chlorophyta), brown algae (Phaeophyta), and red algae (Rhodophyta), are rich sources of bioactive compounds with various biological activities. These macroalgae are well known by seaweeds and have been widely recognized as food, functional food, and potential drug sources for decades. Brown algae are the largest type of seaweed and so far, scientists have identified the therapeutic potential of brown algae-derived secondary metabolites (particularly phloroglucinol-based polyphenols, known as phlorotannins) including, but not limited to antioxidant [6,7], antimicrobial [8], anti-diabetic [9], anti-Alzheimer's disease [10–12], anti-inflammatory [13], neuroprotective [14,15], anti-obesity [16], hepatoprotective [17], monoamine oxidase inhibitor [18], antihypertension [19] and anti-viral [20] activity. *Ecklonia stolonifera* OKAMURA (*E. stolonifera*) is an edible brown alga of the Laminariaceae family that is widely distributed along the Eastern and Southern Korean coast and rich in phlorotannins [19,21]. Dieckol and phlorofucofuroeckol-A (PFF-A) are common phlorotannins in *E. stolonifera* and in our recent study, we had reported human monoamine oxidase (hMAO) inhibition, dopamine D_3R/D_4R receptor agonist effect, dopamine D_1/5-hydroxytryptamine 1A ($5\text{-}HT_{1A}$)/neurokinin 1 (NK_1) receptor antagonist effect [22], and β-secretase and acetylcholinesterase inhibition by dieckol and PFF-A [10,11]. Nonetheless, other promising targets of these phlorotannins are yet to be identified.

Therefore, the main objectives of this study were to: (a) predict prime protein targets of dieckol and PFF-A (Figure 1) via proteocheminformatics modeling (PCM), (b) validate the PCM prediction by evaluating the modulatory effect on predicted receptors via cell-based functional GPCRs assays, and (c) look at the specific binding interactions of test ligands and target receptors via molecular docking simulation.

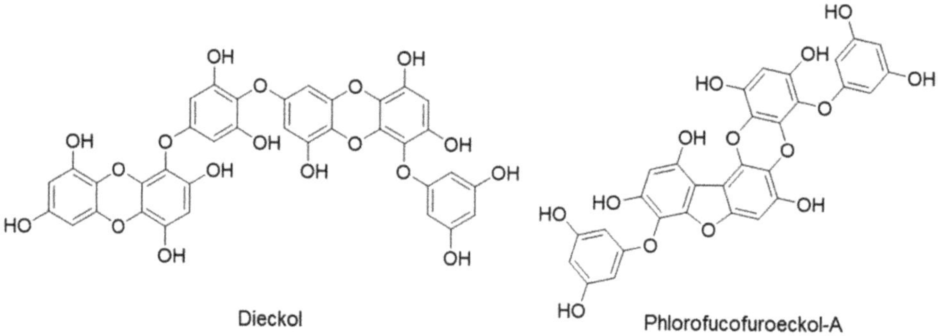

Figure 1. Chemical structures of dieckol and phlorofucofuroeckol-A.

2. Results

2.1. In Silico Target Prediction

Proteocheminformatics (PCM) modeling is a quantitative bio-modeling technique that can predict the affinity and potency of a ligand against multiple different protein targets simultaneously by combining chemical and biological information from the ligand and related targets into a single machine learning model [23]. From in silico PCM modeling, the highest-ranked twenty potential protein targets were predicted for the phlorotannins. Table 1 presents a list of the target proteins with an average score value.

Table 1. List of top 20 protein targets from proteocheminformatics modeling (PCM) prediction of dieckol and phlorofucofuroeckol-A, respectively.

Rank	Dieckol		Phlorofucofuroeckol-A	
	Protein Name	Average Score	Protein Name	Average Score
1	Vasopressin 1A receptor	0.513	Vasopressin 1A receptor	0.797
2			Vasopressin 1B receptor	0.742
3			Oxytocin receptor	0.737
4			B2 bradykinin receptor	0.735
5			B1 bradykinin receptor	0.727
6			Histamine H1 receptor	0.721
7			Serotonin 1D receptor	0.717
8			Type-1 angiotensin II receptor	0.716
9			Dopamine D2 receptor	0.713
10			Cannabinoid receptor 1	0.711
11			Prostanoid EP3 receptor	0.710
12			Rho-associated protein kinase 1	0.710
13			Muscarinic acetylcholine receptor M3	0.709
14			Cholecystokinin A receptor	0.709
15			Serotonin 1A receptor	0.706
16			Neurokinin 1 receptor	0.706
17			Cysteinyl leukotriene receptor 1	0.706
18			Alpha-1D adrenergic receptor	0.705
19			Cholecystokinin B receptor	0.704
20			Serotonin 1B receptor	0.704

As shown in the Table 1, the V_{1A} receptor was predicted as a top target for dieckol and PFFA. For PFF-A, 5-hydroxytryptophan 1A (5-HT_{1A}R), 5-hydroxytryptophan 1B (5-HT_{1B}R), and cannabinoid 1 (CB_1R) receptors were among the predicted top twenty protein targets. Based on this prediction and reported biological activities of the phlorotannins in the literature, we proceeded to validate adenosine A_{2A} receptor (A_{2A}R), alpha-2A adrenergic receptor (α_{2A}AR), alpha-2C adrenergic receptor (α_{2C}AR), δ-opioid receptor (δ-OPR), CB_1R, free fatty acid receptor 1 (FFA_1R or GPR40), glucagon-like peptide-1 receptor (GLP-1), V_{1A}R, 5-HT_{1A}R, and 5-HT_{1B}R cell-based functional assays.

Firstly, the functional effect of dieckol and PFF-A was screened at a 100-μM concentration. As shown in Table 2, dieckol showed an agonist effect on α_{2C}AR (52.4 ± 4.24%) and V_{1A}R (106.73 ± 2.97%) and an antagonist effect on A_{2A}R (55.55 ± 4.03%), δ-OP (66.95 ± 0.92), CB_1R (158.75 ± 17.81%), and GLP-1R (101.0 ± 8.20%).

Likewise, PFF-A showed an agonist effect on α_{2C}AR (83.8 ± 0.07%) and CB_1R (113.8 ± 3.68%) and an antagonist effect on A_{2A}R (66.6 ± 2.26%), δ-OP (73.55 ± 5.44), and GLP-1R (105.7 ± 1.27%). These phlorotannins were either mild active or inactive at other tested protein targets as depicted by the negative and/or low value of % stimulation or inhibition (Table 2).

Based on the functional effect above 50% at 100 μM, the concentration-dependent effect was further tested and compared with the reference agonists and antagonists (Figures 2 and 3 and Tables 3 and 4) followed by molecular docking simulation. Molecular docking simulation of test ligands to the crystal structures of target proteins and comparison with the reference ligands results revealed the mechanism of ligand–target-protein interaction.

Table 2. Agonist and antagonist effect of 100 μM dieckol and phlorofucofuroeckol-A at several GPCRs.

GPCRs	Functional Effect at 100 μM Concentration			
	Dieckol		Phlorofucofuroeckol-A	
	Agonist Effect	Antagonist Effect	Agonist Effect	Antagonist Effect
Adenosine A2A receptor ($A_{2A}R$)	-0.1 ± 1.41	55.55 ± 4.03	-0.7 ± 0.57	66.6 ± 2.26
Alpha-2A adrenergic receptor ($\alpha_{2A}AR$)	13.4 ± 19.87	46.15 ± 20.15	-0.5 ± 0.85	20.95 ± 1.77
Alpha-2C adrenergic receptor ($\alpha_{2C}AR$)	52.4 ± 4.24	-1.2 ± 6.08	83.8 ± 0.07	19.2 ± 9.76
δ-opioid receptor (δ-OPR)	-5.7 ± 0.14	66.95 ± 0.92	14.7 ± 7.35	73.55 ± 5.44
Cannabinoid receptor 1(CB_1R)	-23.3 ± 12.09	158.75 ± 17.18	113.8 ± 3.68	21.35 ± 0.49
Free fatty acid receptor 1 (FFA1R) (GPR40)	0.2 ± 1.56	22.55 ± 5.44	-1.0 ± 0.07	30.15 ± 0.78
Glucagon-like peptide-1 receptor (GLP-1)	-16.3 ± 1.13	101 ± 8.20	-15.5 ± 2.55	105.7 ± 1.27
Vasopressin 1A receptor ($V_{1A}R$)	106.73 ± 2.97	57.77 ± 0.32 [b]	38.45 ± 7.14 [a]	56.90 ± 5.37 [b]
5-hydroxytryptophan 1A ($5\text{-}HT_{1A}R$)	1.75 ± 0.64 [a]	91.0 ± 3.11	1.65 ± 0.49 [a]	77.00 ± 11.03
5-hydroxytryptophan 1B ($5\text{-}HT_{1B}R$)		-7.3 ± 3.96		-18.5 ± 2.69

[a] Value was extracted from our previous study [22]. [b] The test compound induces at least a 25% agonist effect at this concentration, which results in an apparent inhibition.

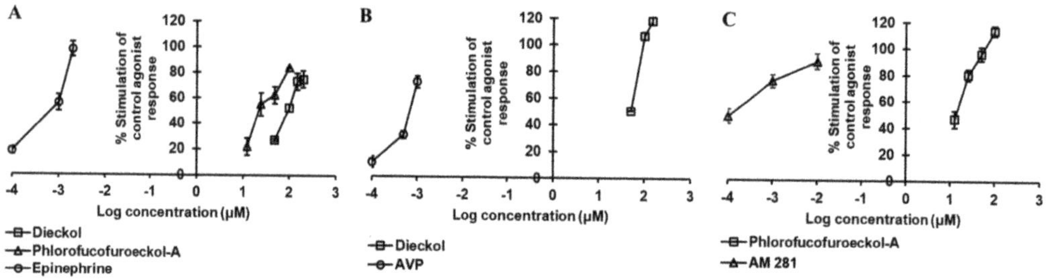

Figure 2. Dose-dependent agonist effect of dieckol and/or phlorofucofuroeckol-A on $h\alpha_{2C}AR$ (**A**), $hV_{1A}R$ (**B**), and hCB_1 (**C**) receptors.

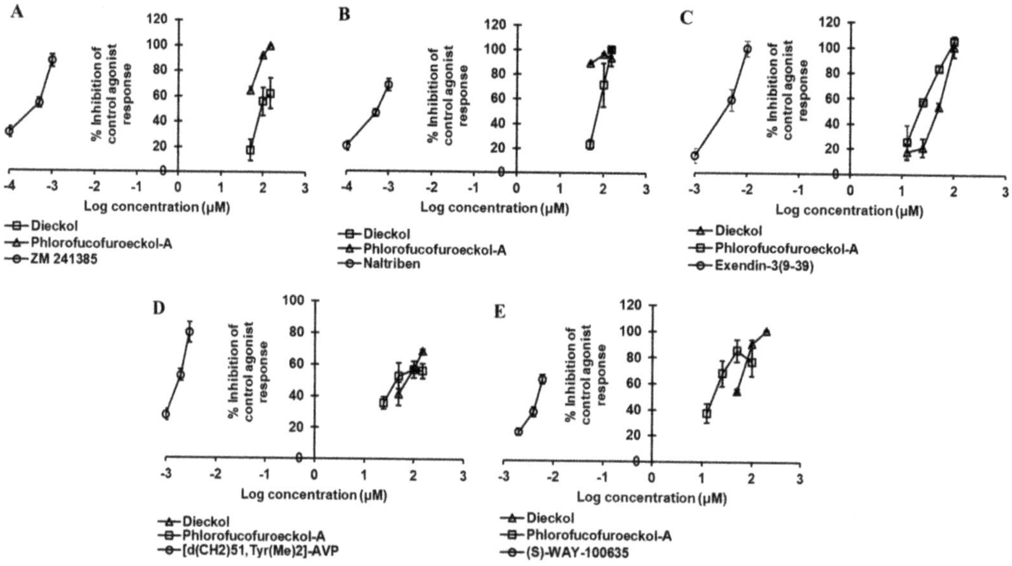

Figure 3. Dose-dependent antagonist effect of dieckol and phlorofucofuroeckol-A against hA_{2A} (**A**), δ-opioid (hδ-OP) (**B**), hGLP-1 (**C**), $hV_{1A}R$ (**D**), and $h5\text{-}HT_{1A}R$ (**E**) receptors.

Table 3. Concentration-dependent agonist effect of dieckol and phlorofucofuroeckol-A at several GPCRs.

Compounds (μM)		Target GPCRs								
		$hA_{2A}R$	$h\alpha_{2A}AR$	$h\alpha_{2C}AR$	hδ-OPR	CB_1R	GPR40	GLP-1	$hV_{1A}R$	$h5\text{-}HT_{1A}R$
Dieckol	12.5	–	–	–	–	–	–	–	–	–
	25	–	–	–	–	–	–	–	–	–
	50	–	–	–	–	–	–	–	50.40 ± 0.42	–
	100	−0.1 ± 1.41	13.4 ± 19.87	52.4 ± 4.24	−5.7 ± 0.14	−23.3 ± 12.09	0.2 ± 1.56	−16.3 ± 1.13	106.73 ± 2.97	1.75 ± 0.64 [c]
	150	–	–	73.0 ± 6.42	–	–	–	–	118.1 ± 2.83	–
	200	–	–	74.77 ± 6.60	–	–	–	–	–	–
EC_{50} (μM) [a]		*NA*	*NA*	98.80 ± 7.71	*NA*	*NA*	*NA*	*NA*	39.12 ± 2.12	*NA*
PFF-A	12.5	–	–	22.03 ± 6.61	–	46.7 ± 6.22	–	–	–	–
	25	–	–	55.0 ± 9.13	–	80.3 ± 4.10	–	–	–	–
	50	–	–	62.27 ± 6.53	–	96.45 ± 5.02	–	–	–	–
	100	−0.7 ± 0.57	−0.5 ± 0.85	83.8 ± 0.07	14.7 ± 7.35	113.8 ± 3.68	−1.0 ± 0.07	−15.5 ± 2.55	38.45 ± 7.14 [c]	1.65 ± 0.49 [c]
	150	–	–	–	–	–	–	–	–	–
	200	–	–	–	–	–	–	–	–	–
EC_{50} (μM) [a]		*NA*	*NA*	23.67 ± 3.32	*NA*	13.42 ± 2.03	*NA*	*NA*	*NA*	*NA*
Reference Drugs, EC_{50} (nM) [b]		9.1	0.74	0.86	4.4	0.21	10000	0.049	0.72	2.5 [c]

[a] The 50% effective concentration (EC_{50}) values of compounds were expressed as mean ± SD, n = 3. [b] EC_{50} values of reference drugs ($hA_{2A}R$: 5′-N-ethylcarboxamidoadenosine (NECA), $h\alpha_{2A}AR$: epinephrine bitartrate, $h\alpha_{2C}AR$: epinephrine, hδ-OPR: DPDPE, CB_1R: CP 55940, GPR40: linoleic acid, GLP−1: GLP-1(7-37), $hV_{1A}R$: AVP, $h5\text{-}HT_{1A}R$: serotonin, $h5\text{-}HT_{1B}R$: serotonin). [c] Value was extracted from our previous study [22]. *NA* No activity. (–) Not tested.

Table 4. Concentration-dependent antagonist effects of dieckol and phlorofucofuroeckol-A at several GPCRs.

Compounds (μM)		Target GPCRs									
		$hA_{2A}R$	$h\alpha_{2A}AR$	$h\alpha_{2C}AR$	hδ-OPR	CB_1R	GPR40	GLP-1	$hV_{1A}R$	$h5\text{-}HT_{1A}R$	$h5\text{-}HT_{1B}R$
Dieckol	12.5	–	–	–	–	–	–	17.87 ± 6.32	–	–	–
	25	–	–	–	–	–	–	21.23 ± 7.31	–	–	–
	50	17.5 ± 8.50	–	–	23.23 ± 4.04	–	–	53.80 ± 3.12	41.53 ± 7.39 [c]	54.7 ± 1.7	–
	100	56.0 ± 11.11	46.15 ± 20.15	−1.20 ± 6.08	71.6 ± 17.85	−1.20 ± 6.08	22.55 ± 5.44	101.0 ± 8.20	57.77 ± 0.32 [c]	91.0 ± 3.11	−7.3 ± 3.96
	150	62.43 ± 12.19	–	–	100.1 ± 1.53	–	–	–	68.80 ± 0.85 [c]	–	–
	200	–	–	–	–	–	–	–	–	100.9 ± 0.57	−8.1 ± 0.85
IC_{50} (μM) [a]		87.18 ± 2.63	*NA*	*NA*	80.46 ± 13.74	*NA*	*NA*	47.19 ± 2.46	82.71 ± 8.73	43.31 ± 3.22	*NA*
PFF-A	12.5	–	–	–	–	–	–	25.63 ± 13.14	–	37.40 ± 2.19	–
	25	–	–	–	–	–	–	57.37 ± 1.15	35.67 ± 3.88	68.20 ± 9.89	–
	50	64.7 ± 2.72	–	–	89.03 ± 0.70	–	–	83.87 ± 2.03	52.80 ± 8.09	85.55 ± 8.41	–
	100	92.2 ± 0.95	20.95 ± 1.77	19.2 ± 9.76	96.47 ± 0.84	21.35 ± 0.49	30.15 ± 0.78	105.7 ± 1.27	56.90 ± 5.37 [c]	77.00 ± 11.03	−18.5 ± 2.69
	150	99.93 ± 0.31	–	–	93.67 ± 6.67	–	–	–	56.07 ± 4.72	–	–
	200	–	–	–	–	–	–	–	–	–	−35.5 ± 4.38
IC_{50} (μM) [a]		< 50	*NA*	*NA*	< 50	*NA*	*NA*	21.56 ± 2.16	42.25 ± 0.41	17.75 ± 3.42	*NA*
Reference Drugs, IC_{50} (nM) [b]		0.41	17	22	9	77	*ND*	4.6	1.9	4.4	23

[a] The 50% inhibition concentration (IC_{50}) values of compounds were expressed as mean ± SD, n = 3. [b] IC_{50} values of reference drugs ($hA_{2A}R$: ZM 241385, $h\alpha_{2A}AR$: RX-821002, $h\alpha_{2C}AR$: rauwolscine, hδ-OPR: naltriben mesylate, CB_1R: AM 281, GLP-1: exendin-3(9–39), $hV_{1A}R$: $[d(CH_2)_5{}^1,Tyr(Me)_2]$-AVP, $h5\text{-}HT_{1A}R$: (S)-WAY-100635, $h5\text{-}HT_{1B}R$: GR55562). [c] The test compound induces at least 25% agonist effect at this concentration, which results in an apparent inhibition. *NA* No activity. (–) Not tested.

2.2. Dieckol and PFF-A as $A_{2A}R$ Antagonists

Dieckol inhibited the 3 nM epinephrine bitartrate response by 17.5%, 56.0%, and 62.43% at a concentration of 50, 100, and 150 μM, respectively, and yielded an IC_{50} value of 87.18 ± 2.63 μM (Table 3 and Figure 3A), while PFF-A inhibited the response of the reference agonist by 64.7%, 92.2%, and 99.93% at a concentration of 50, 100, and 150 μM, yielding an IC_{50} value < 50 μM (Figure 3A).

In the docking simulation, dieckol formed two H-bond interactions with Ile80 and Asp170 (Figure 4B) while four H-bond interactions (His278, Ala59, Ala81, Ser67) were observed for PFF-A (Figure 3C). The binding of reference ligands to the $A_{2A}R$ crystal structure showed the involvement of residues Phe168, Leu249, Asn253, and Met270. The total number of hydrophobic and electrostatic interactions involved in dieckol binding was greater than that of PFF-A binding (Table S2). Interestingly, only one interacting residue (Leu249) was in common with the reference ligand. However, PFF-A had two common interacting residues (Leu249 and Phe168) with reference antagonist ZM241385 (Table S1).

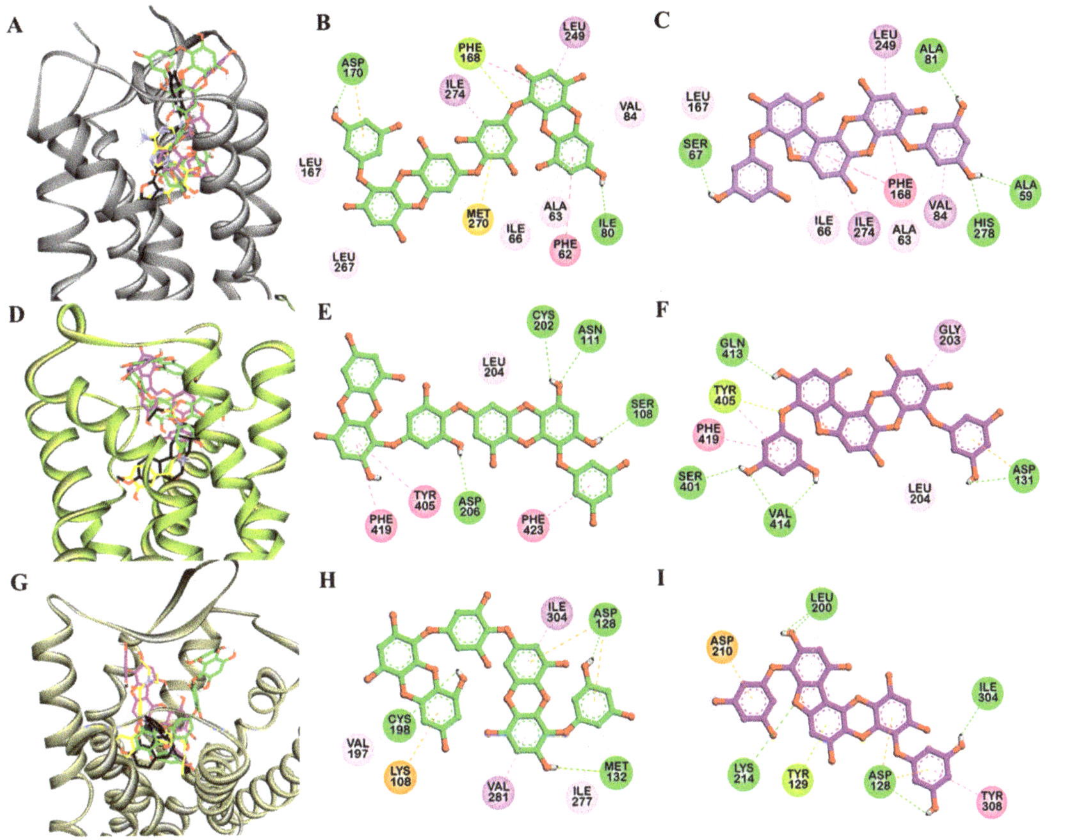

Figure 4. Molecular docking of dieckol and phlorofucofuroeckol-A in the active site of $hA_{2A}R$ (**A**), $h\alpha_{2C}AR$ (**D**), and hδ-OPR (**G**) along with reported agonist (yellow stick) and antagonist (black stick). Detailed $hA_{2A}R$–ligand (**B**) for dieckol and (**C**) for phlorofucofuroeckol-A), $h\alpha_{2C}AR$–ligand (**E**) for dieckol and (**F**) for phlorofucofuroeckol-A), and hδ-OPR–ligand interactions (**H**) for dieckol and (**I**) for phlorofucofuroeckol-A) on a 2D diagram.

2.3. Dieckol and PFF-A as α_{2C}AR Agonists

Evaluation of the concentration-dependent agonist effect of phlorotannins (Table 3 and Figure 2A) at α_{2C}AR depicted dieckol as a moderate agonist (EC$_{50}$: 98.80 ± 7.71 μM) and PFF-A as a good agonist (EC$_{50}$: 23.67 ± 3.32 μM). Even at a 25-μM concentration, PFF-A stimulated the effect of 1 μM epinephrine by 55%. The reference agonist epinephrine had an EC$_{50}$ value of 0.86 nM. To further support the functional effect and delineate the difference in activity between the two phlorotannins, a molecular docking simulation of test ligands and target protein was performed.

As shown in Figure 4D,E, dieckol interacted with Asn111, Ser108, Cys202, Asp206, and Gly203 via H-bond (Figure 2B). Similarly, PFFA also displayed four H-bond interactions with Val414, Asp131, Ser401, and Gln413 (Figure 4F). H-bond interaction with Asp131 was a typical interaction observed for the reference agonist (epinephrine) and PFF-A, but absent in dieckol binding. Between two test ligands, hydrophobic interactions with Phe419, Tyr405, and Leu204 were common (Table S1).

2.4. Dieckol and PFF-A as δ-OPR Antagonists

The dose-dependent antagonist effect at the δ-opioid receptor depicted PFF-A as a potent natural antagonist. As shown in Table 4 and Figure 3B, even at the 50-μM concentration, PFF-A inhibited the effect of 25 nM [D—Pen2, D—Pen5]enkephalin (DPDPE) by 89.03 ± 0.70%, while the effect was 23.23 ± 4.04% for the same concentration of dieckol. Dieckol had an IC$_{50}$ value of 80.46 ± 13.74 μM, but the value was <50 μM for PFF-A. The reference antagonist naltriben mesylate had an IC$_{50}$ value of 9 nM. The binding of dieckol to the crystal structure of 4ej4 (Figure 4G,H) showed an involvement of three H-bond interactions (Asp128, Met132, Cys198) and numerous hydrophobic and electrostatic interactions (Met132 (Sulfur-O, π-alkyl), Lys108 (π-cation, π-Alkyl), Asp128 (π-anion), Val281 (π-sigma), Ile304 (π-sigma), Cys198 (π-sulfur), Ile277 (π-alkyl), and Val197 (π-alkyl)). Likewise, as shown in Figure 4I, PFF-A formed four H-bond interactions with Leu200, Lys214, Ile304, and Asp128 and five hydrophobic and electrostatic interactions with Asp128 (π-anion), Asp210 (π-Anion), Tyr129 (π-lone pair), Tyr308 (π-π stacked), and Leu200 (π-alkyl).

The reference antagonist naltrindole showed an H-bond interaction with aspartic acid residue (Asp128) and numerous hydrophobic interactions with tryptophan residues - Trp284 (π-π-T-shaped), Trp284 (π-alkyl), and Trp274 (π-alkyl). Only Asp128 was a common interacting residue among the test and reference ligands while Tyr308 was observed for PFF-A and reference ligand binding, but not for dieckol (Tables S1 and S2).

2.5. PFF-A as a CB$_1$R Agonist

Only PFF-A showed a full CB$_1$R agonist effect (113.8 ± 3.68%) at the 100-μM concentration. Therefore, the effect at lower concentrations was tested and, as shown in Table 3 and Figure 2C, PFF-A stimulated the effect of 10 nM CP 55940 by 46.7, 80.3, and 96.45% at 12.5, 25, and 50 μM, respectively. Hence, the log concentration vs. % simulation graph yielded an EC$_{50}$ value of 13.42 ± 2.03 μM. Reference agonist CP 55940 had an EC$_{50}$ value of 0.21 nM. To predict the binding affinity and characterize the binding mode of PFF-A and CB$_1$R, molecular docking simulation was performed (Figure 5A). As tabulated in Tables S3 and S4, PFF-A interacted with the active-state CB$_1$R (6kqi) by forming three H-bonds (Ser173, His178, and Met363) and numerous hydrophobic interactions—Phe177, Phe268, Trp279, Val196, Leu193, and Met363. Interactions with Ser173, Phe268, Phe177, Trp279, Val196, and Leu193 are a common observation in the binding of PFF-A and CP 55940 with the active-state CB$_1$R (6kqi). The reference antagonist taranabant interacted with the inactive-state CB$_1$R (5u09) by forming hydrogen-bond interactions with Ser173, Phe189, and Lys192 via the $-CF_3$ group. Likewise, other hydrophobic interactions involved in taranabant–5u09 binding were phenylalanine residues (Phe170, Phe174, Phe189, Phe268, and Phe379), Trp279, His178, Leu192, Leu193, Ile267, and Met363 (Figure 5B).

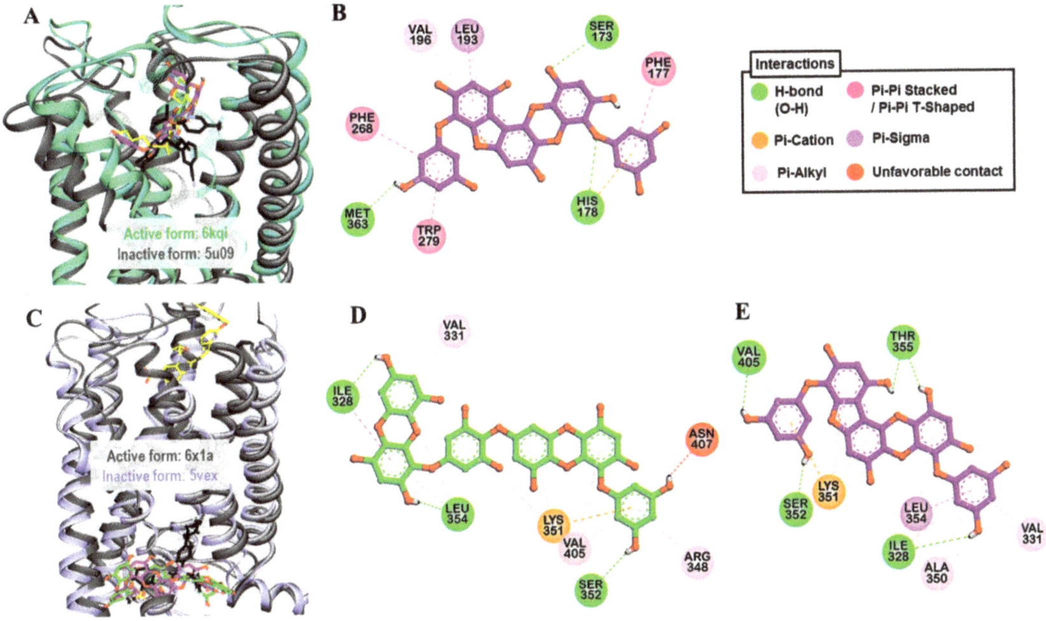

Figure 5. (**A**) Molecular docking of phlorofucofuroeckol-A (purple stick) in an active-state of *h*CB_1R (PDB ID: 6kqi) along with reported agonist (yellow stick). Structure of reported antagonist taranabant docked into the inactive state of *h*CB_1R (PDB ID: 5u09, gray ribbon) is shown as black stick. (**B**) Detailed *h*CB_1R–ligand interactions on a 2D diagram for phlorofucofuroeckol-A. (**C**) Molecular docking of dieckol (green stick) and phlorofucofuroeckol-A (purple stick) in an inactive-state of *h*GLP-1 (PDB ID: 5vex, blue ribbon) along with reported antagonist, NNC0640 (black stick). Structure of reported agonist PF-06882961 docked into the active-state of *h*GLP-1 (PDB ID: 6x1a, gray ribbon) is shown as yellow stick. (**B**,**C**) Detailed *h*GLP-1–ligand interactions on a 2D diagram (**D**) for dieckol and (**E**) for phlorofucofuroeckol-A.

2.6. Dieckol and PFF-A as GLP-1R Antagonists

Results from the functional assay on mouse GLP-1 receptor-expressed βTC6 cells demonstrated dieckol and PFF-A as full antagonists of the GLP-1 receptor. At a concentration of 100 μM, both the compounds inhibited the effect of 0.3 nM GLP-1(7–37) by 100%. However, at the 25-μM concentration, PFF-A inhibited the reference agonist-response by 57.37% and dieckol by 21.23%. Additionally, a dose-dependent response curve yielded IC_{50} values of 47.19 ± 2.46 and 21.56 ± 2.16 μM for dieckol and PFF-A, respectively (Table 4 and Figure 3C). The potency of PFF-A was two-fold higher than that of dieckol. The reference antagonist exendin-3(9–39) had an IC_{50} value of 4.6 nM. From the molecular docking study, hydrogen-bond interactions with Ser352 and Thr355 (Table S3) and hydrophobic interactions with Leu354, Lys351, and Val405 (Table S4) were common observations in test ligands and reference antagonist NNC0640 binding with an inactive-state GLP-1R (5vex) (Figure 5C–E) in our molecular docking simulation. An unfavorable contact between dieckol and GLP-1R receptor was observed via the Asn407 residue.

2.7. Dieckol as Agonist and PFF-A as Antagonist of hV_{1A}R

The agonist effect of dieckol at V_{1A}R was first tested at 100 μM to compare with the effect of PFF-A that we reported earlier [22]. As tabulated in Table 2, dieckol at 100-μM concentration stimulated the percentage agonist effect of 1 μM arginine vasopressin (AVP) by 106.73 ± 2.97% and inhibited the percentage of control agonist response by 57.77 ± 0.32%. In the hV_{1A}R antagonist assay, the 100-μM concentration of dieckol induced at least a 25% agonist effect. In comparison, PFF-A induced a 38.45 ± 7.14% stimulation and 56.90 ± 5.37% inhibition of the control agonist response at 100 μM. Furthermore, the concentration-dependent dose–response curve depicted dieckol as a $hV_{1A}R$ agonist (EC_{50}: 39.12 ± 2.12 μM) (Table 3 and Figure 2B) and PFF-A as an antagonist (IC_{50}: 42.25 ± 0.41 μM) (Table 4 and Figure 3D).

Molecular simulation of dieckol and PFF-A along with reference ligands to a crystal structure of $hV_{1A}R$ predicted that both test ligands bind with high affinity (Figure 6A). Dieckol formed H-bond interactions with Gln131, Ala334, and Asp112, and hydrophobic interactions with Lys128, Met135, Trp204, Ala101, and Ala334 (Figure 6B). Reference agonist AVP formed H-bond interactions with Asp202 (Salt-bridge), Glu54, Asp112, and Ile330 and hydrophobic interactions with Trp204, Ile330, Ala101, Ala334, Val132, and Met135. This shows that dieckol and AVP have numerous residues in common that involve binding with the receptor.

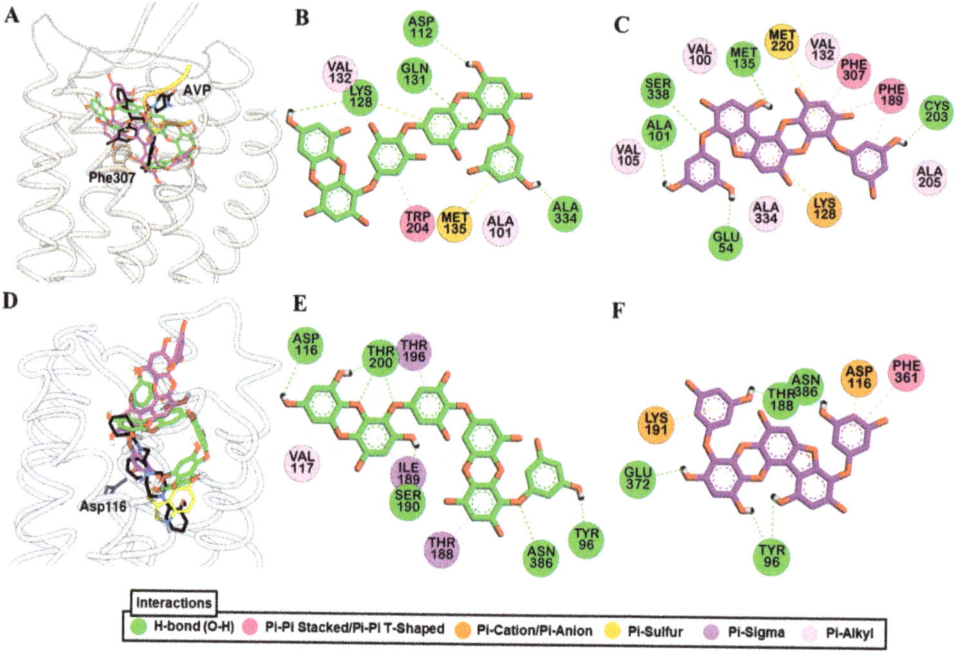

Figure 6. Molecular docking simulation of $hV_{1A}R$ (**A**) and $h5\text{-}HT_{1A}R$ (**D**) binding with dieckol (green stick) and phlorofucofuroeckol-A (purple stick) along with reported agonist (yellow ribbon or stick) and antagonist (black stick). Detailed $hV_{1A}R$–ligand (**B**) for dieckol and (**C**) for phlorofucofuroeckol-A) and $h5\text{-}HT_{1A}R$–ligand interactions (**E**) for dieckol and (**F**) for phlorofucofuroeckol-A) on a 2D diagram.

Likewise, PFF-A bound to the $hV_{1A}R$ via five H-bond interactions (Ser338, Cys203, Met135, Glu54, Ala101) and other hydrophobic interactions with Lys128, Met220, Phe189, Phe307, Val132, Val100, Ala101, Met135, Ala334, Ala205, and Val105 (Figure 6C). Three H-bond interactions with Gln131, Gln108, and Lys128, and hydrophobic interactions with Phe307, Trp204, Val132, Met135, Met220, Ala334, Ala205, Gln131, and Thr333 were observed for SR49059 binding. The docking result shows that, respective to their functional effect, dieckol and PFF-A interact with residues that were involved in the binding of the reference agonist and antagonist (Tables S5 and S6).

2.8. Dieckol and PFF-A as 5-$HT_{1A}R$ Antagonists

An antagonist effect was observed for dieckol and PFF-A in a cell-based functional assay. At 100-μM concentration, dieckol and PFF-A inhibited the response of 30 nM serotonin by 91.0 ± 3.11% and 77.00 ± 11.03%, respectively (Table 2). A concentration-dependent dose–response showed that dieckol and PFF-A inhibited the 50% response of 30 nM serotonin at 43.31 ± 3.22 and 17.75 ± 3.42 μM, respectively (Table 4 and Figure 3E). However, the agonist effect at 5-HT_{1A}R was negligible for both the compounds when tested at the 100-μM concentration. As a result, the EC_{50} value was not determined. Reference drug serotonin had an EC_{50} value of 0.72 nM and antagonist GR55562 had an IC_{50} value of 4.4 nM.

Docking of test and reference ligands to the active site of 5-HT_{1A}R demonstrated that aspartic acid residue Asp116 is one of the important binding residues (Figure 6D). Dieckol formed an H-bond interaction with Asp116, Thr200, Ser190, Asn386, and Tyr96 while PFF-A did with Thr188, Glu372, Tyr96, and Asn386 (Figure 6E,F). Reference ligands serotonin and WAY 100635 formed an H-bond interaction with Asp116 via a salt-bridge. Interactions with Thr200, Phe361, and Val117 were observed for test ligands and serotonin binding (Tables S5 and S6).

3. Discussion

Dieckol and PFF-A are phloroglucinol (1,3,5-trihydroxybenzene)-based polyphenols with a varied number of phloroglucinol units attached via dibenzofuran and dibenzodioxin linkages. Dieckol is a phloroglucinol hexamer and PFF-A is a phloroglucinol pentamer. A structure–activity relationship between phloroglucinol and its oligomers in our recent study [22] showed that more than three repeating phloroglucinol units are necessary for hMAOs inhibition and D_3/D_4 receptor agonist effect. Likewise, oligomerization of phloroglucinol with more than five repeating units is essential for the antagonist effect at D_1, NK_1, and 5-HT_{1A} receptors. Here, although the monomer phloroglucinol is not included in the study, the pentamer (PFF-A) showed better activity than a hexamer (dieckol). An interesting observation in this study is that regardless of the receptors at which these two phlorotannins showed functional effects (except the hV_{1A}R), PFF-A was two-fold more potent than dieckol. In contrary to the findings that the phenolic -OH groups attached to the benzene ring of polyphenols play a vital role in the antioxidant effect [24–26] and that an increase in the number of hydroxyl groups increases antioxidant activity, the functional effect of PFF-A at tested GPCRs was higher than that of dieckol despite having a lower number of hydroxyl groups. The possible reason underlying this might be the structure or orientation of PFF-A that enables it to reach the core active site cavity of receptors where it binds to conserved interacting residues leading to conformational change.

Adenosine is an endogenous autacoid that regulates cellular physiology via adenosine A_1, A_{2A}, A_{2B}, and A_3 receptors. These receptors are expressed in several cells and tissues throughout the body and play a crucial role in regulating the pathophysiology of the human body, suggesting a potential drug target. Of different adenosine receptor subtypes, A_{2A}R is the main receptor subtype in the striatum colocalized with dopamine D_2 receptor and it modulates motor function [27,28]. Activation of A_{2A}R decreases the binding affinity of D_2R for agonists, implying A_{2A}R antagonists as novel therapeutics for Parkinson's disease [29]. At the synapse, A_{2A}R facilitates glutamate release and potentiates NMDA receptor effects. It also stimulates glutamate release in astrocytes by inhibiting glutamate transporter-1 (GLT-1), and the level of A_{2A}Rs in neurons and glia is significantly high in depression and Schizophrenia [30]. Hence, A_{2A}Rs antagonists are effective as antidepressants and anti-anxiety agents. Here, dieckol and PFF-A showed an antagonist effect at hA_{2A}R with IC_{50} values of 87.18 ± 2.63 and <50 μM, respectively. Furthermore, molecular docking simulation showed that dieckol and phlorofucofuroeckol-A strongly interact with the Phe168 residue, which is known as one of the important residues for ligand binding, via pi–pi interaction [31]. Structurally, dieckol and PFF-A are powerful radical scavengers [32] and as such, dieckol, in a recent study [33], protected dopaminergic neuronal cells by preventing α-synuclein aggregation via antioxidant mechanism. In a previous study [34], dieckol suppressed LPS-induced excessive microglial activation and protected neuronal cells by downregulating extracellular signal-regulated kinases, protein kinase B (PKB/Akt), and nicotinamide adenine dinucleotide phosphate hydrogen (NADPH) oxidase-mediated pathways. Likewise, PFF-A inhibited glutamate-induced apoptotic PC12 cell death in a caspase-dependent manner [35].

Similarly, at α_{2C}AR, PFF-A showed a strong agonist effect and formed an H-bond with the Asp131 of α_{2C}AR, which is the conserved active site residue. Adrenergic receptors are targets for epinephrine and norepinephrine and are involved in maintaining homeostasis. Among several types of adrenergic receptors, highly expressed α_2 adrenoreceptors in astrocytes, and in glutamatergic and GABAergic neurons act by increasing intracellular Ca^{2+} levels [36]. The α_{2C}AR subtype mediates cold-induced vasoconstriction, inhibits dopamine release in basal ganglia [37], and serotonin in the mouse hippocampus [38]. Therefore, α_{2C}AR selective ligands have a therapeutic role in neuropsychiatric disorders [38] and α_{2C}AR agonists are implicated in the treatment of neuropathic pain [39–41].

Serotonin (5-hydroxytryptamine, 5-HT) is a monoamine neurotransmitter that plays a crucial role in physiological functions, and of a total of 14 subtypes of 5-HT receptors, the 5-HT_{1A} receptor is a prominent target for the treatment of various neuropsychiatric and neurological disorders, prominently depression [42]. In the functional assay, dieckol and PFF-A showed a good antagonist effect at 5-HT_{1A}R. Furthermore, they interacted with conserved aspartate residue (Asp116) of 5-HT_{1A}R via H-bond and pi–anion binding, respectively.

Vasopressin is an antidiuretic hormone that plays a vital role in the central nervous system (CNS) and peripheral nervous system (PNS). The vasopressin receptor is one of the promising targets for CNS drugs, and vasopressin antagonists represent a novel approach for the treatment of stress, mood, and behavioral disorders [43]. Likewise, as a peripheral role, V_{1A}R is responsible for vasoconstriction, myocardial contractility, platelet aggregation, and uterine contraction [44]. Similarly, in a recent study [45], upregulated vasopressin 1 receptor (V_1R) expression in hepatocytes of ischemia-reperfusion injury mouse model was identified and the V_1R/Wnt/β-catenin/FoxO3a/Akt pathway was highlighted as vital for hepatoprotection.

Cannabinoid CB_1 receptors are among the most abundant GPCRs in the brain and they modulate CNS activity [46]. Cannabinoid CB_1 receptor agonist activation of the CB_1 receptor leads to decreased levels in cellular cAMP via inhibition of adenylyl cyclase. Moreover, CB_1 activation inhibits voltage-gated Ca^{2+} channels and activates K^+ channels, and these overall intracellular signaling activities reduce cellular excitability [47]. Likewise, studies also indicate high expression levels of CB_1R in various types of cancer [48,49]. Interestingly, a new study demonstrated a higher orexigenic effect of the CB_1R agonist AM11101 than tetrahydrocannabinol [50]. This shows that CB_1R agonists could be used as an appetite stimulant in underweight patients. In the present study, only PFF-A showed a promising agonist effect at CB_1R with an EC_{50} of 13.42 ± 2.03 μM. Several reports on PFF-A show neuroprotective effects mainly via antioxidant mechanisms [14,35,51]. Likewise, a recent study suggested the ATF3-mediated pathway as a possible mechanism of PFF-A-induced apoptosis in human colorectal cancer cells [52]. However, it remains unclear whether the neuroprotective and anticancer effect of PFF-A is via CB_1R agonist activity.

The human CB_1 receptor is an important therapeutic target for obesity and obsessive disorders and the mechanism of its transition state (either active or inactive) is vital for understanding the regulatory action of the receptor [53]. A salt bridge between conserved Asp-Arg-Tyr (DRY) motif in the C-terminal region of transmembrane 3 (TM3) and transmembrane 6 (TM6) characterizes the active or inactive conformation of the rhodopsin-like GPCRs [54]. In an inactive conformation of CB_1R, TM6 packs against TM3 and transmembrane 5 (TM5) and G protein-interacting residues—Phe200 (helix III) and Trp356 (helix VI) are obstructed [55]. The reference inverse agonist (taranabant) is bound to the inactive state crystal structure by forming an H-bond interaction between the NH of taranabant and the hydroxyl of Ser383 and the $-CF_3$ group with Ser173, Phe189, and Lys192. This result corroborates the findings of a previous study [56] which concluded that a strong H-bond between the -NH group of taranabant and the hydroxyl of Ser383 was vital for superior affinity to CB_1R. Likewise, the agonist CP55940 formed π–π interactions with Phe170 and Phe268, and two H-bond interactions with Ser173 and Ser383 in a similar fashion, as reported earlier [56]. PFFA also formed a stable pi–pi interaction with Phe268 and an H-bond interaction with Ser173 of the active state crystal structure (6kqi), which could explain the agonist potency of PFFA in vitro.

Among the tested protein targets, CB_1R, GLP-1, and GPR40 are obesity/T2DM related GPCRs and in the functional assays, PFF-A showed a good agonist effect at CB_1R, while both the dieckol and PFF-A showed an antagonist effect at the GLP-1 receptor. Their effect at GPR40 was mild agonist. A gut-derived incretin hormone GLP-1 stimulates insulin and suppresses glucagon secretion, inhibits gastric emptying, and reduces appetite and food intake. In a previous study, intracerebroventricular injection of exendin (9–39), a specific GLP-1 antagonist, blocked the inhibitory effect of GLP-1 on food intake [57]. Hence, GLP-1 agonists represent a new class of antidiabetic agents [58]. In a recent study on the anti-diabetic effect in the zebrafish model [59], dieckol treatment reduced liver glucose-6-phosphate and phosphoenolpyruvate carboxykinase, and enhanced glucose transport and insulin sensitivity via protein kinase B (Akt) phosphorylation. It is of note that dieckol and PFF-A showed a good antagonist effect at GLP-1. Thus, the in vivo effects of these phlorotannins in GLP-1-mediated signaling are urgent.

In conclusion, the present study characterizes the receptors $hA_{2A}R$, $h\alpha_{2C}AR$, hδ-OP, CB_1R, GLP-1, $hV_{1A}R$, and h5-$HT_{1A}R$ as prime protein targets of dieckol and PFF-A. Moreover, the binding mechanism of test ligands with the target proteins strengthens the study and warrants further in vivo studies.

4. Materials and Methods

4.1. Chemicals and Reagents

A transfected Chinese hamster ovary (CHO), Hela, a murine interleukin-3 dependent pro-B (Ba/F3), PC12, and rat basophil leukemia cell lines were obtained from Eurofins Scientific (Eurofins-Cerep, Le Bois I'Eveque, France). Buffers—Dulbecco's modified Eagle medium (DMEM) buffer, 4-(2-hydroxyethyl)-1-piperazineethanesulfonic acid (HEPES) buffer, and Hank's balanced salt solution (HBSS) buffer—were purchased from Invitrogen (Carlsbad, CA, USA). The reference agonists: 5′-*N*-ethylcarboxamidoadenosine (NECA), epinephrine bitartrate, epinephrine, DPDPE, CP 55940, linoleic acid, GLP-1(7–37, arginine vasopressin (AVP), and serotonin, and antagonists: ZM 241385, RX-821002, rauwolscine, naltriben mesylate, AM 281, exendin-3(9–39), $[d(CH_2)_5^1$, Tyr $(Me)_2]$-AVP, (S)-WAY-100635, and GR55562) were obtained from Sigma-Aldrich (St. Louis, MO, USA). All other chemicals and reagents purchased from Merck and Fluka were of the highest available grade unless otherwise stated.

4.2. Isolation of Phlorotannins

Phlorotannins—dieckol and PFF-A were isolated from the ethyl acetate fraction of *E. stolonifera* ethanolic extract, as described previously [11,22].

4.3. In Silico Prediction of Targets

To predict potential protein targets for the phlorotannins, a proteocheminformatics modeling (PCM) in silico target prediction method was employed, as described recently [60]. For full information on the model, readers are further directed to a previous report [61].

4.4. Functional GPCR Assay

The functional assay using transfected cells expressing human cloned receptors, PC12 cells for adenosine A_{2A} receptor, rat basophil leukemia cells for human adrenergic alpha2A receptor, human delta opioid (δ-OP) receptor, CHO cells for adrenergic $alpha_{2C}$ receptor, human cannabinoid CB_1, and vasopressin ($V_{1A}R$), human embryonic kidney 293 (HEK-293) cells for free fatty acid receptor 1 (FFA_1R or GPR40), βTC6 cells for the glucagon-like peptide-1 receptor (GLP-1), Ba/F3 cells for serotonin (5-HT_{1A}), and Hela for 5-HT_{1B} receptors were carried out at Eurofins laboratory (Eurofins-Cerep, Le Bois I'Eveque, France).

The in-house assay protocol and experimental conditions are reported in our previous reports [15,22,62]. The functional effect of dieckol and PFF-A was characterized based on their modulation effect on cytosolic Ca^{2+} ion mobilization using a fluorimetric detection method or by measuring their effect on cAMP modulation using homogeneous time-resolved fluorescence (HTRF) detection.

4.5. *Measurement of cAMP Level*

Functional activity of phlorotannins over $hA_{2A}R$, $h\alpha_{2C}AR$, hCB_1R, GLP-1R, and $h5\text{-}HT_{1B}R$ was determined by measuring their effects on cAMP production by the HTRF detection method using transected cells expressing human cloned receptors.

4.5.1. Functional Activity over $hA_{2A}R$

In brief, the PC12 cells were suspended in HBSS buffer (Invitrogen) complemented with 20 mM HEPES (pH 7.4), 0.2 U/mL ADA, and 100 μM rolipram, then distributed in microplates at a density of 2.10^3 cells/well and preincubated for 5 min at room temperature (RT) in the presence of HBSS (basal control), the test compound, or the reference agonist or antagonist. For stimulated control measurement, separate assay wells contained 3 μM NECA. Following 10 min incubation at RT, the cells were lysed and the fluorescence acceptor (D2-labeled cAMP) and fluorescence donor (anti-cAMP antibody labeled with europium cryptate) were added. After 60 min at RT, the fluorescence transfer was measured at λex = 337 nm and λem = 620 and 665 nm using an EnVision microplate reader EnSpire (PerkinElmer, Waltham, MA, USA). The cAMP concentration was determined by dividing the signal measured at 665 nm by that measured at 620 nm (ratio). Agonist result was expressed as a percent of the control response to 3 μM NECA while the antagonist effect as percent inhibition of the control response to 100 nM NECA. The standard reference agonist was NECA and the antagonist was ZM 241385, which were tested in each experiment at several concentrations to generate a concentration–response curve from which their EC_{50} and IC_{50} values were calculated.

4.5.2. Functional Activity over $h\alpha_{2C}AR$

Briefly, the transfected CHO cells suspended in HBSS buffer (Invitrogen) complemented with 20 mM HEPES (pH 7.4) and 500 μM IBMX were distributed in microplates at a density of 10^4 cells/well in the presence of either of the following: For agonist assay—HBSS (basal control), epinephrine 1 μM (stimulated control) or various concentrations (EC_{50} determination), or the test compounds. For antagonist assay—HBSS (stimulated controls), rauwolscine 10 μM (basal control) or various concentrations (IC_{50} determination), or the test compounds. The reference agonist epinephrine and the adenylyl cyclase activator NKH 477 were added at respective final concentrations of 100 nM and 5 μM. For basal control measurements, epinephrine was omitted from the wells containing 3 μM rauwolscine. After 10 min at 37 °C, the cells were lysed and the fluorescence acceptor (D2-labeled cAMP) and fluorescence donor (anti-cAMP antibody labeled with europium cryptate) were added. After 60 min at RT, the fluorescence transfer was measured at λex = 337 nm and λem = 620 and 665 nm using a microplate reader (Envision, Perkin Elmer). The concentration of cAMP was determined by dividing the measured signal at 665 nm by that measured at 620 nm (ratio). The agonist result are shown as a percent of the control response to 1 μM epinephrine and the antagonist result are expressed as a percent inhibition of the control response to 30 nM epinephrine. Epinephrine and rauwolscine were the standard reference drugs used in each experiment at different concentrations.

4.5.3. Functional Activity over hCB_1R

The transfected CHO cells were suspended in HBSS buffer (Invitrogen) complemented with 20 mM HEPES (pH 7.4). Then, the cells were distributed in microplates at a density of 5.10^3 cells/well in the presence of either of the following: For agonist assay—HBSS (basal control), 30 nM CP 55940 (stimulated control) or various concentrations (EC_{50}

determination), or the test compounds. For antagonist assay—HBSS (stimulated controls), 10 μM AM 281 (basal control) or various concentrations for IC_{50} determination, or the test compounds. Thereafter, the reference agonist CP 55940 and the adenylyl cyclase activator forskolin were added at respective final concentrations of 1 nM and 25 μM. For basal control measurements, CP 55940 was excluded from the wells containing 10 μM AM 281. After 30 min of incubation at 37 °C, the cells were lysed and the fluorescence acceptor (D2-labeled cAMP) and fluorescence donor (anti-cAMP antibody labeled with europium cryptate) were added. The fluorescence transfer was measured at λex = 337 nm and λem = 620 and 665 nm using an Envision microplate reader (PerkinElmer, Waltham, MA, USA) after 60 min at RT. The agonist results are expressed as a percent of the control response to 10 nM CP 55940 and the antagonist results are expressed as percent inhibition of the control response to 1 nM CP 55940. CP 55940 and AM 281 were standard reference drugs that were tested in each experiment.

4.5.4. Functional Activity over GLP-1R

The HBSS buffer (Invitrogen) complemented with 20 mM HEPES (pH 7.4) and 500 μM IBMX was used to suspend and distribute the βTC6 cells at a density of $1.5x10^4$ cells/well. The plate was then incubated for 10 min at RT in the presence of HBSS (basal and stimulated control), the test compound, or the reference agonist and antagonist. In the agonist assay, separate assay wells containing 100 nM GLP-1(7–37) were prepared for the stimulated control measurement, while in the antagonist assay, the reference agonist GLP-1(7–37) was added at a final concentration of 0.3 nM, and separate assay wells contained HBSS for basal control measurements. Following incubation, the cells were lysed and the fluorescence acceptor (D2-labeled cAMP) and fluorescence donor (anti-cAMP antibody labeled with europium cryptate) were added. After 60 min at room temperature, the fluorescence transfer was measured at λex = 337 nm and λem = 620 nm and 665 nm using an Envision microplate reader (PerkinElmer, Waltham, MA, USA). The results are expressed as either a percent of the control response to 100 nM GLP-1(7–37) or a percent inhibition of the control response to 0.3 nM GLP-1(7–37). The standard reference agonist was GLP-1(7–37) and the antagonist was exendin-3(9–39).

4.5.5. Functional Activity over 5-HT_{1B}R

Concisely, a plasmid containing the GPCR gene of interest (5-HT_{1B}) was transfected into Hela cells. The resulting stable transfectants were suspended in HBSS buffer (Invitrogen, Carlsbad, CA, USA) containing 20 mM HEPES (pH 7.4), 400 mM NaCl, 1 mg/mL glucose, and 500 μM IBMX and distributed in microplates at a density of 2×10^4 cells/well. The plates were then incubated for 20 min at RT in the presence of either of the following: HBSS and 0.1% BSA (basal control), serotonin at 10 μM (stimulated control) or various concentrations for EC_{50} determination, or the test phlorotannins. Thereafter, the adenylyl cyclase activator NKH 477 (5 μM) was added and the plates were incubated at 37 °C for 20 min. Then, the cells were lysed and a fluorescence acceptor (D2-labeled cAMP) and fluorescence donor (anti-cAMP antibody with europium cryptate) were added following 60 min incubation at RT. After incubation, the fluorescence transfer was measured using an Envision microplate reader (PerkinElmer, Waltham, MA, USA) and the results are expressed as a percentage of the control response to 10 μM serotonin for the agonist effect and as percent inhibition of the control response to 100 nM serotonin.

4.6. *Measurement of Intracellular [Ca^{2+}] Level*

Functional activity of phlorotannins over human adrenergic α2A (hα_{2A}), human δ-opioid (hδ-OP), free fatty acid receptor 1 (FFA_1R/GPR40), human vasopressin 1A (hV_{1A}), and human serotonin 1A (h5-HT_{1A}) receptors was assessed by measuring their effect on cytosolic Ca^{2+} ion mobilization at the transected cells expressing human cloned receptors using a fluorimetric detection method.

4.6.1. Functional Activity over hα_{2A}AR

The rat basophil leukemia cells were distributed in microplates at a density of 1.1 × 10^4 cells/well after suspending in a HBSS buffer (Invitrogen) containing 20 mM HEPES. Then, the fluorescent probe (Fluo8, AAT Bioquest) mixed with probenecid in HBSS buffer (Invitrogen) complemented with 20 mM Hepes (Millipore) (pH 7.4) was added into each well incubated for 60 min at 30 °C. Thereafter, the assay plates were positioned in a microplate reader (FlipR Tetra, Molecular Device) and we added test compounds, reference agonist/antagonist or HBSS buffer (basal control). Change in fluorescence intensity which varies proportionally to the free cytosolic Ca^{2+} ion concentration was measured. For stimulated control measurements, separate assay wells containing 0.1 µM epinephrine bitartrate were prepared. The agonist effect was calculated as a % of control response to epinephrine bitartrate at 0.1 µM. Similarly, for the antagonist effect, % inhibition of the control response to epinephrine bitartrate at 3 nM was evaluated. Epinephrine bitartrate and RX-821002 were used as reference agonists and antagonists, respectively.

4.6.2. Functional Activity over hδ-OPR

At first, rat basophil leukemia cells were suspended in HBSS buffer (Invitrogen) complemented with 20 mM HEPES, and distributed in microplates at a density of 2.768 × 10^4 cells/well. Thereafter, a mixture of fluorescent probe (Fluo8, AAT Bioquest) and probenecid in HBSS buffer (Invitrogen) complemented with 20 mM Hepes (Millipore) (pH 7.4) was added and plates were incubated for 60 min at 30 °C. Then, the assay plates were positioned in a FlipR Tetra microplate reader (Molecular Device, San Jose, CA, USA) for the addition of the test compound, reference agonist/antagonist, or HBSS buffer (basal control). Change in fluorescence intensity that varies proportionally to the free cytosolic Ca^{2+} ion concentration was measured.

For stimulated control measurements, 1 µM DPDPE was added in separate assay wells. The results are expressed as a percent of the control response to DPDPE at 1 µM or a percent inhibition of the control response to DPDPE at 25 nM. The standard reference agonist and antagonist were DPDPE and naltriben mesylate, respectively.

4.6.3. Functional Activity over FFA_1R/GPR40

In general, transfected HEK-293 cells suspended in DMEM buffer (Invitrogen) containing 1% FCSd were distributed in microplates at a density of 2.10^4 cells/well. Then, the mixture of fluorescent probe (Fluo4 Direct, Invitrogen) and probenecid in HBSS buffer (Invitrogen) complemented with 20 mM Hepes (Invitrogen) (pH 7.4) was added into each well and incubated for 60 min at 37 °C, followed by 15 min incubation at 22 °C. Thereafter, the assay plates were positioned in a CellLux microplate reader (PerkinElmer, Waltham, MA, USA) which was used for the addition of the following: For agonist assay—test compound, reference agonist, or HBSS buffer (basal control). Linoleic acid at 100 µM was added in separate assay wells for stimulated control measurement. For antagonist assay—test compound or HBSS buffer (basal and stimulated control), then, 5 min later, 20 µM linoleic acid. Agonist results are expressed as a percent of the control response to 100 µM linoleic acid while antagonist results are expressed as percent inhibition of the control response to 20 µM linoleic acid.

4.6.4. Functional Activity over hV_{1A}R

Briefly, CHO-V_{1A}R cells were separately suspended in DMEM buffer (Invitrogen, Carlsbad, CA, USA) complemented with 0.1% FCSd and distributed into microplates (4.5× 10^4 cells/well). Then, fluorescent probe (Fluo4, Invitrogen) mixed with probenecid in HBSS buffer (Invitrogen, Carlsbad, CA, USA) supplemented with 20 mM HEPES, pH 7.4 (Invitrogen) was added to each well, allowing to equilibrate with the cells for 60 min at 37 °C, then 15 min at 22 °C. Thereafter, the assay plates were positioned in a CellLux microplate reader (PerkinElmer, Waltham, MA, USA) and dieckol and PFF-A (12.5, 25, 50, 100, and/or 150 µM), reference agonist, or HBSS buffer (basal control) was added. For stimulated control measurements, AVP at 1 μM was added in separate assay wells. The agonist effect on $V_{1A}R$ was calculated as a % of control response to 1 μM AVP. Similarly, for the antagonist effect, % inhibition of the control response to 10 nM AVP was evaluated. AVP and [d(CH_2)$_5$^{1}, Tyr (Me)$_2$]-AVP were used as reference agonist and antagonist, respectively.

4.6.5. Functional Activity over h5-$HT_{1A}R$

In brief, Ba/F3-5$HT_{1A}R$ cells were first suspended in HBSS buffer (Invitrogen, Carlsbad, CA, USA) complemented with 20 mM HEPES buffer (pH 7.4). Then, the cells were distributed into microplates at a density of 1×10^6 cells/well. Subsequently, fluorescent probe (Fluo8, AAT Bioquest) mixed with probenecid in HBSS buffer (Invitrogen, Carlsbad, CA, USA) supplemented with 20 mM HEPES (Invitrogen) (pH 7.4) was added to each well, and the plates were incubated for 60 min at 37 °C. Thereafter, plates were fixed in a FlipR Tetra microplate reader (Molecular Device, San Jose, CA, USA) and dieckol and PFF-A (12.5, 25, 50, 100 and/or 150 μM), reference agonist, or HBSS buffer (basal control) was added. Fluorescence intensity was measured which varied in proportion to the free cytosolic Ca^{2+} ion concentration. Agonist effect on 5-$HT_{1A}R$ was calculated as a % of control response to 2.5 μM serotonin. Similarly, the percentage inhibition of the control response to 30 nM serotonin was calculated for the antagonist effect. Serotonin and (S)-WAY-100635 were used as reference agonists and antagonists, respectively.

4.7. Homology Modeling and Molecular Docking

The primary sequence of the human 5-$HT_{1A}R$ and human $V_{1A}R$ was obtained from UniProt (ID: P08908 and P37288, respectively). Based on the SWISS-MODEL, the 5-HT_{1B} receptor (PDB: 5V54) was selected as a template for homology modeling of human 5-HT_{1A} because it showed a good sequence similarity (0.42), sequence identity (42.97), and quaternary structure quality estimate (QSQE) (0.32) to this receptor. Similarly, μ-opioid receptor (PDB: 4DKL) was selected as a template for homology modeling of human $V_{1A}R$, because it showed a good sequence similarity (0.32), sequence identity (24.54), and QSQE (0.19) to this receptor. The constructed model was refined using the ModRefiner server. Automated docking simulations were carried out with the AutoDock 4.2. program [63]. The structures of dieckol and PFF-A were generated and converted into 3D structures using Marvin Sketch (v17,1,30, ChemAxon, Budapest, Hungary). Structures of dieckol and PFF-A were energy-minimized using a molecular mechanics 2 (MM2) force field. X-ray crystallographic structures of GPCRs were obtained from the RCSB protein data bank (PDB) with respective PDB IDs—$hA_{2A}R$ (3eml) [31], $h\alpha_{2C}AR$ (6kuw), hδ-OP (4ej4) [64], hCB_1R (6kqi) [65], and hGLP-1 [66]. The structures of reported agonists (5′-*N*-ethylcarboxamidoadenosine (NECA), epinephrine, DPI-287, CP 55940, PF-06882961, AVP, and serotonin, and antagonists (ZM241385, RS-79948, naltrindole, taranabant, NNC0640, SR49059, and WAY 100635) were downloaded from PubChem or PDB. For each ligand–protein complex, 10 docking poses were generated using the same grid parameters (size and center) and docking parameters (genetic algorithm and run options). The pose for the lowest binding energy was chosen for the final docking result. When the root-mean-square deviation (RMSD) value between our docking result and the original crystallographic structures of the protein was less than 0.15 nm, we considered our docking protocol to be valid and performed the simulation. Results were analyzed and visualized using Discovery Studio (v17.2, Accelrys, San Diego, CA, USA).

Supplementary Materials: The following are available online at https://www.mdpi.com/article/10.3390/md19060326/s1, Table S1: Hydrogen bonding interaction residues between ligand–GPCRs ($hA_{2A}R$, $h\alpha_{2C}AR$, and hDOP), Table S2: Hydrophobic and electrostatic interaction residues between ligand–GPCRs ($hA_{2A}R$, $h\alpha_{2C}AR$, and hDOP), Table S3: Hydrogen, halogen, or electrostatic bonding interaction residues between ligand–GPCRs (hCB_1R and hGLP-1), Table S4: Hydrophobic interaction residues between ligand–GPCRs (hCB_1R and hGLP-1), Table S5: Hydrogen bonding interaction residues between ligand–GPCRs ($hV_{1A}R$ and h5-$HT_{1A}R$), and Table S6: Hydrophobic and electrostatic interaction residues between ligand–GPCRs ($hV_{1A}R$ and h5-$HT_{1A}R$).

Author Contributions: Bioassays and original draft preparation, P.P.; in silico assays and writing, S.H.S.; in silico assay, S.E.P.; writing—edit, J.H.R.; writing—review and supervision, H.A.J. and J.S.C. All authors have read and agreed to the published version of the manuscript.

Funding: The Basic Science Research Program supported this research through the National Research Foundation of Korea (NRF) funded by the Ministry of Science (2012R1A6A1028677).

Institutional Review Board Statement: Not applicable.

Acknowledgments: We would like to thank Fazlin Mohd Fauzi, Department of Pharmacology and Chemistry, Faculty of Pharmacy, Universiti Teknologi MARA, Selangor Branch, Puncak Alam Campus, 42300 Bandar Puncak Alam, Selangor, Malaysia, for proteocheminformatics modeling.

Conflicts of Interest: The authors declare no conflict of interest.

References

1. Iliopoulos-Tsoutsouvas, C.; Kulkarni, R.N.; Makriyannis, A.; Nikas, S.P. Fluorescent probes for G-protein-coupled receptor drug discovery. *Expert Opin. Drug Discov.* **2018**, *13*, 933–947. [CrossRef]
2. Schlyer, S.; Horuk, R. I want a new drug: G-protein-coupled receptors in drug development. *Drug Discov. Today* **2006**, *11*, 481–493. [CrossRef] [PubMed]
3. Kim, H.R.; Xu, J.; Maeda, S.; Duc, N.M.; Ahn, D.; Du, Y.; Chung, K.Y. Structural mechanism underlying primary and secondary coupling between GPCRs and the Gi/o family. *Nat. Commun.* **2020**, *11*, 3160. [CrossRef]
4. Wang, X.; Wang, Z.-Y.; Zheng, J.-H.; Li, S. TCM network pharmacology: A new trend towards combining computational, experimental and clinical approaches. *Chin. J. Nat. Med.* **2021**, *19*, 1–11.
5. Do Valle, I.F.; Roweth, H.G.; Malloy, M.W.; Moco, S.; Barron, D.; Battinelli, E.; Loscalzo, J.; Barabási, A.-L. Network medicine framework shows that proximity of polyphenol targets and disease proteins predicts therapeutic effects of polyphenols. *Nat. Food* **2021**, *2*, 143–155. [CrossRef]
6. Nakamura, T.; Nagayama, K.; Uchida, K.; Tanaka, R. Antioxidant activity of phlorotannins isolated from the brown alga *Eisenia bicyclis*. *Fish. Sci.* **1996**, *62*, 923–926. [CrossRef]
7. Manandhar, B.; Wagle, A.; Seong, S.H.; Paudel, P.; Kim, H.-R.; Jung, H.A.; Choi, J.S. Phlorotannins with potential anti-tyrosinase and antioxidant activity isolated from the marine seaweed *Ecklonia stolonifera*. *Antioxidants* **2019**, *8*, 240. [CrossRef] [PubMed]
8. Eom, S.-H.; Kim, Y.-M.; Kim, S.-K. Antimicrobial effect of phlorotannins from marine brown algae. *Food Chem. Toxicol.* **2012**, *50*, 3251–3255. [CrossRef]
9. Lee, S.-H.; Jeon, Y.-J. Anti-diabetic effects of brown algae derived phlorotannins, marine polyphenols through diverse mechanisms. *Fitoterapia* **2013**, *86*, 129–136. [CrossRef] [PubMed]
10. Jung, H.A.; Oh, S.H.; Choi, J.S. Molecular docking studies of phlorotannins from *Eisenia bicyclis* with BACE1 inhibitory activity. *Bioorg. Med. Chem. Lett.* **2010**, *20*, 3211–3215. [CrossRef]
11. Yoon, N.Y.; Chung, H.Y.; Kim, H.R.; Choi, J.E. Acetyl- and butyrylcholinesterase inhibitory activities of sterols and phlorotannins from *Ecklonia stolonifera*. *Fish. Sci.* **2008**, *74*, 200. [CrossRef]
12. Seong, S.H.; Paudel, P.; Jung, H.A.; Choi, J.S. Identifying phlorofucofuroeckol-A as a dual inhibitor of amyloid-β25-35 self-aggregation and insulin glycation: Elucidation of the molecular mechanism of action. *Mar. Drugs* **2019**, *17*, 600. [CrossRef]
13. Jung, H.A.; Jin, S.E.; Ahn, B.R.; Lee, C.M.; Choi, J.S. Anti-inflammatory activity of edible brown alga *Eisenia bicyclis* and its constituents fucosterol and phlorotannins in LPS-stimulated RAW264.7 macrophages. *Food Chem. Toxicol.* **2013**, *59*, 199–206. [CrossRef]
14. Ahn, B.R.; Moon, H.E.; Kim, H.R.; Jung, H.A.; Choi, J.S. Neuroprotective effect of edible brown alga *Eisenia bicyclis* on amyloid beta peptide-induced toxicity in PC12 cells. *Arch. Pharm. Res.* **2012**, *35*, 1989–1998. [CrossRef] [PubMed]
15. Paudel, P.; Seong, S.H.; Wu, S.; Park, S.; Jung, H.A.; Choi, J.S. Eckol as a potential therapeutic against neurodegenerative diseases targeting dopamine D3/D4 receptors. *Mar. Drugs* **2019**, *17*, 108. [CrossRef] [PubMed]
16. Jung, H.A.; Jung, H.J.; Jeong, H.Y.; Kwon, H.J.; Ali, M.Y.; Choi, J.S. Phlorotannins isolated from the edible brown alga *Ecklonia stolonifera* exert anti-adipogenic activity on 3T3-L1 adipocytes by downregulating C/EBPα and PPARγ. *Fitoterapia* **2014**, *92*, 260–269. [CrossRef]
17. Lee, M.-S.; Shin, T.; Utsuki, T.; Choi, J.-S.; Byun, D.-S.; Kim, H.-R. Isolation and identification of phlorotannins from *Ecklonia stolonifera* with antioxidant and hepatoprotective properties in tacrine-treated HepG2 cells. *J. Agri. Food Chem.* **2012**, *60*, 5340–5349. [CrossRef] [PubMed]
18. Jung, H.A.; Roy, A.; Jung, J.H.; Choi, J.S. Evaluation of the inhibitory effects of eckol and dieckol isolated from edible brown alga *Eisenia bicyclis* on human monoamine oxidases A and B. *Arch. Pharm. Res.* **2017**, *40*, 480–491. [CrossRef] [PubMed]
19. Jung, H.A.; Hyun, S.K.; Kim, H.R.; Choi, J.S. Angiotensin-converting enzyme I inhibitory activity of phlorotannins from *Ecklonia stolonifera*. *Fish. Sci.* **2006**, *72*, 1292–1299. [CrossRef]
20. Kwon, H.-J.; Ryu, Y.B.; Kim, Y.-M.; Song, N.; Kim, C.Y.; Rho, M.-C.; Jeong, J.-H.; Cho, K.-O.; Lee, W.S.; Park, S.-J. In vitro antiviral activity of phlorotannins isolated from *Ecklonia cava* against porcine epidemic diarrhea coronavirus infection and hemagglutination. *Bioorg. Med. Chem.* **2013**, *21*, 4706–4713. [CrossRef] [PubMed]

21. Kang, H.S.; Chung, H.Y.; Kim, J.Y.; Son, B.W.; Jung, H.A.; Choi, J.S. Inhibitory phlorotannins from the edible brown alga *Ecklonia stolonifera* on total reactive oxygen species (ROS) generation. *Arch. Pharm. Res.* **2004**, *27*, 194–198. [CrossRef]
22. Seong, S.H.; Paudel, P.; Choi, J.-W.; Ahn, D.H.; Nam, T.-J.; Jung, H.A.; Choi, J.S. Probing multi-target action of phlorotannins as new monoamine oxidase inhibitors and dopaminergic receptor modulators with the potential for treatment of neuronal disorders. *Mar. Drugs* **2019**, *17*, 377. [CrossRef] [PubMed]
23. Paricharak, S.; Cortés-Ciriano, I.; IJzerman, A.P.; Malliavin, T.E.; Bender, A. Proteochemometric modelling coupled to in silico target prediction: An integrated approach for the simultaneous prediction of polypharmacology and binding affinity/potency of small molecules. *J. Cheminform.* **2015**, *7*, 1–11. [CrossRef]
24. Burda, S.; Oleszek, W. Antioxidant and antiradical activities of flavonoids. *J. Agric. Food Chem.* **2001**, *49*, 2774–2779. [CrossRef]
25. Dugas, A.J., Jr.; Castañeda-Acosta, J.; Bonin, G.C.; Price, K.L.; Fischer, N.H.; Winston, G.W. Evaluation of the total peroxyl radical-scavenging capacity of flavonoids: Structure- activity relationships. *J. Nat. Prod.* **2000**, *63*, 327–331. [CrossRef]
26. Shibata, T.; Ishimaru, K.; Kawaguchi, S.; Yoshikawa, H.; Hama, Y. Antioxidant activities of phlorotannins isolated from Japanese Laminariaceae. In *Nineteenth International Seaweed Symposium*; Borowitzka, M.A., Critchley, A.T., Kraan, S., Peters, A., Sjøtun, K., Notoya, M., Eds.; Springer: Dordrecht, The Netherlands, 2007; Volume 2, pp. 255–261.
27. Borroto-Escuela, D.O.; Romero-Fernandez, W.; Tarakanov, A.O.; Gómez-Soler, M.; Corrales, F.; Marcellino, D.; Narvaez, M.; Frankowska, M.; Flajolet, M.; Heintz, N. Characterization of the A2AR–D2R interface: Focus on the role of the C-terminal tail and the transmembrane helices. *Biochem. Biophys. Res. Commun.* **2010**, *402*, 801–807. [CrossRef] [PubMed]
28. Fuxe, K.; Agnati, L.F.; Jacobsen, K.; Hillion, J.; Canals, M.; Torvinen, M.; Tinner-Staines, B.; Staines, W.; Rosin, D.; Terasmaa, A. Receptor heteromerization in adenosine A2A receptor signaling: Relevance for striatal function and Parkinson's disease. *Neurology* **2003**, *61*, S19–S23. [CrossRef] [PubMed]
29. Ferre, S.; Von Euler, G.; Johansson, B.; Fredholm, B.B.; Fuxe, K. Stimulation of high-affinity adenosine A2 receptors decreases the affinity of dopamine D2 receptors in rat striatal membranes. *Proc. Natl. Acad. Sci. USA* **1991**, *88*, 7238–7241. [CrossRef] [PubMed]
30. Yamada, K.; Kobayashi, M.; Kanda, T. Involvement of Adenosine A2A Receptors in Depression and Anxiety. *Int. Rev. Neurobiol.* **2014**, *119*, 373–393.
31. Jaakola, V.-P.; Griffith, M.T.; Hanson, M.A.; Cherezov, V.; Chien, E.Y.; Lane, J.R.; Ijzerman, A.P.; Stevens, R.C. The 2.6 angstrom crystal structure of a human A2A adenosine receptor bound to an antagonist. *Science* **2008**, *322*, 1211–1217. [CrossRef]
32. Kang, M.C.; Cha, S.H.; Wijesinghe, W.A.; Kang, S.M.; Lee, S.H.; Kim, E.A.; Song, C.B.; Jeon, Y.J. Protective effect of marine algae phlorotannins against AAPH-induced oxidative stress in zebrafish embryo. *Food Chem.* **2013**, *138*, 950–955. [CrossRef]
33. Cha, S.-H.; Heo, S.-J.; Jeon, Y.-J.; Park, S.M. Dieckol, an edible seaweed polyphenol, retards rotenone-induced neurotoxicity and α-synuclein aggregation in human dopaminergic neuronal cells. *RSC Adv.* **2016**, *6*, 110040–110046. [CrossRef]
34. Cui, Y.; Park, J.Y.; Wu, J.; Lee, J.H.; Yang, Y.S.; Kang, M.S.; Jung, S.C.; Park, J.M.; Yoo, E.S.; Kim, S.H.; et al. Dieckol Attenuates Microglia-mediated Neuronal Cell Death via ERK, Akt and NADPH Oxidase-mediated Pathways. *Korean J. Physiol. Pharmacol.* **2015**, *19*, 219–228. [CrossRef] [PubMed]
35. Kim, J.-J.; Kang, Y.-J.; Shin, S.-A.; Bak, D.-H.; Lee, J.W.; Lee, K.B.; Yoo, Y.C.; Kim, D.-K.; Lee, B.H.; Kim, D.W. Phlorofucofuroeckol improves glutamate-induced neurotoxicity through modulation of oxidative stress-mediated mitochondrial dysfunction in PC12 cells. *PLoS ONE* **2016**, *11*, e0163433. [CrossRef] [PubMed]
36. Gaidin, S.G.; Turovskaya, M.V.; Mal'tseva, V.N.; Zinchenko, V.P.; Blinova, E.V.; Turovsky, E.A. A Complex Neuroprotective Effect of Alpha-2-Adrenergic Receptor Agonists in a Model of Cerebral Ischemia–Reoxygenation In Vitro. *Biochemistry* **2019**, *13*, 319–333. [CrossRef]
37. Bücheler, M.M.; Hadamek, K.; Hein, L. Two α2-adrenergic receptor subtypes, α2A and α2C, inhibit transmitter release in the brain of gene-targeted mice. *Neuroscience* **2002**, *109*, 819–826. [CrossRef]
38. Scheinin, M.; Sallinen, J.; Haapalinna, A. Evaluation of the α2C-adrenoceptor as a neuropsychiatric drug target: Studies in transgenic mouse models. *Life Sci.* **2001**, *68*, 2277–2285. [CrossRef]
39. Fairbanks, C.A.; Stone, L.S.; Kitto, K.F.; Nguyen, H.O.; Posthumus, I.J.; Wilcox, G.L. α2C-Adrenergic receptors mediate spinal analgesia and adrenergic-opioid synergy. *J. Pharmacol. Exp. Ther.* **2002**, *300*, 282–290. [CrossRef]
40. Duflo, F.; Li, X.; Bantel, C.; Pancaro, C.; Vincler, M.; Eisenach, J.C. Peripheral Nerve Injury Alters the α2Adrenoceptor Subtype Activated by Clonidine for Analgesia. *Anesthesiology* **2002**, *97*, 636–641. [CrossRef]
41. Quaglia, W.; Del Bello, F.; Giannella, M.; Piergentili, A.; Pigini, M. α2C-adrenoceptor modulators: A patent review. *Expert. Opin. Ther. Pat.* **2011**, *21*, 455–481. [CrossRef]
42. Chilmonczyk, Z.; Bojarski, A.J.; Pilc, A.; Sylte, I. Functional selectivity and antidepressant activity of serotonin 1A receptor ligands. *Int. J. Mol. Sci.* **2015**, *16*, 18474–18506. [CrossRef] [PubMed]
43. Simon, N.G.; Guillon, C.; Fabio, K.; Heindel, N.D.; Lu, S.-f.; Miller, M.; Ferris, C.F.; Brownstein, M.J.; Garripa, C.; Koppel, G.A. Vasopressin antagonists as anxiolytics and antidepressants: Recent developments. *Recent Pat. CNS Drug Discov.* **2008**, *3*, 77–93. [CrossRef]
44. Narayen, G.; Mandal, S.N. Vasopressin receptor antagonists and their role in clinical medicine. *Indian J. Endocrinol. Metab.* **2012**, *16*, 183–191. [CrossRef] [PubMed]
45. Liu, X.; Luo, G.; Jiang, J.; Ma, T.; Lin, X.; Jiang, L.; Cheng, J.; Tao, R. Signaling through hepatocyte vasopressin receptor 1 protects mouse liver from ischemia-reperfusion injury. *Oncotarget* **2016**, *7*, 69276. [CrossRef]

46. Glass, M.; Faull, R.; Dragunow, M. Cannabinoid receptors in the human brain: A detailed anatomical and quantitative autoradiographic study in the fetal, neonatal and adult human brain. *Neuroscience* **1997**, *77*, 299–318. [CrossRef]
47. Kano, M.; Ohno-Shosaku, T.; Hashimotodani, Y.; Uchigashima, M.; Watanabe, M. Endocannabinoid-mediated control of synaptic transmission. *Physiol. Rev.* **2009**, *89*, 309–380. [CrossRef]
48. Xu, X.; Liu, Y.; Huang, S.; Liu, G.; Xie, C.; Zhou, J.; Fan, W.; Li, Q.; Wang, Q.; Zhong, D.; et al. Overexpression of cannabinoid receptors CB1 and CB2 correlates with improved prognosis of patients with hepatocellular carcinoma. *Cancer Genet. Cytogenet.* **2006**, *171*, 31–38. [CrossRef] [PubMed]
49. Qamri, Z.; Preet, A.; Nasser, M.W.; Bass, C.E.; Leone, G.; Barsky, S.H.; Ganju, R.K. Synthetic cannabinoid receptor agonists inhibit tumor growth and metastasis of breast cancer. *Mol. Cancer Ther.* **2009**, *8*, 3117–3129. [CrossRef] [PubMed]
50. Ogden, S.B.; Malamas, M.S.; Makriyannis, A.; Eckel, L.A. The novel cannabinoid CB(1) receptor agonist AM11101 increases food intake in female rats. *Br. J. Pharmacol.* **2019**, *176*, 3972–3982. [CrossRef]
51. Kim, A.-R.; Lee, M.-S.; Choi, J.-W.; Utsuki, T.; Kim, J.-I.; Jang, B.-C.; Kim, H.-R. Phlorofucofuroeckol A suppresses expression of inducible nitric oxide synthase, cyclooxygenase-2, and pro-inflammatory cytokines via inhibition of nuclear factor-κB, c-Jun NH 2-terminal kinases, and Akt in microglial cells. *Inflammation* **2013**, *36*, 259–271. [CrossRef]
52. Eo, H.J.; Kwon, T.H.; Park, G.H.; Song, H.M.; Lee, S.J.; Park, N.H.; Jeong, J.B. In Vitro Anticancer Activity of Phlorofucofuroeckol A via Upregulation of Activating Transcription Factor 3 against Human Colorectal Cancer Cells. *Mar. Drugs* **2016**, *14*, 69. [CrossRef] [PubMed]
53. D'Antona, A.M.; Ahn, K.H.; Kendall, D.A. Mutations of CB1 T210 produce active and inactive receptor forms: Correlations with ligand affinity, receptor stability, and cellular localization. *Biochemistry* **2006**, *45*, 5606–5617. [CrossRef] [PubMed]
54. Römpler, H.; Yu, H.-T.; Arnold, A.; Orth, A.; Schöneberg, T. Functional consequences of naturally occurring DRY motif variants in the mammalian chemoattractant receptor GPR33. *Genomics* **2006**, *87*, 724–732. [CrossRef] [PubMed]
55. Krishna Kumar, K.; Shalev-Benami, M.; Robertson, M.J.; Hu, H.; Banister, S.D.; Hollingsworth, S.A.; Latorraca, N.R.; Kato, H.E.; Hilger, D.; Maeda, S.; et al. Structure of a Signaling Cannabinoid Receptor 1-G Protein Complex. *Cell* **2019**, *176*, 448–458.e12. [CrossRef]
56. Lin, L.S.; Ha, S.; Ball, R.G.; Tsou, N.N.; Castonguay, L.A.; Doss, G.A.; Fong, T.M.; Shen, C.-P.; Xiao, J.C.; Goulet, M.T.; et al. Conformational Analysis and Receptor Docking of N-[(1S,2S)-3-(4-Chlorophenyl)-2-(3-cyanophenyl)-1-methylpropyl]-2-methyl-2-{[5-(trifluoromethyl)pyridin-2-yl]oxy}propanamide (Taranabant, MK-0364), a Novel, Acyclic Cannabinoid-1 Receptor Inverse Agonist. *J. Med. Chem.* **2008**, *51*, 2108–2114. [CrossRef]
57. Turton, M.; O'shea, D.; Gunn, I.; Beak, S.; Edwards, C.; Meeran, K.; Choi, S.; Taylor, G.; Heath, M.; Lambert, P. A role for glucagon-like peptide-1 in the central regulation of feeding. *Nature* **1996**, *379*, 69–72. [CrossRef]
58. Drucker, D.J.; Nauck, M.A. The incretin system: Glucagon-like peptide-1 receptor agonists and dipeptidyl peptidase-4 inhibitors in type 2 diabetes. *Lancet* **2006**, *368*, 1696–1705. [CrossRef]
59. Kim, E.-A.; Lee, S.-H.; Lee, J.-H.; Kang, N.; Oh, J.-Y.; Ahn, G.; Ko, S.C.; Fernando, S.P.; Kim, S.-Y.; Park, S.-J. A marine algal polyphenol, dieckol, attenuates blood glucose levels by Akt pathway in alloxan induced hyperglycemia zebrafish model. *RSC Adv.* **2016**, *6*, 78570–78575. [CrossRef]
60. Paudel, P.; Seong, S.H.; Fauzi, F.M.; Bender, A.; Jung, H.A.; Choi, J.S. Establishing GPCR targets of hMAO active anthraquinones from *Cassia obtusifolia* Linn seeds using in silico and in vitro methods. *ACS Omega* **2020**, *5*, 7705–7715. [CrossRef]
61. Mohd Fauzi, F.; John, C.M.; Karunanidhi, A.; Mussa, H.Y.; Ramasamy, R.; Adam, A.; Bender, A. Understanding the mode-of-action of *Cassia auriculata* via in silico and in vivo studies towards validating it as a long term therapy for type II diabetes. *J. Ethnopharmacol.* **2017**, *197*, 61–72. [CrossRef]
62. Paudel, P.; Seong, S.H.; Jung, H.A.; Choi, J.S. Characterizing fucoxanthin as a selective dopamine D3/D4 receptor agonist: Relevance to Parkinson's disease. *Chem. Biol. Interact.* **2019**, *310*, 108757. [CrossRef] [PubMed]
63. Goodsell, D.S.; Morris, G.M.; Olson, A.J. Automated docking of flexible ligands: Applications of AutoDock. *J. Mol. Recognit.* **1996**, *9*, 1–5. [CrossRef]
64. Granier, S.; Manglik, A.; Kruse, A.C.; Kobilka, T.S.; Thian, F.S.; Weis, W.I.; Kobilka, B.K. Structure of the δ-opioid receptor bound to naltrindole. *Nature* **2012**, *485*, 400–404. [CrossRef] [PubMed]
65. Shao, Z.; Yan, W.; Chapman, K.; Ramesh, K.; Ferrell, A.J.; Yin, J.; Wang, X.; Xu, Q.; Rosenbaum, D.M. Structure of an allosteric modulator bound to the CB1 cannabinoid receptor. *Nat. Chem. Biol.* **2019**, *15*, 1199–1205. [CrossRef]
66. Song, G.; Yang, D.; Wang, Y.; de Graaf, C.; Zhou, Q.; Jiang, S.; Liu, K.; Cai, X.; Dai, A.; Lin, G.; et al. Human GLP-1 receptor transmembrane domain structure in complex with allosteric modulators. *Nature* **2017**, *546*, 312–315. [CrossRef]

MDPI
St. Alban-Anlage 66
4052 Basel
Switzerland
www.mdpi.com

Marine Drugs Editorial Office
E-mail: marinedrugs@mdpi.com
www.mdpi.com/journal/marinedrugs

www.ingramcontent.com/pod-product-compliance
Lightning Source LLC
LaVergne TN
LVHW070725100526
838202LV00013B/1174